HEALING A[...]
BY RESTORING THE MICROBIOME

THE
KEYSTONE
APPROACH

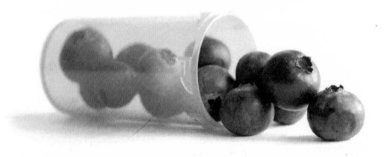

REBECCA FETT

Franklin Fox Publishing
New York

The Keystone Approach: Healing Arthritis and Psoriasis by Restoring the Microbiome

Copyright ©2018 by Rebecca Fett

Published in the United States by Franklin Fox Publishing LLC, New York.

ISBN-13: 978-0-9911269-8-9 (ebook)
ISBN-13: 978-0-9911269-5-8 (print)
ISBN-10: 0-9911269-5-5

www.keystonebook.com

TABLE OF CONTENTS

INTRODUCTION

The world of autoimmune disease is a very different place than it was even five years ago. New evidence is emerging on a daily basis that points to the gut and the microbiome as the origin of a variety of autoimmune diseases. This new paradigm opens up an array of treatment options—options that go beyond merely suppressing the inflammatory response to actually addressing the underlying causes of that inflammation.

The Keystone Approach is your guide to this novel scientific frontier, with a particular focus on dietary changes and specific probiotics. Together, these measures can heal the gut and restore balance to the microbiome. When we do so, we remove the main triggers that drive inflammation in many autoimmune diseases, particularly those conditions in the "spondylarthropathy" family. This family includes

- Psoriasis/ psoriatic arthritis
- Ankylosing spondylitis
- Juvenile idiopathic arthritis
- Crohn's disease

- Ulcerative colitis
- Uveitis

Although these conditions are the main focus of the scientific research discussed in this book, I also cover the latest studies on how diet and gut health impacts other autoimmune diseases, such as rheumatoid arthritis. These research findings are then translated into simple, actionable steps. But first, the story of my own battle against autoimmunity.

A doctor first suspected that I had psoriatic arthritis when I was 18. At the time, my only symptoms were mild back pain and a small patch of psoriasis, but I understood that if I did indeed have psoriatic arthritis, it could become much worse. This form of arthritis affects up to 30 percent of people with psoriasis and can become debilitating.

Six months after the pain began, I noticed that it seemed a little better when I avoided bread and pasta, so I insisted on a celiac test. The test showed that I did have celiac disease, and after completely eliminating gluten from my diet for several months, my psoriasis and back pain mostly resolved. It appeared that I did not have psoriatic arthritis after all.

I went on to complete a degree in biochemistry and molecular biology, and then law school, with only minor aches and pains that I attributed to the physical toll of spending too much time studying.

By my mid-20s, after several years of working long hours at a large law firm in New York, my pain returned with a vengeance. My shoulders, knees, hips, and lower back ached constantly, and joints seemed to dislocate with the slightest provocation. The possibility of psoriatic arthritis was quickly brushed away—I had very little psoriasis, no joint stiffness or swelling, and no blood markers of arthritis. I simply did not fit the old-fashioned textbook definition.

I was given a wide range of diagnoses by various specialists and offered all manner of pain medications. After experiencing severe side effects from these medications, I elected to focus on physical therapy. I hoped that with enough effort and perseverance, my muscles could eventually stabilize my joints. I spent five years religiously devoted to physical therapy, wanting to believe that my recovery was just around the corner.

It was not. By age 30, the pain in my sacroiliac joints (in the lower back) was so severe that I started having great difficulty walking more than a few blocks or sitting for more than 15 minutes. I had pain flare-ups that kept me housebound for weeks at a time and kept me awake much of the night. I tried various injections and anti-inflammatory medications, with little relief.

Around this time, my psoriasis also returned, and a range of other classic symptoms of psoriatic arthritis emerged (such as characteristic nail changes). It became clear that I had probably been suffering from psoriatic arthritis all along.

Understanding the nature of the problem was both a setback and a relief. On one hand, the diagnosis meant that no amount of exercise would ever enable my joints to function normally. It also meant I had wasted many years that I could have spent focusing on the root cause of the pain—a malfunctioning immune system. But on the other hand, a malfunctioning immune system was something I understood all too well, and now I finally had an explanation for my pain.

The precise details of autoimmunity were at this point

already very familiar to me from my immunology studies at university and from my work as a patent litigation attorney for biotechnology companies. As the immunology specialist in lawsuits with billions of dollars at stake, I had actually spent much of the past nine years analyzing the scientific and clinical evidence underpinning the biologics used to treat various autoimmune diseases. My office was filled with boxes of confidential clinical trial reports and FDA submissions, and it was my job to analyze them and talk to experts in the field.

I had essentially spent nine years thinking in great detail about the invisible inflammatory molecules that drive all the damage in autoimmune disease. And now I learned that these same molecules were causing the pain that had taken over my life.

I understood that the new biologic medications were likely my best hope for recovery—if I was willing to take the risks associated with infections and possibly a higher risk of cancer. Although biologics only slightly raise the risk of infection, this was a major obstacle in my particular case. As a teenager, I had undergone surgery that left me with a lifelong susceptibility to serious infections. I had been advised to take preventive antibiotics for life because some common infections carried a 50 to 60 percent mortality rate in my case. I refused the antibiotics but was also reluctant to take any medication that could add to my infection risk. Since my arthritis was progressing slowly and not causing any obvious joint damage, it seemed prudent to exhaust every other option first.

I knew that biologics work so well because they interrupt the specific mediators of inflammation that orchestrate skin and joint damage. Surely there had to be another way to accomplish the same goal. What other factors contribute to elevated inflammatory mediators, and what other factors can reduce them?

As I began to focus more on these questions, I made the difficult decision to pause my legal career and focus on my health. I left New York and moved to a small town by the beach with my husband and two young sons. My new job became scouring the scientific literature for any evidence that diet or lifestyle changes could change the course of my autoimmune disease. I expected to find some clues but was unprepared for the extraordinary amount of good-quality clinical evidence supporting relatively simple strategies.

Perhaps the biggest revelation was the discovery that gut health has a profound impact on the level of inflammation in the skin and joints. A persuasive body of research shows that excess immune activation in the gut is a common feature of psoriasis and several types of inflammatory arthritis, particularly juvenile, psoriatic, and ankylosing spondylitis.[1] Importantly, the degree of gut inflammation appears to determine the severity of these conditions.[2]

In 2016, researchers discovered one factor that could be triggering this immune activation in the gut: a disturbance in the vast community of microbes that make up the microbiome. Those with psoriasis or certain forms of arthritis show characteristic disturbances in the balance of gut bacteria, with an increase in undesirable species and a depletion of species that normally calm the immune system.[3]

Several lines of evidence indicate that this disruption to the microbiome is not just a consequence of inflammation, but a cause. Researchers have found, for example, that a single course of antibiotics doubles the chance of children developing arthritis, while five or more courses of antibiotics triple the risk.[4] It may be that antibiotics deplete the bacteria that regulate the immune system and keep harmful bacteria in check.

These protective bacteria are now regarded as "keystone" species. To scientists studying larger ecosystems, a keystone species is one whose unique role within an ecosystem has a disproportionate effect on the ecosystem as a whole. Mangrove trees growing along a shoreline, for example, provide a habitat for numerous other species, including fish and frogs. Without mangroves, the ecosystem would collapse. The particular gut bacteria that normally regulate our immune system also act as keystone species. Without them, the entire environment of our gut changes. The new paradigm is that this change is a major contributor to autoimmune disease.

The question, then, is how we can take advantage of the newly uncovered link between the microbiome and autoimmunity. Professor Jose Scher of New York University, who led the landmark studies of the microbiome in psoriatic and rheumatoid arthritis, commented that "in 10 or 15 years I think the microbiome will be a key therapeutic option for some of these diseases."[5]

But we don't have to wait that long. Good-quality clinical studies have already demonstrated how to restore the population of immune-regulating keystone species. The strategies to do so are simple and low risk: a high-fiber, vegetable-rich diet, and specific strains of probiotics. Numerous studies performed in the context of inflammatory bowel disease show that these strategies can rapidly shift the balance of the microbiome to an anti-inflammatory state.[6]

My immersion in the latest scientific research also uncovered strong evidence supporting several other strategies that can reduce inflammation. As just one example, the studies clearly show that a Mediterranean diet rich in fish and olive oil can reduce the severity of psoriasis and rheumatoid arthritis.[7] This has long been suspected but has been overshadowed by the recent rise of the "autoimmune paleo diet."

While some aspects of the paleo diet are supported by scientific research, such as the damaging effects of certain grains and refined oils, other aspects are contradicted by research that emerged after the paleo diet rose to prominence.

In particular, several recent studies demonstrate beyond doubt that saturated fats are highly inflammatory.[8] Although the role of saturated fat in heart disease has been called into question, the newest research shows that these fats actually do increase the level of inflammatory mediators. Saturated fats do this by activating certain receptors on the surface of immune cells.[9] Thus the paleo diet's emphasis on coconut oil and animal fat is counterproductive for those with inflammatory diseases such as psoriasis and arthritis.

The Mediterranean diet, in contrast, heavily emphasizes foods that help rebalance the microbiome and otherwise suppress inflammation; such foods include green and cruciferous vegetables, fish, and olive oil. The scientific research also points to strategies to optimize the Mediterranean diet by removing foods that damage the gut and contribute to immune activation, such as wheat.

As I gradually changed my diet and supplement regime to incorporate new strategies supported by the latest evidence, my symptoms began to steadily improve. At first, the only noticeable difference was less fatigue, abdominal pain, and swelling in my hands. After three months, I was experiencing my first pain-free days in more than a decade. The longer I followed the diet and the more elements I tweaked, the more my joint pain improved.

Now, instead of constant and debilitating joint pain, I have only very occasional aches and pains, typically triggered by eating something I know I should not. My psoriasis has also been completely clear for more than a year. In short, I have been able to take control of my health to an extent I never thought possible.

There is clearly an immense gap between the latest research findings and the advice most doctors provide about the connection between diet and inflammation. Despite a vast body of evidence to the contrary, many of us are told that diet has no effect. This gap is not altogether surprising since it reportedly takes at least 10 years for medical research findings to make their way into clinical practice.[10] But we deserve better. I wanted to bridge the gap between the latest discoveries and the people who can benefit from them.

I had already witnessed the power of doing so in the fertility and IVF context with my first book, *It Starts with the Egg*. After receiving countless reports from readers that being able to implement the latest research findings had profoundly changed their lives, I wanted to do the same for those suffering from debilitating autoimmune disease.

With that aim, I thoroughly investigated every last detail of how diet, the microbiome, and many other factors can impact inflammation. I carefully analyzed hundreds of scientific papers, with a particular focus on randomized, controlled clinical studies involving real patients, not animal or test-tube studies. (These scientific papers are listed in the references section, along with information about how to access them online.)

My ultimate goal in writing this book was to distill a vast and complex body of medical research into an easily understood practical guide—to translate the science into a plan of action.

As I developed this systematic plan, I was guided by the recognition that some factors apply generally, such as the beneficial role of fiber and omega-3 fatty acids, while other factors, such as the consumption of sugar and starch, impact different individuals to different degrees. The Keystone Approach is thus designed to help you discover which factors make the most difference in your particular case. There may be one key ingredient to your recovery, such as reducing starch or adding a probiotic, or there may be many small, incremental changes that together produce a dramatic benefit. (To preview the complete plan for your specific autoimmune condition, see chapter 10.)

Importantly, the diet and supplements described in the book are intended to complement, not replace, a conventional medical approach. It is important to tell your doctor about any new supplements and dietary changes. You should also continue with all prescribed medications. Many of the anti-inflammatory strategies at the core of the Keystone Approach, such as fish oil, probiotics, and the Mediterranean diet, have been specifically shown to help patients achieve better results from conventional medicines.[11] Eventually you may be able to work with your doctor to reduce your medications, but that should only happen once you see positive results from your new diet and supplement protocol.

Part 1

The Microbiome and Autoimmunity

CHAPTER 1

UNDERSTANDING THE ROOT CAUSES OF AUTOIMMUNITY

Autoimmune disease reflects a serious malfunction of the immune system. Rather than protecting us from infection, our own immune cells and antibodies mistakenly recognize normal proteins as foreign invaders and launch an attack. But what exactly causes the immune system to become confused and lose the ability to accurately distinguish between normal proteins and foreign antigens? In most cases the cause is some combination of the following factors:

- Damage to the gut barrier
- Immune activation from certain gut microbes or other infections
- Genetics

For decades, these three factors were considered to be mutually exclusive and competing explanations. Yet in just the past few years, more and more evidence has emerged that links these factors together into a unifying theory of autoimmune disease, as this chapter explains.

How the Gut Influences Autoimmunity

Although the precise trigger for autoimmune disease can differ between individuals, there is one common underlying factor that is usually present: a leaky gut. As explained by Dr. Sanford Newmark, a clinical professor at the University of California, San Francisco, "A lot of doctors and people may think that leaky gut itself is sort of a froufrou alternative concept," but "the real name is 'increased intestinal permeability,' and it is a definitive, scientific fact."[12]

It has been known for decades that intestinal permeability is increased in those with inflammatory bowel disease and celiac disease. There is now clear evidence that it is also increased in a variety of autoimmune conditions. Leaky gut is often particularly severe in those with psoriatic arthritis, juvenile arthritis, or ankylosing spondylitis.[13]

A compromised intestinal barrier is a big problem because it forces the immune system into panic mode. Normally, the gut barrier allows the absorption of nutrients from food while preventing bacteria, bacterial toxins, and undigested proteins from crossing into the blood stream. The intestinal lining can achieve this remarkable feat because it is structured as a single layer of epithelial cells joined together by scaffolding proteins called "tight junctions." In healthy people, these junctions are carefully controlled to only allow minute gaps for nutrients to pass through. There is also a protective mucus layer that allows nutrients across, but not proteins or bacteria.

Yet this amazing system is extremely vulnerable to damage. If the epithelial cells, tight junctions, or mucus layer is damaged, large gaps are created. This allows larger particles to cross the barrier. These particles may include bacteria, molecules from bacterial cell walls (such as lipopolysaccharide, also known as endotoxin), and proteins from food that have not yet been broken down into individual amino acids.

When these molecules breach the gut barrier, chaos ensues. Just behind the epithelial cell wall lies a vast army of immune cells in an area called the "gut-associated lymphoid tissue." Up to 70 percent of the immune system resides here, and for good reason. The gut represents a major point at which bacteria and other infections can enter the body. There are in fact billions of bacteria in the gut—some beneficial, some harmful. The immune system normally conducts surveillance for harmful bacteria by taking small samples of the gut contents. There is not supposed to be a deluge of bacteria and their toxins crossing the lining of the intestine to interact with the immune system.[14]

When the intestinal barrier becomes damaged and allows bacterial toxins to cross through the resulting gaps, the immune system is bombarded, triggering immune activation on a massive scale. Critically, the resulting immune activation is not limited to the gut. The end result is systemic inflammation and damage to the skin and joints.[15]

Intestinal Damage in the Spondylarthropathy Family

Although leaky gut appears to be a common element in the development of many autoimmune diseases, there is particularly strong evidence linking gut damage to psoriasis, psoriatic arthritis, and ankylosing spondylitis.[16]

In fact, it has been known for many years that these particular conditions are closely related to Crohn's disease, a form of inflammatory bowel disease. This was discovered in the 1980s when researchers performed colonoscopies on patients with psoriasis, psoriatic arthritis, and ankylosing spondylitis who did not have any bowel symptoms. They found that half of these patients showed visible intestinal inflammation that closely resembled early stage Crohn's disease.[17] Many other researchers have since confirmed these findings.[18]

We now know that patients with psoriasis and psoriatic arthritis have a fourfold higher risk of developing definite Crohn's disease.[19] Many of those with spondyloarthritis also go on to develop some form of inflammatory bowel disease.[20]

The link between psoriatic arthritis, ankylosing spondylitis, and inflammatory bowel disease is in fact so strong that these diseases are now categorized together under the umbrella of the "spondyloarthropathy" family. Other autoimmune diseases within this family that share the same overlap are juvenile arthritis and an inflammatory eye condition called uveitis.

As will be discussed further below, the best explanation for the overlap between these autoimmune diseases is that they all share an origin in the gut.

Immune Activation from the Gut

How exactly can inflammation in the gastrointestinal tract drive autoimmune diseases that primarily affect other parts of the body? For many years, this was a mystery because it was thought that the primary immune cells involved in autoimmunity were "specific responders" (such as B cells and T cells), which recognize specific proteins in the skin and joints. With these cells at the center of the process, it was not clear how leaky gut could influence joint pain or psoriasis. Yet it is now known that other nonspecific "first responder" cells play a key role.[21]

These nonspecific immune cells include mast cells and T

helper 17 cells (Th17 cells). Unlike other immune cells, they do not need to recognize a specific antigen to become activated. Instead, they can be spurred into action by a variety of molecules derived from the gut, including food proteins and bacterial products such as lipopolysaccharide.

Lipopolysaccharide, which is a toxin produced by many species of gut bacteria, is a particularly strong trigger for these nonspecific immune cells. If we have both a compromised intestinal barrier and a lot of gut bacteria producing lipopolysaccharide, this toxin can cross the gut barrier and bind to receptors on the surface of nonspecific immune cells.

When the cells detect the presence of lipopolysaccharide, they switch into "inflammation mode" and start producing chemical mediators that drive the inflammatory response.[22] (These mediators include TNF and Interleukin-17, which are the targets of biologic medications). This process is now thought to be a key mechanism underlying many autoimmune diseases.[23]

To stop this process and halt inflammation, we need to reduce the population of bacteria producing lipopolysaccharide while also addressing the root causes of increased intestinal permeability. These causes include

- Celiac disease
- Food allergy
- A lack of beneficial microbes
- An excess of specific inflammatory gut bacteria or yeast
- Small intestinal bacterial overgrowth (SIBO)

The following chapters provide a step-by-step protocol for addressing each of these factors, with a particular focus on restoring balance between beneficial and potentially harmful gut bacteria. Before we get there, however, it is important to understand more about how the microbiome shapes the immune system, because this guides our decisions as to which microbes we want to encourage, and which we want to suppress.

The Microbiome and Autoimmunity

There is now convincing evidence that we need certain bacteria to calm down our immune system, while other species can actually drive the development of autoimmunity, particularly in individuals with a genetic predisposition.

Beneficial Microbes

New technologies that can rapidly sequence massive amounts of DNA have led to an explosion of new insights into the microbiome. With the revolutionary ability to detect any bacterial species by looking for its DNA signature, scientists can measure the relative abundance of the different species in different individuals.

One of the major findings from this technological leap is the fact that the microbiomes of patients with autoimmune disease often lack certain microbes that are present in healthy individuals. This disparity has been extensively studied in the context of Crohn's and ulcerative colitis. In people with those conditions, there is typically a marked reduction in bacteria with unfamiliar names such as *Faecalibacterium prausnitzii*, *Eubacterium rectale*, and *Roseburia intestinalis*.[24] The more these species are depleted, the more severe the disease and the more likely patients are to relapse.[25]

What these depleted species have in common is that they are part of an important set of bacteria known as *Clostridia* clusters IV and XIVa, which are normally found in healthy humans. The decreased abundance of bacteria in these families, compared to healthy controls, has been described as "one of the major signatures of the microbial dysbiosis in inflammatory bowel disease, especially in (active) Crohn's Disease."[26]

In 2015, the link between these missing microbes and autoimmunity expanded further. In a landmark study, Jose Scher and colleagues at NYU and Memorial Sloan Kettering revealed that patients with psoriatic arthritis also have lower levels of many of the same bacterial species depleted in inflammatory bowel disease (IBD).[27] Other groups have now witnessed a similar phenomenon in psoriasis, juvenile arthritis, and rheumatoid arthritis, with a reduction in various bacterial species that are normally found in healthy individuals.[28]

Notably, in these conditions, many of the missing species also overlap with the species that are depleted in those with IBD.[29] In a study of children with a particular form of juvenile arthritis, for example, *F. prausnitzii* constituted less than 4 percent of total bacterial species in the gut, compared to 10 percent of the microbiota of healthy children.[30] In another study of juvenile arthritis, those children in remission had much higher levels of Clostridium cluster IV bacteria compared to the children with active arthritis.[31] In the same vein, patients with new-onset rheumatoid arthritis were found to have fewer bacteria from Clostridium cluster XIVa.[32]

How Beneficial Microbes Influence Immunity

There is a common characteristic of the particular bacteria that are often depleted in those with autoimmune diseases:

they have an extraordinary ability to set the dial on the immune system to a more tolerant and less reactive state.[33]

The bacteria in Clostridia clusters IV and XIVa are particularly good at directly regulating our immune system.[34] The bacteria do this in part by promoting the development of specialized immune cells called regulatory T cells. As the name suggests, these cells play a vital role in regulating other components of the immune system.

Regulatory T cells are critical to suppressing the aggressive immune cells involved in autoimmune disease.[35] They also produce anti-inflammatory mediators and reduce production of mediators that perpetuate pain and inflammation, such as TNF.[36] In short, regulatory T cells are a key part of the system of checks and balances that normally prevents autoimmunity and keeps inflammation in check.[37]

The extraordinary discovery that certain microbes can calm the immune system in this way sparked a race among researchers to figure out exactly how this happens. How is it that certain bacteria can actually communicate with the immune system to boost the number of regulatory T cells? The race was won in May 2013, with three groups of researchers making the same discovery within weeks of each other.[38] The answer: these bacteria prompt the immune system to make more regulatory T cells by producing a short-chain fatty acid called butyrate. Butyrate acts as an important signaling molecule that encourages immature immune cells to develop into regulatory T cells.

When these microbes are depleted, fewer regulatory T cells are produced, and a powerful control mechanism that typically restrains autoimmunity is compromised.[39]

This is an incredibly important finding, because it helps

us figure out exactly which microbes we need to encourage in order to recalibrate our immune system. In short, we need to do everything we can to boost the population of butyrate-producing species in Clostridia clusters IV and XIVa. In subsequent chapters you will learn how to do this through diet and other strategies, but there is one more aspect of the microbiome to consider first.

Unfriendly Microbes

The depletion of good bacteria in those with autoimmunity is only half the story. An excess of specific harmful bacteria may in fact be just as much of a problem. In 2016 and 2017, a series of paradigm-shifting studies reported that in IBD, psoriasis, and arthritis, there is not only a lower level of protective bacteria but also a higher level of inflammatory species. These inflammatory bacteria include *E. coli*, *Salmonella*, *Prevotella*, *Collinsella*, *Streptococcus*, *Enterococcus*, and *Klebsiella*.[40]

These species cause harm in two ways: firstly, they can damage the gut barrier, rendering it more permeable; secondly, they can activate the specific immune cells involved in autoimmune disease.[41] These particular species appear to switch the immune system into inflammation mode not only by producing large amounts of lipopolysaccharide but also through various other mechanisms.

Interestingly, different forms of arthritis are characterized by overgrowths of different bacterial species. In rheumatoid arthritis, researchers have found an increased abundance of *Prevotella* or *Collinsella*, while spondyloarthritis has been linked to a particularly aggressive form of *E. coli*.

This type of *E. coli* is called "adherent-invasive *E. coli*" because it sticks to intestinal cells and invades the protective mucus layer, which can trigger a massive inflammatory response.[42] It was already known that about half of all Crohn's patients have adherent-invasive *E. coli*, whereas it is found in only 1 percent of the general population.[43] In 2017, researchers found that this type of *E. coli* may also be a major contributor to spondyloarthritis.[44] (The spondyloarthritis group includes psoriatic, juvenile, and ankylosing spondylitis [AS].)

Specifically, a group of researchers at Weill Cornell Medical Center in New York found that patients with both spondyloarthritis and Crohn's disease actually had a much greater number of adherent-invasive *E. coli* than those with just Crohn's disease.[45] When this specific *E. coli* was transferred to mice, it triggered the precise immune response characteristic of spondyloarthritis as well as inflammatory arthritis symptoms.

A separate body of research points to yet another possible culprit in ankylosing spondylitis: *Klebsiella pneumoniae*. This common species of gut bacteria was first suspected of playing a role in AS in the 1980s.[46] Since that time, several groups of researchers have found that patients with AS typically have higher levels of antibodies to *Klebsiella* than healthy controls or those with other forms of arthritis. This has been observed in patients in Japan,[47] the Netherlands,[48] England,[49] and Italy.[50]

Most recently, it was reported that antibodies directed against a specific part of a *Klebsiella* protein were found in 190 of 200 patients with AS (95 percent), 3 of 200 patients with rheumatoid arthritis (1.5 percent), but only 1 of 100 (1 percent) patients with psoriatic arthritis.[51]

By contrast, another collection of studies performed across the world has found that patients with rheumatoid arthritis typically have higher levels of antibodies to an entirely different species, called *Proteus mirabilis*.[52]

To find out whether an overgrowth of pathogenic species is a likely contributor in your particular case, a comprehensive stool analysis may be helpful. In the United States, testing options include Genova Diagnostics, Doctors Data, and GI-Map. At the time of writing, GI-Map appears to be the most sensitive test for detecting the bacterial species involved in autoimmunity. Some of these tests can be ordered by individuals located outside the United States. Similar tests are also available from laboratories located in other countries, such as Therapy Select in Germany.

Microbiome tests are fairly expensive (around $350-$500) but can often be ordered directly without a doctor's prescription. See www.keystonebook.com/testing for further information. Although you do not need a doctor to order these tests (in most places), you may still find that you need the assistance of a functional medicine practitioner to help you interpret the results and treat specific infections. See the Institute of Functional Medicine for a directory of physicians familiar with this approach (www.ifm.org).

Beyond the specific bacterial species implicated in autoimmunity in the studies to date, there is also evidence that a net overgrowth of bacteria in the small intestine can trigger the autoimmune process. This type of overgrowth is actually a recognized medical condition termed small intestinal bacterial overgrowth, or SIBO for short.

What is SIBO

In contrast to the bustling ecosystem in the colon, the small intestine has a relatively low concentration of bacteria. This is a good thing since the walls of the small intestine are highly permeable to allow for nutrient absorption. We do not want a large population of bacteria to be sitting idle in the small intestine, because their toxins would be too readily absorbed into the bloodstream.

Bacterial numbers are usually kept low in the small intestine by the combined effect of stomach acid, bile, and the rapid sweeping away of intestinal contents between meals. The small intestine actually goes through a "cleaning cycle" every couple of hours, but only when the stomach is empty. SIBO can occur when these usual mechanisms fail, whether the result of frequent snacking, acid-blocking medication, stomach acid or enzyme deficiency, celiac disease, hypothyroidism, scar tissue from abdominal surgery, or some other factor.[53]

Whatever the cause, in those with an overgrowth of bacteria (or yeasts) in the small intestine, a steady flow of lipopolysaccharide and other toxins across the thin walls of the small intestine sends a powerful signal to activate the immune system, leading to systemic inflammation. This systemic inflammation can manifest as arthritis, psoriasis, or a variety of other conditions.

A condition sometimes called "bypass arthritis" is a dramatic illustration of the ability of SIBO to cause arthritis. This condition typically arose from a drastic method of weight loss surgery performed from the 1950s to the 1980s, where the small intestine was shortened. The surgery often created "blind loops" where bacteria could overgrow, causing severe SIBO. Up to 20 percent of intestinal bypass patients eventually developed arthritis and skin rashes.[54] This form of arthritis became known as bowel-associated dermatosis-arthritis, or bowel bypass syndrome.[55] Fortunately, studies proved that eradicating the bacterial overgrowth quickly resolved the arthritis and rashes.[56]

Although few studies have directly explored the role of SIBO in contributing to autoimmune diseases, a number of small studies have found SIBO in a significant proportion of patients with psoriasis,[57] rheumatoid arthritis,[58] Crohn's disease,[59] and fibromyalgia.[60] Looking at psoriasis, for example, a group of Russian scientists reported that the average number of bacteria in the small intestine of psoriasis patients was approximately 3000 times higher than in the control group.[61]

Another study found that one-third of patients with plaque psoriasis had fragments of DNA in their bloodstream from bacteria that are hallmarks of SIBO.[62] (*E. coli, Klebsiella pneumonia, Enterococcus faecalis, Proteus mirabilis, Streptococcus pyogenes*, and *Shigella*.)[63] Patients with DNA from these bacteria in their bloodstream had much higher levels of inflammation. Most persuasively, it was reported in 2018 that **treating SIBO can dramatically improve psoriasis**.[64]

There are also studies providing indirect evidence of SIBO playing a role in ankylosing spondylitis and juvenile arthritis. When researchers in Sweden took samples of fluid from the small intestine of those with ankylosing spondylitis, they found much higher levels of antibodies to species associated with SIBO (*Klebsiella, E. coli*, and *Proteus mirabilis*).[65] A noteworthy study published in the *Journal of Rheumatology* in 2017 also found that children with juvenile arthritis have much higher levels of antibodies to lipopolysaccharide, which suggests an overgrowth of undesirable species in the small intestine, where lipopolysaccharide can more easily cross into the bloodstream.[66] Another 2017 study found that MS patients with more severe symptoms typically had higher levels of *Streptococcus* in the small intestine.

SIBO Diagnosis

SIBO becomes an even more likely culprit if, in addition to psoriasis or arthritis, you also have the other common signs and symptoms of the condition. SIBO often manifests as either chronic constipation or diarrhea. It is found in up to 80 percent of people with IBS and is now regarded by some experts as the most common cause of the syndrome.[67]

Other classic symptoms of SIBO include multiple food sensitivities, histamine intolerance, nausea, bloating after meals, abdominal pain, eczema, and rosacea. If you have any of these common symptoms of SIBO, or a major risk factor such as celiac disease, endometriosis, or a history of food poisoning or abdominal surgery, it may be worth taking a breath test to help determine if SIBO is involved. The test can be ordered by your doctor, or you can order it yourself (e.g. from www.lifextension.com. Additional testing services are listed at www.keystonebook.com/testing).

The SIBO breath test involves drinking a lactulose and/or glucose solution and collecting breath samples over several hours using an in-home kit. These tests are far from perfect: they are sometimes difficult to interpret and miss many cases of true SIBO (detecting only around 60 percent of cases).[68] Yet a clear positive result can provide useful information.

SIBO is traditionally treated with antibiotics, but for many people this is not a long-term solution. In fact, within nine months of antibiotic treatment, 40 percent of patients relapse, most likely because the underlying causes of SIBO remain.[69] A better approach is to support the normal mechanisms that prevent SIBO in healthy individuals. Strategies to do so are described in chapter 3. For some people with SIBO, carefully chosen probiotics and prebiotics can also be extremely helpful, as discussed in chapter 2. The following chapters also explain how reducing intake of sugar and starch can help address overgrowths of pathogenic species of bacteria and yeasts, including in the small intestine.

Bacteria Beyond the Gut

Although the main focus of this book is the gut microbiome, some surprising research suggests that particular bacteria in other parts of the body can also trigger certain autoimmune diseases. Psoriasis, for example, has a particularly strong connection to *Streptococcal* throat infections, while some limited studies have raised suspicions that some cases of rheumatoid arthritis are linked to urinary tract or periodontal infections. Knowing about these unusual links may further help you tackle the autoimmune response.

Psoriasis and Strep Throat

The link between psoriasis and strep was first suggested after many physicians noted that psoriasis flares often follow episodes of strep throat infections (typically about two weeks later).[70] More recently it has been found that those with chronic psoriasis and psoriatic arthritis often have higher levels of antibodies to *Streptococcus pyogenes*, the species that causes strep throat.[71] There is also some degree of cross-reactivity between streptococcal antigens and human skin proteins.[72] Thus the prevailing theory is that a low-level, chronic infection with streptococcal bacteria in the tonsils can drive the autoimmune reaction, with exacerbations in psoriasis following exacerbations in the streptococcal infection.

Interestingly, there is even stronger evidence for a link between *Streptococcus* and those cases of psoriasis with an earlier age of onset (before age 40) and with either a family history of psoriasis or certain genetic markers.[73] Thus it may be that *Streptococcus* only triggers psoriasis and psoriatic arthritis in those with a genetic predisposition.

If flares of strep throat make psoriasis much worse, it stands to reason that reducing the low-level chronic infection could also make the baseline level of psoriasis much better. That is exactly what the studies have now found. Most persuasively, a 2012 randomized study found a major reduction in psoriasis after patients had their tonsils removed[74] (ranging from a 30 percent to 90 percent reduction in disease severity). In these patients, there was a close correlation between the degree of improvement in psoriasis and the reduction of T-cells that recognized peptides common to both *Streptococcus* and skin proteins.[75] As of 2018, the consensus appears to be that tonsillectomy significantly improves psoriasis in about 75 percent of cases associated with strep throat.[76] Less drastic measures include frequent gargling with warm salt water or peroxide-based mouthwash, and using *S. salivarius K12* oral probiotic lozenges[77] (see www.keystonebook.com/K12).

It is worth noting that *Streptococcus* species are also typically found in the gut, particularly in the small intestine. As noted above, *Streptococcus* is one of the most common types of bacteria found to be elevated in those with SIBO. A gut microbiome analysis can also help identify whether you have an overgrowth of streptococcal species in the gut. If you do, it is highly likely that these bacteria could continue to perpetuate psoriasis and psoriatic arthritis in much the same way as streptococcal infections in the throat. Thus it is important to focus on rebalancing the gut microbiome and treating SIBO, even if you suspect that recurrent strep throat could be a major contributor in your case.

Rheumatoid Arthritis and Infections Beyond the Gut

Entirely different bacteria in the oral microbiome may potentially trigger some cases of rheumatoid arthritis (RA). Population studies have noted that individuals with serious gum disease (periodontitis) are more likely to develop rheumatoid arthritis. More recently, researchers have found that the *gingivalis* bacteria that often cause gum disease also produce an enzyme that could potentially trigger RA.[78] Good dental care is therefore important if you have RA.

Although the evidence is quite limited, some have also suggested a link between *Proteus mirabilis* urinary tract infections and rheumatoid arthritis.[79] Supporting this idea, elevated levels of specific antibodies against *Proteus* bacteria have indeed been found in RA patients in 16 different countries.[80] But even if *P. mirabilis* is a contributing organism, we should bear in mind that this species is also commonly found in the gut. In fact, it is thought that the majority of *P. mirabilis* urinary tract infections actually originate in the gastrointestinal (GI) tract,[81] suggesting that the gut microbiome should remain our primary focus.

Understanding Our Enemies

Whether we view the overarching problem as SIBO, or an overall imbalance between good and bad bacteria, the fact remains that there is a fairly short list of bacterial species we are most concerned about keeping under control. The exact same species that are common culprits in SIBO have also been directly linked to ankylosing spondylitis, psoriasis, rheumatoid arthritis, inflammatory bowel disease, and other autoimmune conditions: [82]

- *Escherichia coli*
- *Klebsiella pneumonia*
- *Enterococcus faecalis*
- *Proteus mirabilis*
- *Streptococcus pyogenes*

These bacteria produce immune-activating toxins such as lipopolysaccharide, along with bacterial proteins that may confuse the immune system by closely resembling our own proteins. They have the net effect of encouraging the immune system to shift toward a more inflammatory state by promoting the proliferation of Th17 cells, which play a direct role in autoimmunity.

There is likely a constant fight for real estate in our gut between the beneficial microbes that calm the immune system, and these unfriendly microbes that antagonize it. As explained by Ivaylo Ivanov, Assistant Professor of Microbiology and Immunology at Columbia University in New York, it is "probably the ratio, the combination of bacteria in the gut that will determine whether you will get disease or not."[83] Our goal, then, is to restore the ratio—to combat autoimmune disease by boosting the protective species and controlling the harmful species. Before we get there, however, it is important to acknowledge one of the major culprits responsible for getting us into this mess: antibiotics.

The Problem with Antibiotics

Due to widespread use of antibiotics, "our microbiome has changed significantly over the past century, and especially over the past 50 years," says NYU microbiologist Martin Blaser.[84] The destruction caused by antibiotics to our resident gut bacteria is actually reflected in a strong link between antibiotic use and the development of autoimmunity.

Juvenile arthritis provides the clearest example. In a recent study published in the journal *Pediatrics*, any recent antibiotic use doubled the chance of children developing arthritis, while five or more courses of antibiotics tripled the risk.[85]

There is also a correlation between exposure to antibiotics and development of a range of other autoimmune diseases, including asthma[86] and Crohn's disease.[87] This effect is even more pronounced in children, and the risk increases with repeated exposure and broader-spectrum antibiotics.

The best explanation for the impact of antibiotics on autoimmunity is that antibiotics wipe out protective bacteria that regulate the immune system while allowing a small number of rare bacterial species to flourish.

While the reasons for this are not fully understood, there is strong evidence that antibiotics have a disproportionate effect on the beneficial butyrate-producing bacteria. As one example, a randomized, placebo-controlled trial published in 2015 used new genome-sequencing technology to analyze the microbiome of 66 healthy adults up to a year after a course of antibiotics.[88] The researchers found that antibiotics "showed a severe and long-term impact on the health-associated butyrate-producing microbial community of the gut."

Antibiotics do not just wipe out the beneficial species we need to maintain a well-calibrated immune system. They also allow the unfriendly species to take over. This is well illustrated in the context of antibiotic-associated diarrhea. A significant proportion of patients that receive broad-spectrum antibiotics can develop severe diarrhea that persists even after the antibiotics are stopped. This condition is most often due to an overgrowth of certain bacteria and yeasts that are able to take advantage of a decimated ecosystem by expanding rapidly. Although the most notorious culprit in causing antibiotic-associated diarrhea is *C. difficile*, it is not the only type of infection that can occur. In fact, when we look at the other species that are most often responsible (such as *Klebsiella*), there is significant overlap with the "bad guys" seen in SIBO and autoimmune conditions.[89]

It is therefore evident that antibiotic use encourages our familiar enemies to expand and take over, while decimating the population of good bacteria. For anyone suffering from autoimmune disease, this provides a powerful reason to do everything you can to avoid using antibiotics. At a practical level, this means becoming vigilant about controlling minor infections at the first sign. For example, if you are prone to sinus infections, it will be important to do everything possible to minimize sinus congestion during allergy season or when you catch a cold. If you are prone to bacterial throat infections, consider gargling with warm salt water or antiseptic mouthwash at the first sign. For urinary tract infections, if you catch them early enough, a simple probiotic supplement can be effective.[90] The important point is to do what you can to combat any infection before it develops into something that requires antibiotics.

If you do find yourself with an infection that requires antibiotics, there may be value in asking your doctor for antibiotic injections rather than pills. When antibiotics are administered by injection rather than taken orally, they may be more effective against infections while having less impact on the gut microbiome.[91]

This also raises the question of antibiotics in the food supply. Modern farming often involves giving healthy animals a variety of antibiotics to encourage rapid weight gain. In the United States, the Department of Agriculture tests meat and poultry to check that antibiotic residues are below a certain level. The overall results of this testing are available online, and the vast majority of tested samples are compliant. The wide variety of antibiotics found in meat violating the standards is not entirely reassuring, but the total dose is still negligible compared to a prescription for antibiotics.[92] If you want to err on the side of caution, choose beef and chicken labeled "organic" or "no antibiotics." This is less important for lamb, which almost never tests positive for antibiotics.[93]

While no one can undo a past littered with antibiotics, it is possible to limit our exposure to antibiotics in the future. By avoiding unnecessary antibiotic prescriptions, and perhaps reducing exposure to trace amounts of antibiotics in our food, we can halt further depletion of our anti-inflammatory microbes. Yet the more important question is how to dial back the damage that has already been done, and how to restore balance to the microbiome. That is the subject of the next two chapters.

CHAPTER 2

REBALANCING THE MICROBIOME WITH PROBIOTICS

Probiotics are one of the best tools we have to rebalance the microbiome. While we cannot simply take a supplement to replace the bacteria that are depleted, new research suggests that probiotics can actually shift the balance of the microbiome as a whole—both lowering the abundance of harmful species and raising the level of beneficial species. The right probiotics can ultimately make the microbiome of someone with autoimmune disease more closely resemble that of healthy individuals.

Using Probiotics to Support Our Beneficial Microbes

Only certain species of probiotics possess the remarkable ability to boost the population of other important species already present in our microbiome. We know, for example, that *L. Rhamnosus GG* (sold as Culturelle®) has this property, because a 2016 study found that it significantly increased the population of butyrate-producing bacteria such as *Roseburia* and *Blautia*.[94] In infants given *L. Rhamnosus GG*, the boost to these other beneficial species resulted in higher butyrate levels and greater immune tolerance (reflected in reduced rate of cow's milk allergy).

The best explanation for how certain probiotics can help other good bacteria thrive is by way of "cross-feeding."[95] In short, different bacteria are good at performing different steps in the fermentation of fiber to short-chain fatty acids such as butyrate. Probiotic species that are good at early steps in the process effectively feed the downstream butyrate-producing bacteria.[96]

Bifidobacteria species appear to be particularly good at cross-feeding the butyrate-producers.[97] Bifidobacteria are in fact critical to the development of a healthy microbiome. These species are among the first to colonize the human gut, typically constituting 95 percent of the total bacterial population in healthy breast-fed infants. The population then drastically declines, making up only 3 to 6 percent of the microbiome by middle age.[98] Common Bifidobacteria species found in healthy humans include *B. longum*, *B. breve*, *B. bifidum*, and *B. infantis*.[99] These species are also readily found in probiotic supplements.

One of the defining characteristics of Bifidobacteria is the production of acetate (whereas Lactobacilli primarily produce lactate). Acetate is important because it is the preferred food source of many of the butyrate producers. If we want to truly help the butyrate-producers flourish, we therefore need to look at the whole ecosystem. It is important to not only provide sufficient dietary fiber, but also ensure adequate numbers of Bifidobacteria, to turn that fiber into a more useable energy source.[100] Bifidobacteria are therefore considered keystone species, because they have a disproportionately large influence on the bacterial ecosystem as a whole.[101]

When it comes to choosing a probiotic supplement to support the butyrate-producing species, the recommended Bifidobacteria species include

- *B. infantis*
- *B. longum*
- *B. breve*

Any Bifidobacteria strain will likely be able to perform the cross-feeding function, but these three species have other anti-inflammatory benefits, as will be discussed further below. *Lactobacillus rhamnosus* GG (found in Culturelle) is another good choice for promoting butyrate-production and thereby calming the immune system.

Using Probiotics to Suppress Harmful Species

The second way in which probiotics can help rebalance a microbiome in disarray is by inhibiting the growth of harmful bacteria such as *Klebsiella, E. coli, Streptococcus,* and other species implicated in inflammatory diseases.[102] Almost all probiotics will combat these pathogens to some degree, by competing with the harmful species for nutrients. Lactobacilli and Bifidobacteria are also generally helpful in suppressing pathogenic bacteria and yeast purely as a function of their general metabolism. That is because these species naturally produce acids that will change the acidity of the gut and thereby suppress many harmful species.

Against this backdrop, some probiotic species appear to have a particularly good ability to inhibit the growth of pathogenic bacteria: [103]

- *B. breve*
- *B. infantis*
- *B. longum*
- *L. rhamnosus*
- *L. plantarum*

A probiotic supplement including some combination of these species is a good starting point in the fight to reclaim territory from the pathogens that contribute to inflammation. Yet there are even more potent options available, if we take advantage of the fact that even within the same species, some very specific strains of probiotics have pathogen-fighting properties that exceed that of other strains.

For example, within the *L. reuteri* species, the strain *L. Reuteri DSM 17938* appears to be especially good at outcompeting pathogens. As a result, this particular strain (sold as BioGaia Protectis®) is often given to preterm infants to prevent serious infections.[104] As further evidence of its ability to suppress pathogens, the strain helps reduce the number of episodes and duration of infectious diarrhea in young children attending day care centers.[105] A recent study also suggests that this strain is effective in combating constipation-dominant SIBO by reducing the population of methane-producing bacteria in the small intestine.[106]

Within the *L. rhamnosus* species, the Culturelle® strain *L. rhamnosus GG* also has a slight edge in preventing opportunistic infections after antibiotics.[107] It also outperformed many other probiotics in a study focused on reducing the severity and duration of infectious diarrhea in children.[108] This strain is a particularly good choice because it helps calm inflammation, boost the butyrate producers, and restore the gut barrier.

Culturelle and BioGaia Protectis are therefore good options to consider. These products are widely available in many countries and are relatively inexpensive.

Advanced Pathogen-Fighting Probiotics

For a more aggressive approach to combating overgrowths of harmful bacteria or yeasts, we can turn to even more potent probiotics. Namely, the pathogen-fighting probiotics that have been proven effective in preventing or treating serious infections such as post-antibiotic *C. difficile* infection and adherent-invasive *E. coli*. These probiotics are

- BioK+® (*L. acidophilus CL1285, L. casei LBC80, L. rhamnosus CLR2*)
- Mutaflor® (*E. coli Nissle 1917*)
- Florastor® (*S. Boulardii CNCM I-745*)

These products are typically more expensive and not as widely available as other probiotics, but they are supported by persuasive evidence from multiple randomized clinical trials.[109] These pathogen-fighting strains are exceptionally good at combating overgrowths of harmful bacteria because they have the unique ability to produce specific antimicrobial compounds. They can also block other organisms from adhering to the gut lining, which makes it more difficult for the harmful species to take up residence.

If testing shows you have an overgrowth of inflammatory

species such as *Candida, E. coli, Streptococcus,* or *Klebsiella,* it may be worth using one of these advanced pathogen-fighting options for one or two months to help clear the overgrowth. When it comes to choosing between these options, each has different advantages and availability in different countries.

Bio-K+

Bio-K+ contains three proprietary strains: *L. acidophilus CL1285, L. casei LBC80,* and *L. rhamnosus CLR2.* It is available in capsules or beverage form in WholeFoods and other health food stores in the United States and Canada. It is unfortunately more difficult to obtain in other countries.

The strains were originally isolated in the 1970s from the stools of a healthy infant. Dr. Francois-Marie Luquet isolated a variety of bacterial strains then identified three strains with the strongest antimicrobial activity against various pathogenic bacteria. After several years of research to optimize culture conditions and gastrointestinal survival of the strains, the Bio-K+ product was developed.[110]

Since that time, it has been used extensively in hospitals to prevent *C. difficile* infections. Following an outbreak of potentially fatal *C. difficile* infections in one hospital in Montreal in 2004, doctors began providing Bio-K+ to all patients there treated with antibiotics.

Multiple randomized, double-blind, placebo-controlled trials have now confirmed that Bio-K+ reduces the risk of developing the infections that cause antibiotic-associated diarrhea.[111] For example, one study found that 44 percent of patients treated with antibiotics alone developed diarrhea and 24 percent developed *C. difficile* infection, whereas of the patients taking two capsules per day of Bio-K+, only 15 percent developed diarrhea and only 1 percent developed *C. difficile* infections.[112]

These findings are important because beyond *C. difficile*, many of the other infections that cause diarrhea in those taking antibiotics correspond to the infections that contribute to systemic inflammation, such as *Klebsiella, E. coli,* and *Candida*.[113] The strains found in Bio-K+ may therefore be helpful to combat overgrowths of these pathogens.

Laboratory studies have also found that the strains used in Bio-K+ have strong antimicrobial activity against *E. coli O157:H7, Salmonella, Staphylococcus, Listeria,* and *Enterococcus faecalis,* all of which are strongly inflammatory.[114]

Bio-K+ has many other advantages, including a long history of use in hundreds of thousands of patients. The beverage formulations are certified gluten free and available in dairy, rice, or soy fermented drinks. Although soy is known for containing compounds that compromise gut health, these compounds are drastically reduced in fermented foods and unlikely to pose a risk in the very small amounts likely found in the Bio-K+ drinks.[115] For those with celiac disease, the gluten-free certification likely outweighs the risk from consuming a small amount of soy, given the concern of unlabeled gluten being found in probiotics.[116]

Another advantage of Bio-K+ is that the strains have demonstrated survival in the gastrointestinal environment.[117] The manufacturer also performs extensive quality control to verify strain identity and potency in each batch of the final product. These factors, along with its proven effects in protecting against serious gut infections, make Bio-K+ a good choice for a short-term pathogen-fighting protocol.

Mutaflor

Mutaflor contains an extensively studied strain of *E. coli*, called *E. coli Nissle 1917*. This particular strain was originally isolated from a soldier in World War I who escaped a severe outbreak of diarrhea affecting his regiment. The strain is thought to have protected the soldier from infection by *Shigella*. Unlike many other strains of *E. coli*, *Nissle 1917* does not produce any known toxins or elicit an inflammatory response.[118]

Soon after the strain was isolated, it became apparent that it could not only help prevent infections but also treat other intestinal conditions. It began being used as a probiotic supplement in Europe in the 1920s, under the trade name Mutaflor. Since then, research has confirmed the value of this particular probiotic strain in the treatment of diarrhea, constipation, and ulcerative colitis.

In patients with ulcerative colitis, two clinical studies have found that Mutaflor shows efficacy in maintaining remission equivalent to the gold standard medication treatment, mesalazine.[119] As a result of these studies, Mutaflor is actually one of the few probiotics licensed as a medicine in Europe. A clinical trial in Crohn's disease also reported a lower relapse rate after 12 months of receiving steroid treatment in combination with Mutaflor.[120]

Importantly, there is good reason to believe that in these conditions, Mutaflor works in part by suppressing pathogenic *E. coli*. [121] As discussed previously, there is a growing body of research linking many cases of Crohn's, ulcerative colitis, and spondyloarthritis to a particularly aggressive form of *E. coli*, called "Adherent-invasive *E. coli*" (AIEC). Researchers have now found that *E. coli Nissle 1917* can effectively inhibit the adhesion and invasion of various AIEC strains isolated from patients with Crohn's disease.[122] In laboratory studies, *E. coli Nissle 1917* can in fact outcompete a range of pathogenic *E. coli* strains.[123] It also appears to be particularly good at inhibiting the growth of *Klebsiella* and preventing invasion by *Salmonella, Yersinia, Shigella, Listeria,* and various other species known to cause serious gut infections.[124] When given to newborns, *E. coli Nissle 1917* colonizes the gut and reduces infection by pathogenic bacteria.[125]

Beyond suppressing harmful bacteria, *E. coli Nissle 1917* may also directly calm inflammation and help repair the gut barrier.[126] Mutaflor is readily available in capsule form in Europe, Canada, Australia, and the United Kingdom. Unfortunately, the FDA barred Mutaflor from sale in the United States in 2011 because it does not fall within the technical definition of a "dietary ingredient," unlike other probiotic species that have long been included in foods such as yogurts.[127] To be sold in the United States, Mutaflor would therefore have to be approved as a drug, which is a long and expensive endeavor. Until the situation is resolved, many people in the United States have resorted to ordering online from Canadian pharmacies.

Florastor

Saccharomyces boulardii is a species of yeast distantly related to baker's yeast. In recent years, it has become a popular probiotic, particularly in the context of treating *Candida* yeast and preventing the opportunistic infections that often arise after antibiotic use. Although there are now many products available containing *S. boulardii*, it is important to note that all of the clinical studies showing efficacy in combating pathogens have been performed with a specific strain, known as *S. boulardii CNCM I-745* or the Biocodex strain. This particular strain is sold under the trade name Florastor.

The Biocodex strain of *S. boulardii* was discovered in Southeast Asia in 1920 by the French microbiologist Henri Boulard. He was searching for new strains of yeast to use in fermentation and happened to be visiting an area during a cholera outbreak. He noticed that people drinking a tea made from the skins of lychees were able to resist the cholera infection. Eventually, he isolated a specific strain of yeast from the surface of the lychees and found that it was this yeast that conferred protection against cholera.[128]

Since that time, more than 50 randomized clinical studies have been performed to investigate the extraordinary properties of this strain, with many showing that it can protect against a variety of infections.[129]

For example, numerous controlled trials have found that those taking *S. boulardii* during antibiotic treatment are about 50 percent less likely to develop antibiotic-associated diarrhea, which is usually caused by opportunistic infections.[130] A 2017 study found that taking *S. boulardii* in conjunction with antibiotics leads to less overgrowth of *E. coli*.[131]

Supplementing with *S. boulardii* does not just prevent gastrointestinal infections but can also help reduce the severity of infections that are already established.[132] Studies have found that *S. boulardii* can reduce the severity of infectious diarrhea, which is often caused by pathogens such as *E. coli* or *Salmonella*.[133] It has also been shown to directly inhibit other specific pathogens most often associated with inflammation and SIBO.[134] One way in which *S. boulardii* can reduce the severity of gut infections is by blocking or breaking down the toxins they produce, such as lipopolysaccharide.[135]

Furthermore, *S. boulardii* is particularly well known for its activity against a variety of species of *Candida* yeast.[136] In addition to suppressing the growth of *Candida,* it helps stop *Candida* adhering to surfaces and forming a biofilm to protect itself.[137] The ability to combat *Candida* is invaluable because *Candida* overgrowths in the GI tract are very common and highly inflammatory.[138] Higher levels of intestinal *Candida* are often seen in those with Crohn's disease and ulcerative colitis.[139] It has been suggested that inflammation in the gut makes it easier for *Candida* to colonize, which then triggers further inflammation in a vicious cycle.[140] Supplementing with *S. boulardii* could be one step toward breaking this cycle. (Additional supplements to combat *Candida* are discussed in chapter 3.)

In addition to suppressing harmful bacteria and yeasts, *S. boulardii* can also help restore the intestinal barrier. This was evident from a study of patients with Crohn's disease who still show abnormal intestinal permeability even when the disease is in remission. When a group of patients took *S. boulardii* for three months, their intestinal permeability improved.[141]

The effect of *S. boulardii* in Crohn's disease does not end there. It also significantly reduces symptoms and the risk of relapse. When patients with Crohn's disease in remission took *S. boulardii* for six months, only 6 percent relapsed, compared to 38 percent not taking the probiotic.[142] In another placebo-controlled study, *S. boulardii* significantly reduced the severity of Crohn's disease in those with continuing moderate symptoms.[143] Again, this likely occurs by suppressing pathogens that would otherwise antagonize the immune system. *S. boulardii* may therefore be able to play a similar role in dialing back other related autoimmune diseases.

S. boulardii is not suitable for everyone, however. Isolated cases of *S. boulardii* entering the bloodstream and causing infection have been reported in seriously ill patients and those with central venous lines.[144] This probiotic should probably also be avoided by those with an allergy or hypersensitivity to baker's yeast (*Saccharomyces cerevesiae*), because the two are closely related.

If you decide to try *S. boulardii*, it is best to choose the Florastor brand if you can because this product contains the specific strain used in the clinical trials discussed above. The dose used in most studies is 500–1000 mg per day, which corresponds to two to four capsules per day.

Probiotics and SIBO

The value of probiotics in treating small intestinal bacterial overgrowth (SIBO) is hotly debated. Some take the view that if SIBO is caused by an excess of bacteria in the small intestine, adding further bacteria in the form of probiotics is counterproductive. In addition, those with SIBO often find that probiotics can worsen symptoms such as bloating and histamine reactions, at least in the short term.

The alternate view is that the inflammation and damage caused by SIBO are often driven by particular species of unfriendly bacteria, and probiotics can be a key weapon in suppressing those species in the long term. Probiotics may also combat SIBO in other ways, such as improving the speed of transit through the digestive system, which reduces the opportunity for bacterial overgrowth.

The clinical studies that have been done so far do indicate that probiotics can be somewhat helpful in treating SIBO. For example, we saw earlier that the BioGaia Protectis strain of *L. reuteri* appears to be effective in combating methane-dominant SIBO. Another study found that four weeks of treatment with a probiotic combination that included several Bifidobacteria and Lactobacillus species was able to eradicate SIBO in a quarter of patients.[145] A similar probiotic combination was able to produce a clinical improvement in 80 percent of patients with SIBO, whereas only 52 percent of patients taking antibiotics improved.[146] Other probiotic species that have been found helpful for SIBO include *Bacillus clausii* and *Bacillus coagulans*.[147] These species are not necessarily the best choices for those with autoimmunity though, because they can be somewhat inflammatory.

Two other types of probiotics are often recommended to those with SIBO: soil-based organisms and so called "D-lactate-free" probiotics. There is little to no clinical evidence supporting the use of soil-based organisms and these products should be considered high-risk, given the possibility that they can colonize the gut long term.

The benefit of D-lactate-free probiotics may also be over-sold. The supposed advantage of these probiotics is based on the fact that in some cases, SIBO can involve an excess of D-lactate.[148] Although the body has mechanisms to quickly metabolize lactate, extreme excess is thought to cause fatigue, weakness, and cognitive impairment.[149] Companies have therefore marketed probiotics that produce very little D-lactate as more suitable for those with SIBO. Yet the original studies linking D-lactate to SIBO were done in the context of severe SIBO caused by surgical shortening of the small intestine. This is a very unique situation and the findings cannot be extrapolated to ordinary SIBO. Very little is known about the role of D-lactate in producing symptoms of SIBO in those with intact digestive systems. Nevertheless, if you do notice worsening fatigue or cognitive impairment with Lactobacillus probiotics, note that Bifidobacteria species typically produce very little D-lactate.

In the end, our choice of probiotic in the context of SIBO should focus on the ultimate goal of reducing the burden of pathogens in the small intestine. Bifidobacteria are likely helpful in this context, but we may see even more benefit from the specialist pathogen-fighting strains discussed above: BioGaia Protectis, Mutaflor, Bio-K+, and Florastor. These have all been studied extensively in clinical trials and have been found to suppress a range of pathogens that are common culprits in causing SIBO. They also share the important properties of reducing overall inflammation and helping repair the gut barrier, which are the other key goals of probiotic treatment.

For more advanced treatment of SIBO and pathogen overgrowth, some people may still find that they also need to supplement with bile, digestive enzymes, and other supplements. These strategies are covered in chapter 3.

Using Probiotics to Restore the Integrity of the Gut Barrier

Probiotics that suppress harmful species of yeast and bacteria will go a long way toward healing leaky gut, because pathogen overgrowth is often one of the root causes of increased intestinal permeability.[150] By addressing the cause of the problem, we give the natural repair mechanisms a chance to work.

Yet probiotics can also help directly support the healing process itself. That is because butyrate is in fact the main energy source for the cells lining the intestines. It powers the repair and regeneration of every component of the intestinal barrier.[151] Because probiotics such as Bifidobacteria and *L. rhamnosus GG* help support butyrate production, they can therefore help reverse leaky gut.[152] Other strains of probiotics can also promote repair and regeneration of the intestinal lining in more direct ways. *E. coli Nissle 1917* and *B. infantis*, for example, have both been found to produce compounds that directly boost the production of tight junction proteins.[153]

Overall, the probiotics that are particularly good at reversing leaky gut include[154]

- *B. infantis*
- *B. breve*
- *L. rhamnosus GG*
- *E. coli Nissle 1917*
- *L. plantarum*
- *L. acidophilus*

Anti-inflammatory vs. Inflammatory Probiotics

All the beneficial effects of probiotics discussed so far have the net effect of reducing inflammation. But probiotics can also directly modulate the immune system, for better or worse. That is because different probiotics can shift the dial on the immune system in different directions. Some can reduce the production of inflammatory mediators, which makes the immune system more tolerant and less likely to overreact to perceived threats. Other probiotics activate components of the immune system that fight infection, but in the process may increase the production of inflammatory mediators.

Probiotics that are known to be anti-inflammatory include[155]

- *B. infantis*
- *B. breve*
- *B. longum*
- *L. rhamnosus GG* (Culturelle)
- *L. reuteri DSM 17938* (BioGaia Protectis)
- *B. infantis 35624* (Align)
- *E. coli Nissle 1917* (Mutaflor)
- *S. boulardii CNCM I-745* (Florastor)
- *L. acidophilus*

At the cellular level, these probiotics have been shown to reduce a wide variety of inflammatory mediators, including the mediators involved in psoriasis and arthritis.[156] Clinical studies also show that these probiotics can reduce the severity of inflammatory conditions such as ulcerative colitis, allergy, and eczema.[157]

In contrast, certain other probiotics can tend to promote immune activation and could potentially undermine our efforts to lower inflammation. There are two main ways in which this can occur in the autoimmune context. The first is by activating immune cells called T helper 17 cells (Th17 cells), which produce powerful inflammatory mediators. The second is by producing large amounts of histamine, which can trigger the innate immune system.

Th17 cells, IL-17, and Probiotics

Th17 cells are specialized helper immune cells that have recently been recognized as playing a significant role in driving autoimmune disease.[158] Th17 cells produce a cytokine called Interleukin 17 (IL-17). This is an immune-stimulating mediator that ordinarily plays an important role in combating gut infection but can also orchestrate the inflammation involved in some autoimmune diseases, particularly ankylosing spondylitis, psoriatic arthritis, and psoriasis. In fact, the newest generation of biologics used to treat these conditions (such as Cosentyx and Taltz) actually work by blocking IL-17.

Given that IL-17 plays a key role in driving inflammation, it stands to reason that we should try to minimize anything that boosts IL-17. Some species of bacteria and yeasts are very strong inducers of IL-17. This includes *Klebsiella*, *Candida albicans*, *Campylobacter*, *Enterococcus*, and other common gut pathogens, but also species occasionally found in probiotic supplements, such as *B. adolescentis*.[159]

Research in this area has only just begun, so for many species of probiotics, we have no information about how they influence Th17 cells and IL-17 production. Yet we do know that some probiotics can actually calm inflammation by reducing IL-17 production, while many others have very little direct effect on IL-17. At the time of writing, the best available information we have is as follows:

Mild suppressors of IL-17:[160]

- *L. rhamnosus GG*
- *B. longum subspecies infantis 35624*
- *L. acidophilus*
- *L. reuteri DSM17938*

Little to no direct effect on IL-17:[161]

- *B. breve*
- *B. infantis*
- *B. longum*
- *B. lactis*
- *L. rhamnosus*
- *L. casei*
- *S. boulardii*

Possible inducers of IL-17:[162]

- *B. bifidum*
- *B. coagulans*

Strong inducers of IL-17:[163]

- *B. adolescentis*
- *Klebsiella pneumoniae*
- *Enterococcus faecalis*
- *Campylobacter jejuni*
- *Candida albicans*
- *Citrobacter species*
- *Salmonella species*
- *Streptococcus*

Until more is known, the most cautious approach is to strictly avoid probiotics that contain *B. adolescentis*. What is less clear is whether we need to avoid probiotic combinations that contain *B. bifidum*. On its own, this species appears to be a mild-to-moderate inducer of IL-17 in laboratory studies.[164] But in at least one animal study, a probiotic combination that included *B. bifidum* decreased IL-17 production overall (and also suppressed experimental inflammatory bowel disease and rheumatoid arthritis).[165] *B. bifidum* is particularly good at combating infections, so in real life it may ultimately lower IL-17 levels by suppressing other inflammatory bacteria or yeasts.

A similar effect has been seen with *B. breve* and *L. casei*. On their own, these species have no direct effect on IL-17 production. But in the real-world context, they significantly reduce the IL-17 triggered by other infections.[166]

Ultimately, the major cause of high levels of IL-17 in those with autoimmune disease is likely to be the overgrowth of species such as *Klebsiella*, *E. coli*, *Streptococcus*, and *Candida*. Addressing these overgrowths with pathogen-fighting probiotics is probably one of the best tools we have to naturally lower IL-17. Other strategies that can help reduce IL-17 production include getting adequate amounts of vitamin A, vitamin D, and omega-3 fats, along with supporting our resident butyrate-producing microbes.[167]

Histamine production by probiotics

The second way in which probiotics can potentially promote inflammation is by producing histamine. Some species of bacteria produce large amounts of histamine by degrading dietary amino acids. In sensitive individuals, this histamine then activates mast cells, which triggers an increase in intestinal permeability, along with a variety of allergy-like symptoms such as itching, flushing, fatigue, and headaches.

The probiotic species typically regarded as the worst when it comes to histamine production are *S. thermophilus* and *L. bulgaricus*.[168] There is unfortunately a lack of reliable data about histamine production by many other species. Even within the same species, different strains may produce different amounts of histamine. We do know that in general, Bifidobacteria are less likely to produce histamine than Lactobacilli. Within the Lactobacilli species, *L. acidophilus* and *L. rhamnosus* are not typically histamine producers.[169]

The fact that a probiotic combination contains some histamine-producing species is not necessarily a deal-breaker, however. Other strains in the combination may be good at degrading histamine, and the combination as a whole may be good at suppressing histamine-producing bacteria naturally resident in your gut. The high-potency combination probiotic VSL#3, for example, contains the high-histamine producers *S. thermophilus* and *L. bulgaricus*. Some people will tolerate this probiotic, while others will not. (Note that researchers have recently raised quality concerns with VSL#3, following a change in manufacturing.[170])

If you find you are particularly sensitive to histamine-producing strains of probiotics, the root cause may be an overgrowth of histamine-producing or immune-stimulating microbes in your gut. Recent studies have found that certain gut microbes can produce a significant amount of histamine. This includes *E. coli* and *Morganella morganii*.[171] (Overgrowths of these particular species can be detected on stool tests such as the GI-Map.) Other pathogens in the gut can also stimulate the immune system itself to release histamine. This includes *Candida* yeast, for example. The net effect is that an overgrowth of pathogens can heighten sensitivity to additional histamine from probiotics. Yet probiotics that combat these pathogens may be part of the long-term solution to histamine intolerance.

Probiotic Buyers Guide

There are many factors to weigh when choosing a probiotic, but perhaps the best place to start is by identifying products containing the species we want, without any that could spur inflammation. We can then consider whether to choose a probiotic containing mild strains, or more potent pathogen-fighters.

Level 1 Probiotics

At the introductory level, it is best to choose a probiotic combination that includes at least one of the preferred Bifidobacteria species, namely:

- *B. infantis*
- *B. longum*
- *B. breve*

These species excel at cross-feeding the butyrate producers, restoring the gut barrier, and calming inflammation. Recommended products with these species and no inflammatory species include:

- **Jarrow-dophilus Allergen Free**
- **Klaire Labs Ther-Biotic Metabolic Formula**
- **Probiotic Pearls Digestion and Immunity**

These particular combination products also contain lactobacillus strains that may provide some further help in suppressing harmful bacteria and restoring the gut barrier. For example, *L. acidophilus* is known for its ability to combat leaky gut, while three of the specific strains used in the Jarrow Allergen Free combination are particularly good at suppressing *E.coli* (namely, *L. plantarum LP01, L. rhamnosus LR-04,* and *B. breve BR-03*).

Culturelle Health & Wellness and **BioGaia Protectis** are also good entry-level probiotics. These single-strain lactobacillus probiotics have been studied extensively and are typically well tolerated by even the most sensitive individuals, including newborn infants.

All of these Level 1 probiotics are good options for long-term maintenance, to continue supporting your beneficial microbes while deterring undesirable species. If, however, you do not see sufficient improvement, or you already know you have a significant pathogen overgrowth, you may need one of the more potent probiotics detailed below.

Level 2 Probiotics

For stronger activity against the undesirable bacteria that can drive inflammation, we can select a probiotic with a higher potency and broader range of Bifidobacteria species. Good options include:

- **Gut Pro and Gut Pro Infant**
- **Jarrow Bifidus Balance**
- **Renew Life Adult 50 Plus Go Pack**
- **Kirkman Bifido Complex**

Because these probiotics contain *B. bifidum*, they may be slightly more effective than the level 1 probiotics at combatting pathogens. Yet once pathogen overgrowth is brought under control, this potent species is likely no longer required. Because *B. bifidum* may theoretically spur immune activity, it may be preferable to return to a milder level 1 probiotic for ongoing maintenance. (You can of course continue taking a level 2 probiotic long-term, if you find that you respond well).

Level 3 Probiotics

For those with particularly severe inflammation, an overgrowth of persistent species such as *E.coli*, *Candida*, or *Klebsiella*, or a diagnosis of SIBO, you may see the greatest improvement by starting with 30 to 60 days of treatment with one of the advanced pathogen-fighting probiotics:

- **BioK+**
- **Mutaflor**
- **Florastor**

This intensive treatment phase is intended to suppress the harmful species that are notoriously difficult to combat. Once you see a significant improvement in symptoms, you can then revert to a level 1 or 2 probiotic for long-term use. (You may also decide to continue taking a level 3 probiotic for an extended period of time if you prefer.)

Other Factors Influencing Probiotic Choice

Within each of the levels above, the choice of probiotic may be dictated by other factors unique to your particular circumstances. If you are located in Europe, for example, you may have easy access to BioGaia, Mutaflor, and Florastor, but difficulty obtaining certain other products. For individuals who are sensitive to even trace amounts of dairy, most of the probiotics listed above will be suitable, with the exception of Pearls Digestion & Immunity and Jarrow Bifidus Balance.

If you find that you need to avoid fillers containing starch, prebiotics or maltodextrin, preferred options include:

- Klaire Labs Ther-Biotic Metabolic Formula (level 1)
- Probiotic Pearls Digestion and Immunity (level 1)
- BioGaia Protectis (level 1)
- Gut Pro and Gut Pro Infant (level 2)
- Kirkman Bifido Complex (level 2)
- Renew Life Adult 50 Plus Go Pack (level 2)
- Florastor (level 3)
- BioK+ (level 3)

In the end, the probiotics identified in this chapter are good options to consider, but some experimentation may be needed to find what works best for you. For up-to-date information on available products and links to online stores, see www.keystonebook.com/probiotics.

Prebiotics

An optional add-on strategy to maximize the effect of your probiotic is to include a daily prebiotic fiber supplement. Prebiotics are typically forms of soluble fiber that are intended to preferentially feed beneficial bacteria. They can have a dramatic effect on the balance of species in the gut, with much bigger boosts to beneficial bacteria than we can produce with probiotics or diet alone.

The problem is that the resulting changes to the microbiome are quite unpredictable. Many prebiotics can feed unwanted species, too, and help these species multiply alongside the beneficial species we are trying to boost. In this way, prebiotics are similar to fertilizer. Fertilizing a lawn can help grass grow, but it may also help the weeds grow.

It may be that we can get the best results from prebiotics

by doing some "weeding" first. That is, by spending several months focused on other measures to suppress harmful species, such as pathogen-fighting probiotics, supplements, and dietary changes, before introducing a prebiotic to help the beneficial species maintain the upper hand. Even with this strategy of holding off until some balance is restored, prebiotics will remain a high-risk but high-reward proposition. We can improve the odds somewhat by choosing particular prebiotics that have a greater chance of favoring the right bacteria. While there are a wide variety of prebiotic supplements available, the following section describes five commonly available options.

Acacia Fiber

One of the most well-tolerated prebiotics currently available is acacia fiber, also known as gum arabic or acacia gum. Derived from the sap of the African acacia tree, this form of soluble fiber is sold as Heather's Tummy Fiber™ and Renew Life™ Organic Clear Fiber, among other products. Acacia fiber can very effectively stimulate the beneficial Bifidobacteria, increase butyrate levels, and improve leaky gut.[172] The balance of the evidence suggests that it does not encourage significant growth of undesirable species.[173] (Although one laboratory study did report that *Klebsiella* could ferment a similar type of carbohydrate, so it is best avoided by those with ankylosing spondylitis or a known *Klebsiella* overgrowth.)[174]

In human studies, acacia fiber typically causes little to no gas or bloating even at high doses, unlike most other prebiotics.[175] When used for several weeks, it has a remarkable ability to reduce both diarrhea and constipation, likely due in large part to its ability to promote beneficial bacteria.[176] The optimal dose of acacia fiber is thought to be 10 to 15 grams per day, which is approximately two measuring table-spoons. However, it may be better to start at a much lower dose, such as ½ a teaspoon per day, and increase the dose over the course of several weeks.

Galactooligosaccharides (GOS)

Another form of prebiotic often used to boost beneficial bacteria is galactooligosaccharides, or GOS for short. On their own, GOS do little to support the butyrate producers, but they may be helpful for getting the best response from a Bifidobacteria probiotic.

These indigestible carbohydrates are actually a major component of human breast milk, where they are present solely to feed important beneficial bacteria in the infant.[177] With this context, it is perhaps unsurprising that galac-tooligosaccharides are fairly selective for Bifidobacteria.[178] Bifidobacteria are among the predominant bacteria present in newborns, and it makes sense that human breast milk evolved to include a prebiotic that feeds these species but not potential pathogens.

GOS may even suppress some pathogens. When preterm infants were given a formula supplement with GOS, the total abundance of common pathogens dropped significantly (while the Bifidobacteria increased from 5 percent of total bacteria to over 30 percent).[179] Another recent study found that supple-menting with GOS could reduce the level of *Streptococcus*, a common contributor to both SIBO and psoriasis.[180] Yet this same study found that GOS can also suppress some of the butyrate-producing species and increase the abundance of *Prevotella*, which has been linked to rheumatoid arthritis.[181] Therefore the effects of GOS may be somewhat unpredictable and it is likely more appropriate for those with psoriasis than RA.

Most of the studies finding a benefit of GOS have used a dose of 8 to 15 grams per day, but it appears that GOS can boost Bifidobacteria even at a much lower dose of 2.5 grams per day,[182] which is similar to the amount found in a single-serve sachet of Bimuno™, the most well-known GOS prebiotic supplement.

Partially Hydrolyzed Guar Gum

Partially hydrolyzed guar gum is an alternative prebiotic that is often well tolerated by those with significant intestinal symptoms. This prebiotic is sold as Sunfiber™ and Nutrisource Fiber™, for example.

Partially hydrolyzed guar gum clearly enhances the growth of beneficial bacteria such as Bifidobacteria and the butyrate producers.[183] As we would expect, it also strongly boosts butyrate levels.[184] Yet there is conflicting and limited information available concerning its impact on undesirable bacteria.[185]

We do know that in human studies, partially hydrolyzed guar gum has been found useful in treating conditions involving bacterial overgrowth, such as irritable bowel syndrome.[186] The results are likely to differ between individuals though. Dr. Allyson Siebecker, a physician who specializes in treating SIBO, reports that some patients are "prebiotic responders" and do very well with prebiotics such as partially hydrolyzed guar gum, whereas these prebiotics may worsen symptoms for others.[187]

Psyllium

Psyllium husk is yet another alternative prebiotic that feeds beneficial butyrate producers, apparently without significantly feeding *E. coli* or *Klebsiella*.[188] Yet it has a major drawback. Unfortunately, the plants used to grow psyllium are very good at absorbing lead from the soil. As a result, psyllium fiber supplements often contain high levels of lead and probably should not be used long term.

Fructooligosaccharides (FOS)

The least desirable prebiotics for those with gut-related autoimmune conditions are those made up of chains of fructose molecules, called fructans. Fructans include short chains of fructose, known as fructooligosaccharides (FOS), or long chains, known as inulin. These prebiotics are well known for their ability to profoundly boost beneficial bacteria.[189] Yet fructans are not suitable for everyone.

These prebiotics not only feed the beneficial bacteria but may also feed undesirable bacteria such as *Klebsiella*, *Streptococci*, and *E. coli*.[190] It is therefore best to avoid prebiotics containing large amounts of inulin or FOS.

Fructans are also found in onion, asparagus, leeks, garlic, green banana, and some probiotic supplements. The smaller amount found in these sources is less concerning than a concentrated prebiotic supplement and may not be a problem for everyone. Nevertheless, some people may benefit from limiting high-fructan foods, at least in the short term and as part of a broader program to suppress the population of inflammatory microbes.

CHAPTER 3

ADDITIONAL STRATEGIES TO COMBAT BACTERIAL OVERGROWTH

Probiotics and diet should be the cornerstones of a long-term strategy to combat an excess of undesirable bacteria. Yet there are several other approaches that can provide further help to tackle specific pathogens or SIBO, including supporting proper digestion and the short-term use of natural antimicrobial supplements. The conventional medical approach to treating SIBO with antibiotics is also one option to consider.

The Conventional Approach

The standard treatment for SIBO is an antibiotic called Rifaximin (Xifaxan). Unlike other antibiotics, Rifaximin is not absorbed into the bloodstream. Instead, it stays in the gut where it can target the bacteria that cause SIBO. This particular antibiotic is not as detrimental to the overall microbiome as other antibiotics because its activity is largely limited to the small intestine. It needs bile to dissolve, so becomes poorly soluble and loses effectiveness when it arrives in the large intestine. As a result, Rifaximin can target over-growth in the small intestine without significantly harming the good bacteria in the large intestine.

Nevertheless, this antibiotic is not a magic solution for SIBO. Rifaximin is very expensive, often not covered by insurance, and relapses after treatment are incredibly common. In fact, within nine months, 40 percent of patients relapse, most likely because the underlying causes of SIBO are not addressed.[191]

Yet it cannot be questioned that at least in the short term, Rifaximin often works quite well. In a recent study in three patients with psoriasis who tested positive for SIBO by glucose breath test, treatment with a combination of Rifaximin and a prebiotic (guar gum) for 12 days eradicated the bacterial overgrowth and significantly improved psoriasis.[192] The redness of psoriasis plaques was reduced by 43 percent just from this very brief treatment regime.

Another common method of treating SIBO is to use various natural antimicrobial supplements, such as oregano oil and grapefruit seed extract. Many of these antimicrobials will indeed suppress the bacteria involved in SIBO, but they can also cause significant destruction to the population of beneficial microbes. In the long term this may actually exacerbate SIBO and allow harmful bacteria to flourish.

For long-term control of SIBO while preserving the beneficial species in the large intestine, a better starting point is to focus on restoring the normal mechanisms that prevent bacterial overgrowth in healthy individuals. The first way to do this is through meal spacing.

Meal Spacing

One of the most important mechanisms that normally keeps bacteria numbers low in the small intestine is the cleaning cycle that sweeps away the bacteria and debris between meals. This is termed the migrating motor complex (MMC). The MMC is a very specific pattern of gastrointestinal muscle activity that differs significantly from the normal activity during digestion. It involves coordinated waves to push debris along the small intestine. A small amount of bile is also secreted to act as soap and help the cleaning function. The entire cycle takes about two hours, culminating in a burst of activity that produces the rumbling noises many people mistake for hunger pangs.

Importantly, the MMC cleaning process shuts down when food is ingested. The small intestine effectively has two modes of operation: digesting and cleaning. If food is eaten too frequently during the day, the small intestine will remain in digesting mode and the MMC will never get the chance to clean away food residue and bacteria.

To give the MMC as much opportunity as possible to do its important job, it is best to eat only at defined meal times. Dr. Mark Pimental, a gastroenterologist who has led much of the research on SIBO, recommends spacing meals at least four to five hours apart, with no snacking.[193] (Drinking water or other noncaloric beverages between meals is not a problem.) It may not be realistic to space your meals properly every single day, but the more often you can, the better.

The MMC also significantly slows down during sleep, so it is best to eat dinner several hours before bed, if possible. An example meal schedule would be to eat at 8 a.m., 1 p.m., and 6 p.m. Alternatively, you may find it easier to eat four smaller meals, say at 8 a.m., 12 p.m., 4 p.m., and 8 p.m.

If you find it difficult to stick to an eating schedule and maintain steady energy levels without snacking, it is possible that you are relying too heavily on carbohydrates for fuel. Try to include at least 30 grams of protein in each meal, along with a source of fiber and fats such as avocado or olive oil. It may also take some time to adjust to a new eating schedule.

Digestive Support

In healthy people, the combined action of stomach acid, enzymes, and bile salts also plays a key role in preventing bacterial overgrowths. Bile not only acts as a detergent to clean the small intestine, but it also directly suppresses many undesirable species, including *Streptococci*, *Klebsiella*, *E. coli*, and other species that produce lipopolysaccharide.[194] Bile in fact reduces our exposure to lipopolysaccharide in another way as well—by reducing the amount of lipopolysaccharide absorbed from the small intestine.[195]

Producing adequate stomach acid and digestive enzymes is also essential to preventing bacterial overgrowth. If you do not produce enough, digestion will slow and food can sit and ferment in the upper digestive system, leading to SIBO.

Some people therefore benefit tremendously from supplementing with enzymes, acid, or bile. Several physicians have reported that bile supplementation alone can significantly improve psoriasis in many cases.[196]

Unfortunately, it is difficult to know whether you are producing sufficient bile, acid, and enzymes, so some element of trial and error is inevitable. A good starting point is a bile supplement such as ox bile or Jarrow Bile Factors, taken at the end of meals. The next step would be to consider adding a supplement containing a combination of betaine HCL, pepsin, and pancreatin. (See www.keystonebook.com/supplements.)

Prokinetics

Gastroenterologists who specialize in SIBO often emphasize that long-term control of bacterial overgrowth in the small intestine depends on supporting motility as much as possible, particularly where scar tissue or a history of food poisoning is involved. To that end, doctors often prescribe medicines or natural agents to stimulate the cleansing activity of the migrating motor complex.

Prescription options include low-dose erythromycin or low-dose naltrexone. Low-dose naltrexone has other potential benefits and is discussed in chapter 9. Nonprescription options include ginger and a herbal combination called Iberogast. Iberogast is often regarded as the best choice, because it is well tolerated and continues working long term. Used in Europe for the past 40 years to treat all manner of digestive complaints, Iberogast has been shown to increase motility in the small intestine.[197] In controlled clinical trials, it has also been proven effective for irritable bowel syndrome and conditions associated with delayed stomach emptying.[198] In addition, the safety of Iberogast has been studied extensively in clinical trials, with no serious side effects, despite use by an estimated 25 million people over the past 50 years.[199] To support the migrating motor complex, Iberogast is best taken two hours after each meal.

Together, the combination of meal spacing, digestive supplements, and prokinetics can provide a powerful boost to the natural mechanisms that sweep the small intestine clear of excess bacteria. These three steps alone provide a good starting point to begin tackling milder cases of bacterial overgrowth, without any risk of harming the overall microbiome. The same three steps are also important to prevent SIBO from returning after more aggressive treatment, such as with antibiotics or natural antimicrobials.

Natural Antimicrobials

The next phase of combating either SIBO or particular inflammatory bacteria such as *Klebsiella* or *Streptococcus* is a short-term treatment with one or more natural antimicrobial compounds. It may or may not be necessary to go down this path, depending on how well you respond to diet, probiotics, and other measures.

If you do decide to use natural antimicrobials, it is best to keep the treatment period short (typically one month) and to choose compounds that do the least damage possible to the beneficial species of gut bacteria. To that end, it is important to avoid broad-acting antimicrobials, such as grapefruit seed extract and oregano oil, and instead choose the most targeted and specific options.

When it comes to suppressing the microbes most often implicated in SIBO and autoimmunity, without harming the overall microbiome, the best options are **lactoferrin**, **allicin**, and **berberine**. For the best results, all three of these can be taken half an hour before meals for 30 days. If you have a sensitive stomach, it may be best to start each supplement separately and begin with a single capsule each day.

Note that many people report an initial phase of feeling worse after beginning antimicrobial compounds, with symptoms such as fatigue, stomach pain, or nausea. This may be caused by an immune reaction to the dying bacteria and yeasts and should only last for one or two weeks.

Lactoferrin

Lactoferrin is an iron-transport protein that plays a key role in defending against infection. It is present in high concentrations in tears, saliva, and breast milk. Because human and bovine lactoferrin are quite similar, this protein can also be purified from cow's milk and is therefore readily available in supplement form.

Lactoferrin works in part by strongly binding to iron, making that iron unavailable to pathogenic bacteria but still usable by our own cells. This mechanism of action targets undesirable bacteria while leaving many beneficial species untouched.[200]

Lactoferrin is particularly effective against *Klebsiella* and *E. coli*, for example.[201] It not only inhibits the growth of these species but also helps break down the biofilms that *E. coli* and *Klebsiella* produce to shield themselves from our immune system. In addition, lactoferrin stops harmful bacteria from sticking to and invading intestinal cells, including the specific type of aggressive *E. coli* implicated in Crohn's disease.[202]

Importantly, lactoferrin can suppress harmful bacteria without harming important anti-inflammatory species such as Bifidobacteria. Researchers have actually found that it can boost the number of Bifidobacteria, especially *B. breve* and *B. infantis*.[203] In human trials, giving lactoferrin-supplement formula to infants prevents serious infections while increasing Bifidobacteria levels.[204]

Lactoferrin supplements may not be suitable for those with severe dairy allergy because the protein is purified from cow's milk and trace amounts of whey or casein may therefore be present in the final supplement. The amount of these other proteins is likely to be minute, however, so the benefits of lactoferrin may outweigh this concern for those with only minor sensitivities to dairy.

Lactoferrin supplements are typically available in a dose of 250 milligrams per capsule and the usual dose is two to four capsules per day, before meals. Recommended brands include Jarrow and Life Extension.

Allicin

Garlic has been used to treat gastrointestinal complaints and infections for thousands of years.[205] The primary compound in garlic responsible for this infection-fighting ability is allicin, which forms when garlic is cut or crushed.

To obtain a sufficient amount of allicin to suppress harmful bacteria and yeasts, a supplement is typically more convenient than consuming large amounts of fresh garlic. An allicin supplement also allows us to avoid the fructans found in fresh garlic, which cause intestinal symptoms for many people with bacterial overgrowth.

Although allicin can combat a range of infections, this compound is particularly good at conquering the specific bacteria that have been implicated in psoriasis, rheumatoid arthritis, psoriatic arthritis, and ankylosing spondylitis (namely *Streptococcus pyogenes*, *Proteus mirabilis*, *E. coli*, *and Klebsiella*).[206] Allicin can also combat other inflammatory species that may contribute to inflammation, including *Enterococcus faecalis*, *Helicobacter pylori*, and *Citrobacter freundii*.[207]

In addition, allicin has potent antiviral and antifungal

activity. Studies have found that it kills *Candida* yeast almost as effectively as the prescription antifungal fluconazole.[208]

Helpfully, allicin appears to be relatively selective for harmful species of bacteria and has much less effect on beneficial species such as Lactobacilli and Bifidobacteria.[209] We do not yet know how allicin impacts the broader microbiome, but initial laboratory and animal studies indicate that it may actually increase the overall diversity and boost the all-important butyrate-producing species.[210]

The preferred supplement option is AlliMax, because it contains stabilized allicin rather than merely a garlic extract intended to result in allicin production in the body. AlliMax does contain a small amount of maltodextrin, which can potentially feed unwanted microbes, but the powerful antimicrobial effect of the supplement likely outweighs the presence of maltodextrin. Other alternative brands include Garlinase and Pure Encapsulations GarliActive, although these products contain garlic extract rather than allicin, so they may be less effective and more likely to cause unpleasant side effects.

Berberine

Berberine is a compound found in several medicinal herbs, including goldenthread, goldenseal, Oregon grape, and barberry. These herbs have been used in traditional Ayurvedic and Chinese medicine for centuries, typically to treat gastrointestinal infections. More recently, berberine has become a popular treatment option for SIBO, diabetes, and high cholesterol.[211] Most importantly for our purposes, berberine has been found to kill or inhibit a variety of inflammatory species of gut microbes, including *Klebsiella*, *Streptococcus*, and many other species that produce lipopolysaccharide.[212] Berberine is particularly active against *Candida* yeast and *E. coli*.[213]

Perhaps the most exciting prospect in the use of berberine is the potential to not only suppress these harmful species but to actually *increase* the population of beneficial species. In a series of animal studies published in 2017 and 2018, berberine was found to boost the population of important butyrate-producing species.[214] This led to a reduction in inflammatory mediators and an improved gut barrier.

From these extraordinary properties, we would expect berberine to be incredibly helpful in autoimmune diseases driven by disruptions to the microbiome. Although we do not yet have any human clinical trials in this area, the results of animal studies are very promising. Two studies published in 2017 found that in animal models of arthritis, berberine reduces joint inflammation and prevents bone erosions.[215] Additional studies have suggested that berberine may be useful in a variety of other autoimmune diseases that have been linked to gut bacteria and Th17 cells, such as multiple sclerosis and Behcet's disease.[216]

Even setting aside this new encouraging research, berberine has a long history of use in successfully treating gastrointestinal complaints such as SIBO and *Candida*, so there is particularly good reason to try this supplement if testing reveals you have an overgrowth of yeast or bacteria.

When it comes to potential side effects, the major concern with berberine is its interaction with other medications. Because berberine may slow down the activity of specific liver enzymes, it is best avoided by those taking medications that are metabolized by Cytochrome P450 enzymes (a list of these medications can be found online by searching for

"Flockhart table").[217] Do not take berberine if you are pregnant or nursing.

Berberine also has other potential effects to be mindful of. Some of these effects may actually be helpful, such as the ability to lower cholesterol and to lower blood sugar levels in those with diabetes.[218] Berberine may also lower blood pressure in some individuals.

The typical dose of berberine is 500 milligrams, three times per day. Recommended brands include Thorne and Metagenics Candibactin-BR. Since berberine may occasionally cause nausea or stomach upset, many practitioners recommend working up to this dose, starting with one capsule, once per day.

Yeast-Targeting Supplements

Yeasts are a natural part of the human ecosystem and may or may not cause problems depending on their abundance and the particular species present. Nevertheless, if testing reveals that you do have a *Candida* overgrowth in your digestive system, it is worth treating because an excess of *Candida* can contribute to leaky gut and activate the inflammatory response.

The question is how best to combat yeast without harming the microbiome. Typical yeast-fighting supplements contain a myriad of broad-acting antimicrobials that also harm beneficial bacteria and are therefore best avoided. Safer options include allicin, berberine, and the probiotic Florastor (*S. boulardii*), which are known to have strong activity against *Candida* without causing significant collateral damage. In order for these supplements to work well, it may also be necessary to add a biofilm-targeting enzyme combination, such as Candex, Klaire Labs Interface, or Kirkman Biofilm

Defense. *Candida* is known to produce a robust biofilm layer that can shield it from both the immune system and antifungal compounds.[219] Using enzymes to break down this layer is therefore useful in combating *Candida* while posing little risk to the overall microbiome.

Part 2

Using Food as Medicine

CHAPTER 4

A MICROBIOME-RESTORING DIET

For better or worse, the food we eat has a profound impact on our gut microbes. That is because different species of resident microbes prefer different types of carbohydrates and other nutrients. Those species that are given a steady supply of their preferred food will multiply and out-compete other species. Our goal then is to adopt a way of eating that gives the beneficial species the upper hand.

Feeding the Good Species

In previous chapters we saw that the most important beneficial microbes for preventing and calming autoimmune disease are the Bifidobacteria and the butyrate-producing species in Clostridia clusters IV and XIVa. If we want these microbes to out-compete the less desirable species, the key is to feed them their preferred food: fiber.

For millennia, a diet rich in fibrous plants has nurtured these important bacteria in the human microbiome. We have co-evolved alongside fiber-loving bacteria with the net result that we have come to depend on them as much as they depend on us. We provide the bacteria with energy in the form of fermentable prebiotic fiber, and in return they produce butyrate and other key compounds that calibrate our immune system and teach it to tolerate the body's own proteins.

If instead we adopt a diet based on highly processed grains and sugars, we effectively starve our most important gut bacteria, while allowing unwanted species to take over. This sets the stage for the immune system to lose its equilibrium and shift toward an inflammatory state.

The lack of fiber in the modern diet is likely a major factor in the geographic distribution of inflammatory disease.[220] Diseases such as arthritis and inflammatory bowel disease are much more prevalent in societies with highly processed and low-fiber diets, and virtually nonexistent in traditional hunter-gatherer societies. There are obviously many factors contributing to this disparity (such as the use of antibiotics) but there is clear evidence pointing to fiber as a major issue. It is beyond question that fiber shapes the microbiome toward butyrate production, and butyrate is essential in fine-tuning the immune system and protecting against inflammation.

This effect can be seen when comparing the microbiome of individuals following Western-style diets to those with diets similar to our ancient ancestors. Children living in a rural village in Burkina Faso, for example, have a high-fiber diet based largely on vegetables, legumes, and millet. These children have very different microbiomes from European children, resulting in butyrate levels four times higher.[221]

In one 2015 study, switching to a high-fiber, low-fat "African-style" diet for two weeks not only doubled butyrate levels in the colon but also reduced immune activation.[222]

The reverse effects were seen when 20 rural Africans were switched to a "Westernized" diet with less fiber: lower levels of beneficial bacteria and butyrate production, and higher intestinal inflammation.

Population-based studies have also linked high-fiber diets to a lower risk of immune-related diseases such as ulcerative colitis and Crohn's disease.[223] The beneficial effects of high-fiber diets can similarly be seen in measurements of inflammatory markers in the blood of otherwise healthy individuals.[224] For example, women consuming at least 25 grams of total fiber per day have significantly lower levels of inflammatory markers such as TNF.[225]

When it comes to feeding the microbiome, not just any fiber will do. The term "fiber" simply refers to carbohydrates that are resistant to digestion. For our purposes, the key is to include more *fermentable* fiber, which is typically soluble fiber.[226] Moreover, when it comes to feeding beneficial bacteria, the forms of soluble fiber found in fruit and vegetables are even more effective than the fiber found in grains and legumes.[227] In one long-term human study, a significant increase in beneficial bacteria was associated with higher fruit and vegetable intake, while there was no clear benefit from the fiber found in grains.[228]

Cruciferous vegetables such as broccoli, cabbage, cauliflower, and kale are particularly good at feeding the beneficial bacteria.[229] Apples, pears, and oranges are also good choices because they contain substantial amounts of soluble fiber. Apples actually contain a specialized form of soluble fiber called pectin, which has been shown to strongly boost butyrate production.[230] These fruits and vegetables are just examples of some of the best options to choose. The key to encouraging a healthy and diverse microbiome is to consume a wide variety of produce and to make nonstarchy vegetables the foundation of most meals.

The Power of Polyphenols

Fiber is not the only tool we have for promoting the growth of beneficial microbes. The polyphenols found in certain fruits are also extremely helpful. Several different groups of researchers have found that cranberry, pomegranate, and Concord grape extract dramatically enhance the growth of *Akkermansia muciniphila*.[231] This beneficial species helps maintain a strong gut barrier, and it is also one of the major species depleted in those with psoriatic arthritis and other autoimmune conditions.[232]

In these studies, fruit polyphenols not only boosted beneficial *Akkermansia* but also lowered serum inflammatory markers, including TNF, IL-6, and lipopolysaccharide. Because the polyphenols found in cranberries, pomegranate, and Concord grapes are somewhat different, the fact that all three were effective in increasing the abundance of *Akkermansia* has led researchers to suggest that related polyphenols from a wide variety of fruits may have the same effect. The fruits with the highest levels of similar polyphenols are those that are darkly pigmented, such as blackberries, blueberries, black currants, and black plums.

Suppressing the Harmful Species

At the same time as feeding the good species of fiber and polyphenols, we want to avoid feeding the harmful species too much of their favorite foods: **starch** and **sugars**. For some people with autoimmune disease, eliminating these components from the diet produces extraordinary results, even where biologic medications have failed.[233]

Eliminating starch appears to be particularly useful for those with ulcerative colitis, Crohn's, ankylosing spondylitis, psoriatic arthritis, and other forms of arthritis that impact the spine and sacroiliac joints. These conditions are closely related to one another and also happen to have the strongest link with starch-loving bacteria (namely *E. coli*, *Streptococcus*, and *Klebsiella*). There are fewer reports of this approach helping rheumatoid arthritis and other autoimmune conditions, but it may still be worth trying, particularly if testing shows bacterial overgrowth in the gut.

For those who do respond to eliminating starch, the results can be life changing. As explained by one man with ankylosing spondylitis, "In the months before I began the [no-starch] diet, my daily pain was about a 5 out of 10, with no easy days to speak of. Some days, I would flare up to an 8 or 9. After two weeks on the diet I was down to 0–1. At six months I couldn't detect any pain or inflammation at all. This completely astonished me."[234]

The Origins of the Low-Starch Diet for Arthritis

Although most rheumatologists do not acknowledge the role of carbohydrates in contributing to inflammation, there is actually a long history of doctors using low-starch and low-carbohydrate diets to treat arthritis, with great success. In one of the earliest studies, published in 1922, 150 arthritis patients at Toronto General Hospital were put on a low-carbohydrate diet and 80 percent improved, with some making a full recovery.[235] Several other physicians in the 1920s and 1930s reported similar success treating arthritis with a carbohydrate-restricted diet.[236] Even at that time, the doctors suspected a link between carbohydrate consumption, gut bacteria, and arthritis.[237]

This approach faded into the background until the 1980s, when Dr. Alan Ebringer, a London rheumatologist, reported success in treating ankylosing spondylitis with a low-starch diet.[238] The story began when one of his patients was placed on a low-carbohydrate diet for weight loss. Four months later, his back pain was gone. Dr. Ebringer performed further research and eventually settled on a theory: starch provides nutrients for the growth of a particular species of gut bacteria called *Klebsiella pneumoniae*, and this bacteria triggers ankylosing spondylitis. Starve the bacteria of starch, and the trigger for inflammation is removed.

With some initial evidence supporting this theory,[239] a low-starch diet began being used as a first-line therapy for ankylosing spondylitis at the Middlesex Hospital in London in the 1990s.[240] After several years, Dr. Ebringer reported that it was helpful in about half of patients with ankylosing spondylitis.[241] There are now vast online communities of people following this diet who report a full or partial recovery after several months of strictly avoiding starch, and significant pain flares from even minor lapses. (See, for example, the "NSD and Diet Related" forum at KickAS.org and the Facebook group "The Low/No Starch Diet for Ankylosing Spondylitis," where hundreds of people have shared their extraordinary success stories.)

The Current Science on the Low-Starch Diet

The exact reason why this way of eating is so effective has not been conclusively established, but all lines of evidence point to gut bacteria as playing a key role.

Even in healthy individuals, between 10 percent and 20 percent of starch consumed can escape digestion. The percentage is likely even greater in those with gut inflammation and damage, because the cells lining the small intestine are responsible for producing starch-degrading enzymes. With fewer healthy cells left to provide these enzymes, more starch will survive the digestive process. The starch that remains in the gut can fuel the growth of both good and bad bacteria but appears to particularly favor the growth of several harmful species. *Klebsiella*, for example, produces specific starch-degrading enzymes to allow it to take full advantage of any starch in our diet.[242]

The connection between *Klebsiella*, starch, and ankylosing spondylitis remains somewhat controversial. This is because several groups of researchers have been unable to find higher levels of *Klebsiella* in the large intestine in AS patients. Yet there is clear evidence that those with AS often have elevated antibodies to *Klebsiella*.[243] There are two possible explanations for this apparent contradiction. It could be the case that the *Klebsiella* is present only as small intestinal overgrowth and is thus not being detected in analysis of the microbiome of the large intestine.

Another explanation is that those with AS do not necessarily have higher levels of *Klebsiella* but rather have a heightened immune response to this species, likely due to genetic reasons. (Research has implicated the HLAb27 gene in the immune responses to *Klebsiella*.) It may be that both factors are at play. In other words, individuals with ankylosing spondylitis may have an overgrowth of *Klebsiella* limited to the small intestine **and** an exaggerated immune response to this overgrowth. This immune response to *Klebsiella* then drives the autoimmune process, perhaps due to cross-reactivity between the antibodies to *Klebsiella* and the proteins that are often attacked by the immune system during AS. [244]

But the value of reducing starch and other carbohydrates goes far beyond AS and *Klebsiella*. Successful results have been seen in psoriasis, psoriatic arthritis, ulcerative colitis, and Crohn's disease.[245] This could be because the low- starch diet also reduces overgrowths of other particularly harmful species in the small or large intestine, such as *E. coli*.

Although *E. coli* is a normal resident in the human gut, a rare and aggressive form called "adherent-invasive *E. coli*" is not only more likely to be found in those with spondyloarthritis or inflammatory bowel disease, but it also appears to trigger the precise immune response characteristic of these autoimmune diseases.[246]

This discovery lends support to the no-starch diet because adherent-invasive *E. coli* happens to be particularly good at multiplying and invading cells in the presence of maltodextrin, a carbohydrate that forms when starch is broken down by our digestive enzymes.[247] Thus, in some cases, the no-starch diet may work so well because it starves these invasive *E. coli*.

In other cases, the low-starch diet may reduce inflammation by reducing a net overgrowth of bacteria in small intestinal overgrowth (SIBO). Most dietary approaches to treating SIBO involve the reduction or elimination of starch, along with lactose and excess sugars.[248]

Starch and Inflammatory Bowel Disease

Perhaps the clearest evidence we have on the value of reducing starch and sugars in the treatment of autoimmune disease comes from recent studies performed in the context of inflammatory bowel disease. These studies involved a particular formulation of the low-starch diet known as the "specific carbohydrate diet" (SCD). The SCD diet eliminates starch and two-unit sugars (lactose and sucrose) while allowing simple sugars in fruit and honey. By reducing carbohydrates that need more processing by enzymes before they can be absorbed, the SCD diet aims to reduce the amount of carbohydrates that can remain in the intestine to feed harmful bacteria.[249]

Several groups of researchers have now found this diet to be very effective at reducing intestinal and systemic inflammation, particularly in children.[250] It does not work in all cases, but when it does work, patients often make a full recovery, with serious intestinal inflammation and damage disappearing in a matter of months. As a result, the SCD diet is now being used by several top hospitals as a first-line treatment for pediatric Crohn's disease and ulcerative colitis. One of these hospitals is Seattle Children's, where Dr. David Suskind has noted that "the specific carbohydrate diet (SCD) often times works with amazing end results for our patients. At Seattle Children's, we have seen great improvements and the disappearance of symptoms altogether for some."[251]

Perhaps one of the most interesting findings from the recent studies using SCD to treat inflammatory bowel disease is the changes that occur in the microbiome. In 2017, doctors analyzed how the microbiome changed in 10 children with Crohn's disease or ulcerative colitis who were following the SCD diet.[252] After three months, eight of the 10 children were in clinical remission, with no remaining intestinal or systemic inflammation.

The children's gut bacteria also changed substantially. There was an overall increase in microbial diversity and an increase in the peacekeeping microbes that are typically depleted in those with autoimmune diseases (the butyrate producers). The diet also reduced overgrowths of *E. coli* and *Klebsiella* in the two patients with these bacterial overgrowths.

Researchers at the University of California witnessed similar changes to the microbiome in adults with Crohn's following the SCD: an increase in overall diversity and a specific increase in bacteria associated with immune regulation (such as *F. prausnitzii*).[253]

Although these studies were focused on inflammatory bowel disease, they are highly relevant to other related autoimmune diseases. As explained previously, inflammation in the gut is at the heart of the other autoimmune diseases in the same family as Crohn's and ulcerative colitis (namely psoriasis, psoriatic arthritis, ankylosing spondylitis, juvenile arthritis, and uveitis). All of these conditions show similar changes to the microbiome, the pattern of immune activation, and intestinal inflammation.

The body of research to date strongly suggests that avoiding starch and sugar can reduce inflammation by rebalancing the microbiome. These simple dietary changes appear to starve the harmful species while allowing room for the beneficial species to recover. For some, this could make a tremendous difference to the severity of symptoms. There are, however, no guarantees of success; the only way to know how you will respond is to perform the experiment.

The Overall Keystone Diet

Before delving into the details of exactly how to reduce your consumption of starch and sugar, we should set the stage with some broader dietary principles that will also help reduce inflammation.

The most important overarching strategy is to **lean toward a Mediterranean diet**, emphasizing fish, olive oil, and non-starchy vegetables. This dietary pattern has a proven ability to lower inflammation. An immense body of research has found that the specific fats found in fish and olive oil can reduce inflammation in the skin and joints.[254] As chapter 5 explains, in those with psoriasis or arthritis, a higher consumption of fish and olive oil directly correlates with milder symptoms.[255]

The Mediterranean diet is also anti-inflammatory because it is nutrient dense. Several large-scale studies have found that the more closely children and adults adhere to the Mediterranean diet, the less likely they are to have nutrient deficiencies.[256] You may expect that vitamin deficiencies are relatively uncommon in modern times, but more than 40 percent of the United States population is deficient in vitamin A, vitamin C, vitamin E, and magnesium.[257]

A deficiency in any one of these micronutrients is especially problematic for anyone with psoriasis or arthritis, because they play key roles in controlling inflammation. A deficiency in magnesium, for instance, has been found to significantly increase inflammation.[258] While modern processed foods often contain very little magnesium, it is found in large amounts in leafy greens, fish, avocado, and seeds.

Many other vitamins and minerals likely play equally important roles in regulating inflammation. Vitamins B12,

C, E, and K are particularly anti-inflammatory, as are other minerals such as selenium, manganese, and zinc.[259] The best sources of vitamin B12, selenium, and zinc are fish, lamb, and grass-fed beef. The best sources of vitamins C, E, K, and manganese are leafy green vegetables. In short, the vitamins and minerals we need most to reduce inflammation are found in abundance in the foods at the core of the Mediterranean diet.[260]

Extraordinary Antioxidants

The anti-inflammatory effect of the Mediterranean diet is also a product of its heavy emphasis on antioxidants. Clinical trials have confirmed that those who follow a Mediterranean diet have a significantly higher antioxidant intake than those on a standard modern diet.[261]

People with psoriasis and arthritis actually have a much greater need for antioxidants because the cells at the site of inflammation in the skin and joints produce vast amounts of reactive oxygen molecules.[262] The usual antioxidant defenses cannot keep up with all of these reactive molecules, and oxidative damage occurs.[263] This damage further increases inflammation and a vicious cycle ensues.[264]

Fortunately, a greater intake of antioxidants from fruit and vegetables reduces oxidative damage and lowers the specific inflammatory mediators that drive psoriasis and arthritis.[265] Fruits and vegetables not only contain antioxidant vitamins such as vitamins C and E, but they also contain hundreds of other antioxidant compounds such as polyphenols and carotenoids.[266] These compounds are important because they can help fine-tune the immune system—boosting our protection from infections while reducing inflammation.

The anti-inflammatory effect of fruit and vegetables is most pronounced for cruciferous vegetables, such as broccoli, Brussels sprouts, cauliflower, collard greens, cabbage, and kale.[267] The more often these are eaten, the more inflammation is kept under control.[268] Olive oil, avocados, and brightly colored fruits are also prime sources of antioxidants.

Color is a good key to antioxidant content because the phytochemical antioxidants are often deeply pigmented. As a result, red lettuce and red cabbage are better than standard varieties, as are purple cauliflower, purple carrots, and black grapes. Dark green is another good clue to high antioxidant content, with kale triumphing over most other vegetables.

Unsurprisingly, the lowest antioxidant vegetables are white or pale in color: potato, celery, cucumber, and iceberg lettuce. The lowest antioxidant fruits are also pale, including banana and pear.

Coffee, tea, and red wine are additional common sources of antioxidants in the Mediterranean diet, but their benefit is more open to debate. Although wine is often touted as anti-inflammatory, the impact on people with autoimmune disease is not clear. In small amounts, alcohol consumption appears to reduce the severity of rheumatoid and psoriatic arthritis, while more than one drink per day worsens symptoms.[269] There is also some evidence that alcohol may contribute to intestinal permeability and the growth of harmful gut bacteria.[270] Alcohol also increases the risk of serious side effects from medication such as NSAIDs and methotrexate.

Coffee is another rich source of antioxidants, and drinking coffee has been correlated with lower inflammatory markers in four studies, while one study reported higher inflammatory markers with "moderate-to-high" coffee intake.[271] There does not appear to be any association between coffee intake and risk of developing psoriasis, rheumatoid arthritis, or other autoimmune conditions.[272] Thus the balance of evidence suggests that having one or two cups of coffee per day is not problematic and may even lower inflammation.

Many traditional Mediterranean diets also include antioxidant-rich herbal teas made from plants not typically available elsewhere in the world. We can probably reap similar benefits from drinking green tea, which is a potent source of antioxidants and has been found to reduce joint inflammation.[273]

In sum, there are several key components of the Mediterranean diet that we can incorporate to start tackling inflammation. Before focusing on what foods to reduce or eliminate from your diet, it is helpful to concentrate on adding more fish, olive oil, and nonstarchy vegetables. Doing so will allow you to reap the benefits of anti-inflammatory fats, antioxidants, and a wide array of vitamins and minerals that are critical to healing and balancing the immune system. This then sets the stage for the next component of the Keystone Diet, which is reducing starch and sugars.

Comparing the Keystone Diet to Other Healing Diets

The starch-lowering component of the Keystone Diet has much in common with other healing diets, such as the Specific Carbohydrate Diet (SCD), the Gut and Psychology Syndrome (GAPS) Diet, the Wahl's Protocol, and the basic low-starch diet adopted by many with ankylosing spondylitis. Like these protocols, the Keystone Diet seeks to minimize the foods that encourage the growth of pathogenic organisms, while providing as many nutrients as possible to encourage healing and reduce inflammation. Yet there are some major differences to note between the Keystone Diet and these other diets, which are generally tailored to quite different autoimmune diseases.

Perhaps most importantly, the Keystone Diet seeks to minimize saturated fat whereas paleo-based healing diets strongly encourage the consumption of saturated fat through coconut oil or animal fats such as ghee and lard. As chapter 5 explains, new studies show that saturated fats are particularly harmful for those with autoimmune diseases driven by mediators such as TNF and the immune response to bacterial toxins.[274] Long-chain saturated fats in palm oil and animal fat are especially good at boosting TNF, for example. The saturated fats in coconut oil can also help shuttle bacterial toxins across the gut barrier.[275]

Saturated fats are therefore especially problematic for those with autoimmune diseases such as psoriasis, psoriatic or rheumatoid arthritis, or ankylosing spondylitis. By contrast, the fats typically used in the Mediterranean diet are strongly anti-inflammatory and help suppress the inflammatory mediators involved in these conditions.

For these reasons, the Keystone Diet encourages the use of oils that are rich in monounsaturated fats, such as olive oil and avocado oil, as the only added fats. Fish that is rich in omega-3 fatty acids is also emphasized, along with other animal proteins that are lower in saturated fat, such as chicken, pork, turkey, and leaner beef.

Finally, there is an optional troubleshooting phase that involves eliminating nightshades and common allergens (such as dairy, nuts, and eggs). This is done on a short-term basis in order to identify possible food sensitivities. In this respect, there is some overlap with the autoimmune paleo (AIP) diet. The AIP diet otherwise differs significantly from the Keystone Diet because it encourages consumption of starches such as sweet potato, cassava, and plantains, along with animal fats and coconut oil. If you are already following the AIP diet, transitioning to the Keystone Diet will primarily involve replacing starches with nonstarchy vegetables and switching to leaner proteins and olive oil.

With that broader context in mind, we can now begin to focus on the specifics of the first element of the Keystone Diet: cutting back on sugar and starch in order to rebalance the microbiome.

CHAPTER 5

THE LOW-STARCH
DIET IN PRACTICE

To reduce the overgrowth of inflammatory gut bacteria, it can be incredibly helpful to avoid foods that contain significant **starch** and **sugars**. Many individuals with ankylosing spondylitis find that they get the most benefit from avoiding starch very strictly. In practice, this means not only completely eliminating all grains and legumes but also root vegetables and bananas. Yet individuals with autoimmune conditions other than ankylosing spondylitis can often make dramatic improvements by removing grains and legumes and continuing to eat fruits and vegetables with moderate amounts of starch. To reflect these different possible approaches, the low-starch diet is therefore divided into basic, intermediate, and advanced levels.

Level 1: The Basic Low-Starch Diet. This introductory level is based on removing the "worst offenders." These are foods that are almost entirely starch or sugar, have very low nutrient density, and can potentially damage the gut barrier (such as wheat, oats, potatoes, and corn). Level 1 is the recommended starting point for those with rheumatoid arthritis or mild psoriasis and for anyone who needs a more gradual approach to reducing starch.

Level 2: The Intermediate Low-Starch Diet. In addition to eliminating grains and legumes, level 2 removes the starchiest vegetables, nuts, and seeds, along with high-lactose dairy. This level still includes some starch in the form of fruits and vegetables with low to moderate starch levels such as bananas, winter squash, and carrots. It also includes some nuts and seeds. This level is the recommended starting point if you have inflammatory bowel disease, psoriatic arthritis, juvenile arthritis, or moderate or severe psoriasis.

Level 3: The Advanced Low-Starch Diet. The advanced version of the low-starch diet is intended for those with ankylosing spondylitis, who typically find that they need to keep starch intake very low to control inflammation. This level builds upon the intermediate level by also removing moderately starchy fruits, vegetables, nuts, and seeds. The net result is a greater focus on animal proteins and low-carbohydrate vegetables such as salads and leafy greens. This level may also be needed by some people with psoriatic arthritis, particularly in cases involving the spine or sacroiliac joints.

Whichever level you start with, it is important to note that your starch tolerance may change significantly over time as your microbiome rebalances and your gut heals. Once you have built a healthy population of good bacteria, and suppressed the population of bad bacteria, you may be able to consume more starch without triggering inflammation. Furthermore, as the gut lining heals, your capacity to break down starch is likely to improve, which could further increase your tolerance. Thus, after following the intermediate or advanced low-starch diet for an extended period of time (such as six months), you may be able to step down a level and expand your diet without reigniting inflammation.

Note that each level of the low-starch diet focuses on the choice of carbohydrate-containing foods, namely namely fruits, vegetables, seeds, nuts, and to some extent dairy and grains. At all levels of the low-starch diet you are encouraged to consume lean animal proteins and healthy fats, such as avocado and olive oil. The rationale for emphasizing these particular protein and fat sources is covered in chapter 6.

A printable summary of each level is available at www. keystonebook.com/low-starch

Level 1: The Basic Low-Starch Diet

The basic level starts to dial back the damage to the gut by reducing fuel for harmful microbes and eliminating foods that directly damage the gut lining, such as gluten-containing grains.

This basic level is the recommended starting point for those with either rheumatoid arthritis or mild psoriasis because these two conditions are less likely to require a stricter avoidance of starch. You may also choose to start with the basic level as an introductory phase to get used to reducing your reliance on starchy foods and begin to observe how these foods impact your symptoms. In addition, the basic level can be used as a long-term maintenance program once you have healed your gut and microbiome.

There are four components to the level 1 low-starch diet: eliminating gluten-containing grains, eliminating other starchy foods that can directly damage the gut barrier or trigger inflammation (such as corn, soy, and potatoes), reducing "safe starches" to no more than two servings per day, and avoiding added sugar.

1. Eliminate all gluten-containing grains

The extraordinarily high prevalence of celiac disease in those with autoimmune disease provides good reason to eliminate gluten, at least for a short-term trial. Celiac disease is not only incredibly common in those with arthritis or psoriasis, but it also often goes undiagnosed for decades. That is because many doctors incorrectly believe that celiac disease always produces gastrointestinal symptoms, so they don't think to test for the condition. We now know that up to two-thirds of cases of celiac disease are asymptomatic.[276] We also know that those with psoriasis are twice as likely to have celiac disease as the rest of the population.[277] Up to 40 percent of children with juvenile arthritis also have celiac antibodies.[278]

In individuals with celiac disease, gluten has a particularly severe impact on intestinal inflammation and immune activation. The levels of celiac antibodies also correlate with psoriasis and psoriatic arthritis severity. Those with the highest levels of celiac antibodies have greater psoriasis activity and more joint stiffness.[279] The only way to reduce these antibodies is to strictly eliminate gluten.

As we would expect, a gluten-free diet can have a major positive impact. In one clinical study of psoriasis patients with elevated anti-gliadin antibodies, 75 percent saw a significant improvement on a gluten-free diet.[280] Others have since confirmed these findings.[281] Similarly, in a study of patients with rheumatoid arthritis, 40 percent of patients saw a significant improvement in joint pain after one year of following a dairy-free and gluten-free diet.[282]

Although the benefit of avoiding gluten is most dramatic for those with celiac antibodies, frequent gluten consumption is likely problematic for all individuals with autoimmune disease because of its adverse impact on intestinal permeability.

Several studies have now found that gluten increases intestinal permeability in everyone, not just those with celiac disease.[283] This occurs in a variety of ways, but the major mechanism is by triggering disassembly of the tight junction complex that holds intestinal cells together.[284] This effect is more extensive and long lasting in celiac patients but still occurs in those without celiac.

Importantly, the increased permeability in those without celiac disease may still be enough to allow an increased level of bacterial by-products to cross the gut barrier and cause widespread immune activation.[285] This was shown in a recent study on a group of patients having no antibodies or evidence of celiac disease but who had some symptoms of gluten sensitivity.[286] These patients had a very high level of bacterial by-products in the bloodstream and elevated markers of immune activation and intestinal cell damage. These signs all reduced significantly after six months of following a gluten-free diet, demonstrating that gluten can in some cases contribute to leaky gut and widespread immune activation even without celiac disease.

Even though gluten is best avoided by those with autoimmunity, regardless of whether or not you have celiac disease, it is useful to get tested for celiac antibodies and/or a genetic predisposition to celiac disease, because that will determine how careful you need to be to avoid accidental gluten exposure. If you have celiac disease, the activation of autoimmunity can be quite severe from consuming even a minuscule amount.[287] Those without celiac disease do not need to be as vigilant about avoiding gluten.

Gluten Contamination for Celiacs

If you do have celiac disease, even gluten-free grains should be approached with caution because there is widespread gluten contamination in products labeled gluten-free.[288] Studies have reported that one-third of products made from gluten-free grains contained gluten above the limit set by the FDA for gluten-free labeling.[289] In a 2014 study, five out of eight breakfast cereals labeled gluten-free contained gluten above the limit.[290]

The contamination of grains and seeds with gluten may occur at any point in the supply chain, from farming to harvest to grain processing to food manufacture. If you test positive for celiac antibodies, this frequent contamination means there is value in avoiding all grain products, even those marked gluten-free.

For those with celiac disease, there is also particular value in avoiding **quinoa**, **oats**, and **corn** because these grains contain proteins similar to gluten that, in some individuals, can activate an immune response in the same way.[291] (Additional problems with these particular foods are discussed further below.)

Avoiding contaminated and cross-reactive grains can dramatically improve the health of those with celiac disease. This effect was recently reported by a group of gastroenterologists at Johns Hopkins and Massachusetts General Hospital. The doctors found that when individuals with celiac disease who showed symptoms even on a strict gluten-free diet removed all grain and seed products except for unprocessed rice, 80 percent had a complete resolution of symptoms.[292]

2. Eliminate other gut-damaging foods

Many advocates for the paleo diet suggest that even gluten-free grains, pseudo-grains, and legumes can damage the gut barrier and should be strictly avoided by those with autoimmune disease. This proposition is somewhat controversial, but there is persuasive evidence with respect to the following foods:

- Corn
- Peanuts
- Soy
- Quinoa
- Potatoes

These foods are worth avoiding because they are not only high in starch and relatively low in nutrients, but they also contain "antinutrients" that are potentially damaging to intestinal cells. These antinutrients include lectins (in the case of peanuts, corn, soy, and potatoes), saponins (in the case of quinoa and soy), and glycoalkaloids (in potatoes).

Lectins are proteins that stick to carbohydrates on cell surfaces. Plants likely evolved these proteins as a self-defense strategy—a form of chemical warfare against animals and fungi to protect the plant's embryo (i.e., seed) from being eaten. While lectins are found in many plant foods, the specific lectins found in peanuts, soy, corn, and potatoes are the most problematic because these particular lectins not only survive cooking and digestion but also can cross the gut barrier and activate immune cells, triggering inflammation.[293] They also increase intestinal permeability.[294]

In addition to lectins, potatoes contain another type of gut-damaging compound called glycoalkaloids. In laboratory and animal studies, potato glycoalkaloids were found to disrupt the intestinal barrier.[295] Potatoes are therefore among the first of the starchy foods we should try to eliminate.

Quinoa and soy also earn their place on the list of foods to avoid by virtue of another type of antinutrient that can damage the gut barrier. They contain saponins, which are soap-like molecules that can make holes in cells that lead to cell death and potentially contribute to leaky gut.[296] In animal and laboratory studies, quinoa and soy saponins have been found to kill intestinal cells and increase intestinal permeability.[297] While there is currently no direct evidence that the same thing happens in humans, it is best to err on the side of caution, particularly given our overarching goal of reducing starch intake.

It should be noted that the potential harm associated with foods such as corn, soy, and potato depends significantly on the amount consumed. Small amounts present in supplements, medications, and sauces may not be worth worrying about, particularly at the basic level when you are not strictly avoiding starch. Fermentation also significantly reduces antinutrients such as lectins, so fermented soy products such as tempeh, miso, and soy sauce may be less problematic.[298]

Another category of potentially gut-damaging foods that you may choose to minimize or eliminate at this stage is the nightshade family of fruits and vegetables. In addition to white potatoes (but not sweet potatoes or yams), nightshades include

- Tomatoes
- Bell peppers/capsicum/sweet peppers

- Chili peppers (and derivative spices such as cayenne, paprika, and chipotle)
- Eggplant

These foods are known for worsening arthritis symptoms
for many people, likely because they contain compounds that
can potentially damage the intestinal cells and activate the
immune system, as discussed in further detail in chapter 7. You
may decide to start avoiding these foods right away, or hold off
and see how you respond to other dietary changes first.

3. Limit other starchy foods to no more than two servings per day

Level 1 of the low-starch diet allows for two small servings per day of starchy foods. This is intended to keep the
diet as broad as possible without providing excess starch for
unfriendly microbes. One serving is equivalent to 1 cup of
sweet potato, or ½ cup per day of rice, beans, or lentils. Yet
this limit is only an approximate guide. Individual tolerance levels vary greatly, and you may find you do well with
an even higher starch intake, particularly when you have
healed your gut and are following this basic level as a long-
term maintenance diet. Conversely, you may find that your
inflammation does not improve significantly while you continue to include starch in your diet, in which case you can
then progress to the intermediate or advanced level.

If you do tolerate moderate amounts of starch in your diet,
the best use of your daily quota is likely starchy vegetables
such as sweet potatoes, parsnips, and yams because these vegetables come with the added bonus of fiber, vitamins, minerals, and antioxidants. Other starches to consider include

- Soaked and pressure-cooked beans
- Well-cooked lentils and split peas
- White rice (including rice noodles)
- Plantains

Not everyone will tolerate beans or lentils, but they have the particular advantage of being very high in soluble fiber and therefore may help support our beneficial microbes. The key to getting the most benefit from legumes is to properly prepare them to eliminate lectins and other antinutrients. Unlike soy and peanut lectins, the lectins found in legumes such as navy or kidney beans can be largely eliminated by cooking for a sufficient length of time.[299] Several hours of boiling or 45 minutes of pressure-cooking was found to abolish lectin activity in red kidney beans.[300] The same is likely true for other similar beans.[301] Some lectin activity is still found in commercially canned beans, so these should be cooked further before use.

Soaking beans for 12 to 24 hours before cooking is also recommended. This helps eliminate other indigestible carbohydrates that cause gas and bloating and allows for more even cooking. According to proponents of the Specific Carbohydrate Diet, the legumes that are easiest to digest are navy beans, lentils, peas, split peas, adzuki beans, and lima beans.

Rice is another relatively safe starch option for many people, although there are some reports of individuals with celiac disease cross-reacting to rice. At least from the perspective of antinutrients such as lectins, white rice is the best choice because the antinutrients are concentrated in the bran—the outer protective layer that is present in brown rice but removed to produce white rice.

A particular type of white rice called glutinous or sticky rice may be even better than standard white rice. This distinct species grown in Southeast Asia contains highly branched starch (amylopectin). This type of starch is more accessible to digestive enzymes and therefore a greater proportion is absorbed before it feeds undesirable gut bacteria. The rapid digestion of glutinous rice is reflected in its much higher glycemic index, which measures the rise in blood glucose shortly after a food is consumed.[302] Sushi rice also has a higher glycemic index than conventional rice and is therefore more easily digested.

Whichever starches you choose to include, it is important to remain mindful of quantities and limit intake to two small servings per day, at least until you determine your own personal starch tolerance.

4. Cut back on sugar

Many people with autoimmune conditions see significant improvement just by reducing their overall sugar intake. In fact, several studies have reported a link between excess sugar consumption and a variety of autoimmune conditions, including inflammatory bowel disease and rheumatoid arthritis.[303] As one example, the large-scale Nurses Health Study found that women who consumed at least one sugared soda per day had a 63 percent increased risk of developing rheumatoid arthritis.[304]

The inflammatory effect of sugar is likely due in large part to its impact on the microbiome, because sugar readily feeds undesirable bacteria and yeasts. We should therefore try to limit overall sugar intake, whether in the form of table sugar or other natural sweeteners such as maple syrup and honey. At the intermediate and advanced levels, this also means moderating fruit intake, but at the basic level the goal is simply to reduce added sugars.

TABLE 1: Summary of the Basic Low-Starch Diet

ALLOWED	AVOID
All fruits	Grains other than rice
Vegetables	Corn
(except corn and nightshades)	Soy
Well-cooked legumes	Peanuts
(except soy and peanuts)	Quinoa
White rice	Nightshades (potato, tomato,
Nuts and seeds	peppers)
Dairy	Added sugars
Meats	
Fish	
Eggs	
Olive oil	
Avocado oil	

If you find that you do not improve sufficiently after following the basic level for several months, you can either progress to the intermediate or advanced low-starch diet, or experiment with eliminating common allergens, namely nuts, eggs, and dairy (see chapter 7). Laboratory testing may be useful to guide your choice at that point. For example, if testing for gut pathogens finds an overgrowth of *E. coli*, a stricter approach to starch and sugars may be warranted. If, however, allergy testing finds IgE or IgG antibodies to certain foods, eliminating those foods may be the next best step.

Level 2: The Intermediate Low-Starch Diet

The intermediate level is the recommended starting point for those with psoriatic arthritis, juvenile arthritis, inflammatory bowel disease, moderate or severe psoriasis, SIBO, or a known pathogen overgrowth. This level builds on the basic level by further reducing starches and focusing more heavily on nonstarchy fruits and vegetables.

In addition to eliminating the gut-damaging foods that are removed with the level 1 low-starch diet, at level 2 you will remove **all grains, starchy legumes, a few very high starch vegetables, and most dairy**.

What remains is a relatively low-carbohydrate diet that heavily emphasizes vegetables and lean proteins along with a moderate intake of fruit, olive oil, and perhaps some nuts and seeds. This is an incredibly nutrient-dense diet that provides everything you need to build a healthy microbiome, heal the gut barrier, and allow the immune system to reestablish its normal equilibrium.

Legumes and Vegetables on the Intermediate Low-Starch Diet

Although level 2 excludes starchy legumes such as lentils and dried beans, you can continue to include legumes with a green edible pod, such as green beans and sugar snap peas. Tofu is relatively low starch but is best avoided due to the gut-damaging effects of soy lectins.

Most vegetables are included in the intermediate low-starch diet, with the exception of the very high starch vegetables such as sweet potatoes (see Table 2). Although these very high starch vegetables are typically root vegetables, not all root vegetables are off limits. You can continue to include carrots, radishes, rutabaga, celeriac, and beets, for example. Pumpkin and spaghetti squash can also be lower in starch, although this is quite unpredictable.

TABLE 2: Vegetables and Legumes on the
Intermediate Low-Starch Diet

ALLOWED Low starch (under 0.5g starch per 100g)	ALLOWED Moderate starch (0.6–2g starch per 100g)	LIMIT (2–5g starch per 100g or F: high fructan)	AVOID (more than 5g starch per 100g or *nightshade)
Artichoke heart	Beansprouts,	Acorn squash[T]	Beans (other
Arugula/rocket	mung	Asparagus[F]	than green
Asparagus	Beetroot	Broccoli[F]	string beans)
Bok choy	Brussels	Butternut	Black eyed peas
Cabbage (all	sprouts	squash[T]	Chickpeas
varieties)	Collard greens	Frozen peas	Corn
Carrots	Green beans	Garlic[F]	Eggplant*
Cauliflower[T]	Mustard leaves	Leek[F]	Lentils
Celeriac[T]	Pumpkin[T]	Onion[F]	Parsnip
Celery	Rutabaga[T]		Peppers*
Collard greens	Snow peas		Plantains
Cucumber	Spaghetti		Potato
Endive	squash[T]		Split peas
Kale	Sugar snap		Sweet potato
Kohlrabi	peas		Taro
Fennel	Swede[T]		Tomato*
Lettuce			Yam
Mushrooms			Yucca/cassava
Pak choi			
Radicchio			
Radish			
Shallots			
Snow peas			
Spinach			
Spring mix			
Spring onion			
Scallion			
Summer squash			
Turnip			
Watercress			
Zucchini			

T: starchy if unripe. Test with iodine. F: high fructan
(individual tolerance varies). *: nightshade

Note that all tables can be downloaded in printable
format at www.keystonebook.com/low-starch

Throughout this chapter, the categorization of foods as low, moderate, or high starch is based on McCance and Widdowson's "The Composition of Foods Integrated Dataset 2015," which is published by the Department of Health in England. This data, also referred to as the UK food composition tables, is based on a vast set of analytical tests and scientific publications. Yet the data is not always reliable, due to the unpredictability of starch content in certain foods.

For some fruits and vegetables, the starch content varies dramatically depending on growing conditions and whether they were picked ripe. This includes pumpkin, winter squash, avocados, apples, pears, and stone fruit. These foods may be starchy when unripe and then become quite low in starch as they ripen and the starches are converted to sugars.

If in doubt, you can test these and other foods with iodine solution, sold as antiseptic in pharmacies. A drop of iodine will turn blue-black or dark brown on foods that contain a significant amount of starch but remain light orange on nonstarchy foods. Outside its peak season, pumpkin often tests very starchy in this way, in contradiction to the official data that reports pumpkin as having little to no starch.

In addition to avoiding vegetables that are very high in starch, some people may find that they need to limit their intake of vegetables that are high in fructans, such as onion, garlic, asparagus, and leeks. Fructans are chains of fructose molecules, also known as fructooligosaccharides or inulin. These carbohydrates are indigestible to humans but readily fermentable by gut bacteria. The effects of fructans on the microbiome likely vary greatly between individuals. Fructans definitely encourage the growth of beneficial species and boost butyrate levels, but theoretically an excess may also

worsen overgrowths of species such as *Klebsiella* and *E. coli.*
Many individuals with SIBO are also sensitive to fructans.
The best solution is likely to eat these vegetables occasionally
and not in excessive portions. You can also add garlic flavor
to recipes without adding any fructans by warming olive oil
with sliced garlic and then discarding the garlic solids. To
add onion flavor to recipes, use the green parts of scallions,
also known as spring onions.

Fruits on the Intermediate Low-Starch Diet

All fruit is allowed at the intermediate level, but you may
find you need to moderate your overall fruit consumption,
particularly when it comes to fruits that are particularly high
in fructose or are moderately starchy, such as bananas.

People with significant gut damage often have difficulty
absorbing large amounts of fructose.[305] Given our overarching
goal of choosing carbohydrates that are quickly and easily
absorbed to avoid feeding bacteria in the small intestine, it is
best to limit fruit intake to **two or three small servings per
day**. You may be able to eat more fruit than this by focusing
on fruits that are naturally lower in fructose, such as oranges,
honeydew melon, and cantaloupe. Even so, these fruits contain other sugars such as sucrose, and so you may need to
experiment somewhat to determine your own personal limit.

It is particularly important to be mindful of portion size
when it comes to dried fruit. Raisins, dates, prunes, and other
dried fruits are very concentrated sources of fruit sugars,
including fructose and sucrose. Dried fruits often also contain substantial amounts of fructans, which are indigestible
and highly fermentable by gut microbes.

TABLE 3: Fruits on the Intermediate Low-Starch Diet

Low starch and lower fructose	LIMIT (high fructose or fructans)	LIMIT (2–5g starch per 100g)
Avocado	Apples	Banana (less starch when ripe)
Blueberries	Apricot	Citrus peel for baking
Cantaloupe	Cherries	Custard apple
Clementine	Dates	Durian
Dragon fruit	Figs	Sapodilla
Grapes	Grapefruit	Unripe pear
Honeydew melon	Guava	
Kiwi fruit	Mango	
Lemon	Nectarine	
Lime	Peach	
Lychee	Plums	
Orange	Prunes	
Paw paw/papaya	Raisins	
Pineapple	Ripe pear	
Pomegranate	Watermelon	
Raspberries		
Rhubarb		
Rockmelon		
Starfruit		
Strawberries		
Tangerine		

Sweeteners on the Intermediate Low-Starch Diet

Although it is best to minimize all added sugars, when a small amount of sweetener is needed, what is the best choice? The Specific Carbohydrate Diet recommends honey because it contains primarily fructose and glucose rather than sucrose. Fructose and glucose do not need to be broken down by enzymes before they are absorbed, so they are less likely to remain in the gastrointestinal tract and feed undesirable bacteria and yeasts.

Yet honey is still a concentrated source of fructose and should only be used occasionally. Given that many people with intestinal inflammation can only absorb a small amount of fructose each day, it is probably better to use that daily quota for whole fruit, which provides a multitude of vitamins as well as polyphenols and fiber to feed our beneficial microbes.

An alternative option for a natural sweetener is brown rice syrup, which is composed of single glucose subunits, along with maltose and maltotriose. Maltose is simply two glucose units joined together, while maltotriose is three. These molecules are broken down and absorbed very rapidly, so they are unlikely to fuel bacterial overgrowth when used in reasonable amounts. In fact, the glycemic index, which rates how quickly a food impacts blood glucose levels, indicates that the sugars in brown rice syrup are absorbed almost as quickly as pure glucose.

One concern with brown rice syrup is potential arsenic contamination, because rice naturally absorbs arsenic from soil. To minimize arsenic levels, it is best to buy rice syrup from reputable companies that test for and publish their arsenic levels. Rice that is grown in California is also typically safer than rice grown in other parts of the United States. For those in the United States, Lundberg Farms is the best option and their rice crops consistently test below the regulatory limits for arsenic.

Certain noncaloric sweeteners such as stevia and monk-fruit extract can also be used. It is better to avoid significant amounts of sweeteners made from sugar alcohols (such as mannitol, xylitol, erythritol, and sorbitol), because these can be readily fermentable by gut bacteria and have unpredictable effects on the microbiome.[306] Artificial sweeteners such as acesulfame potassium and sucralose may also perturb the microbiome and encourage the growth of pathogens such as *E. coli*, although research in this area is only just beginning.[307]

Nuts and Seeds on the Intermediate Low-Starch Diet

Most tree nuts are relatively low starch and are good sources of vitamins and minerals. The most significant concern with nuts is that they are highly allergenic. Thus it can be helpful to eliminate nuts from your diet for one or two months and then monitor your reaction when you reintroduce them.

The nuts with the lowest starch content include pine nuts, walnuts, and macadamias. Many people who follow the low-starch diet also report tolerating blanched almond flour, which is particularly useful for baking. Other good flour replacements for baking include coconut flour and ground flax seed.

TABLE 4: *Nuts and Seeds on the Intermediate Low-starch Diet*

ALLOWED (low starch)	LIMIT (2–5g starch per 100g)	AVOID (more than 5g starch per 100g)
Brazil nuts	Almonds	Cashew nuts
Coconut flour	Chia seeds	Chestnuts
Coconut milk	Chocolate	Peanuts
without additives	Cocoa	Pumpkin seeds
Desiccated coconut	Hazelnuts	Quinoa
Flax seeds	Hemp seeds	Sunflower seeds
Macadamias	Pistachios	Tigernuts
Pecans		
Pine nuts		
Sesame seeds		
Tahini paste		
Walnuts		

Dairy on the Intermediate Low-Starch Diet

Many people with autoimmune disease do best when they completely avoid dairy products, particularly products derived from cow's milk. There are two main reasons why dairy is so often problematic. The proteins found in dairy are highly allergenic and often trigger inflammatory immune responses, especially in individuals with celiac disease or rheumatoid arthritis[308] (although some people with cow's milk allergies find that they do not react to goat or sheep's milk, perhaps because they have not yet had sufficient exposure to develop a sensitivity).

The second problem with dairy is lactose, which is often poorly absorbed and can provide fuel for harmful microbes. If you do not appear to have a sensitivity to the proteins found in dairy and would like to include dairy in your diet, the best option is homemade yogurt that has been fermented for at least eight hours to reduce the lactose content.

Many healing diets also recommend the use of dairy-based fats such as ghee, which contains little to no milk protein and is therefore thought to be safe for those with dairy sensitivities. Yet the type of fat found in ghee is highly inflammatory, as discussed in chapter 6, and is not recommended as part of the Keystone Diet.

When looking for a low-starch replacement for dairy milk, options include coconut milk, hemp seed milk, flax seed milk, and nut milks such as almond and macadamia. Avoid products that contain added starches and thickeners such as carrageenan and maltodextrin. The thickeners that are less concerning are guar gum, gellan gum, locust bean gum, and gum arabic. Some of these gums are prebiotics that are fermentable by gut microbes, but they do not appear to preferentially encourage the growth of harmful species, unlike maltodextrin and carrageenan.[309]

Miscellaneous Items on the Intermediate Low-Starch Diet

At the intermediate level, it is worth looking for hidden sources of starches in foods such as deli meats and yogurts. In addition to checking the ingredients of packaged foods, you can consult the nutritional information for a rough approximation of starch content. Simply subtract the grams of fiber and sugars from the total carbohydrate content and the remaining grams of carbohydrates are typically starches. (This is not always accurate, for example in products that contain other nonstarch polysaccharides, but it gives general guidance.)

Products that are usually safe include fresh and dried herbs, tea, coffee, gelatin, and collagen peptides. Collagen peptides are the best option for protein powder for smoothies, because they are not only low starch but also contain the precise amino acids needed for healing the skin, joints, and gastrointestinal tract (gelatin has these same benefits).

TABLE 5: Miscellaneous Foods and Additives on the Intermediate Low-starch Diet

ALLOWED	BEST AVOIDED
Baking soda	Arrowroot
Bicarbonate of soda	Carrageenan
Cellulose	Chicory
Coffee	Dextrose
Collagen peptides	Fructooligosaccharides
Cream of tartar	Inulin
Gelatin	Maize
Guar gum	Maltodextrin
Gum arabic	Xanthan gum
Herbs	
Hypromellose	
Magnesium stearate	
Pectin	
Spices	
Tea	

Level 3: The Advanced Low-Starch Diet

The advanced level is the recommended starting point for those with ankylosing spondylitis or uveitis. It may also be the right level for those with psoriatic arthritis that impacts the spine or sacroiliac joints. These particular conditions have the strongest connection to gut bacteria that thrive on starch. As a result, sometimes it is necessary to keep starch intake extremely low for several months for pain to begin subsiding.

Level 3 provides a more aggressive approach to combating harmful microbes with a stricter avoidance of starch and other carbohydrates and a heavy emphasis on meats, fish, olive oil, and the very-low-starch vegetables.

At level 3, the allowed vegetables are those with less than 0.2 grams of starch per 100 grams, which include salad vegetables, greens, mushrooms, and cabbage. (See the full list in the table below.) The allowed fruits are those that are low in starch and do not have an excess of fructose or fructans. Even then, fruit intake is limited to one or two small servings per day, to keep total sugar intake very low. The net result is that carbohydrates will typically be below 50 to 60 grams per day (or much lower if you exclude fruit and adopt a ketogenic version of the diet). To ensure adequate energy with such a low-carbohydrate intake, make sure that each meal includes at least 30 grams of protein and some fat, such as a tablespoon of olive oil.

TABLE 6: Advanced Level Low-Starch Diet

ALLOWED VEGETABLES (0–0.2g starch per 100g)	ALLOWED FRUITS (2 servings per day)	ALLOWED NUTS, SEEDS (2 tablespoons per day)	ALLOWED OTHER
Arugula	Avocado	Chia seeds	Baking soda
Cabbage	Blueberries	Coconut (milk,	Brown rice
Celery	Cantaloupe	fresh, flour, or	syrup
Courgette	Clementine	desiccated)	Coffee
Cucumber	Dragon fruit	Flax seeds	Collagen
Endive	Grapes	Macadamia nuts	peptides
Fennel	Honeydew melon	Pine nuts	Gelatin
Kale	Kiwi fruit	Walnuts	Herbs
Kohlrabi	Lemon		Tea
Lettuce	Lime		
Mushrooms	Orange		
Radicchio	Papaya		
Radish	Paw paw		
Scallions	Pineapple		
Spinach	Raspberries		
Spring mix	Rhubarb		
Spring onions	Rockmelon		
Summer squash	Starfruit		
Watercress	Strawberries		
Zucchini	Tangerine		

The advanced approach likely represents a dramatic shift from your usual diet, but it offers the best chance of producing rapid results. It also has the advantage of simplicity. You will be starting from scratch with a relatively short list of basic ingredients. Once you start to see results from this approach, you can then expand your diet and determine how much starch you can tolerate.

After following this advanced level for three to six months, you may decide to introduce additional vegetables that typically contain only very small amounts of starch, such as carrots and Brussels sprouts. You can also experiment with reintroducing small portions of the fruits that are higher in fructose and fructans, as listed in the table for the intermediate level (such as apples, pears, apricots, and cherries).

Note that the advanced level does not include asparagus, onion, leek, broccoli, or cauliflower, despite the fact that they are quite low in starch. These vegetables (and garlic, which is somewhat starchy) are omitted from the "safe list" because they contain a significant amount of fructans such as inulin, which can potentially feed both beneficial and harmful microbes. The most cautious approach is to omit high-fructan foods during the initial stage of the advanced low-starch diet, but you may find that you can reintroduce them without any problems.

During the initial stage when you are trying to keep starch intake very low to determine how you respond, it may be worth testing certain fruits and vegetables with iodine. A drop of dilute iodine solution (sold as antiseptic in pharmacies) will turn blue-black or dark brown on foods that contain a significant amount of starch.

Some proponents of the low-starch diet for ankylosing spondylitis suggest an even more extreme approach to vegetables: limiting the diet to those that contain no starch, rather than allowing trace amounts. Based on the UK food composition data, this would allow lettuce, cucumbers, mushrooms, and cabbage but exclude kale, zucchini, and spinach. The concern with this approach is that it becomes more difficult to ensure adequate fiber intake.

A high-fiber diet is imperative because fiber not only supports our beneficial microbes, as discussed earlier, but also helps suppress the harmful bacteria. In the study comparing the microbiomes of children in Africa with a high-fiber diet to children in Europe, the African children had significantly lower levels of harmful bacteria such as *Klebsiella* and *E. coli*.[310] Fiber from vegetables may also interfere with the ability of *E. coli* to adhere to and invade intestinal cells.[311] A vegetable-rich diet is therefore one of the best ways to arm our defenses against bacteria that can trigger autoimmunity.

Avoiding Other Hidden Starches at the Advanced Level

At level 3 it may be worth avoiding even small amounts of starches that are hidden in unexpected places. If you decide to try baking (using blanched almond meal, coconut flour, or ground flax as the flour replacement), note that conventional baking powder usually contains cornstarch, for example. To avoid this, you can make your own baking powder using bicarbonate of soda and cream of tartar. (Half a teaspoon of cream of tartar plus a quarter of a teaspoon of bicarbonate of soda is equivalent to one teaspoon of baking powder.)

When it comes to spices, the UK food composition tables indicate that most spices do not contain starch, but some followers of the low-starch diet report reacting to spices, perhaps because unlabeled starches are used during the manufacturing process. Ginger and mustard do contain some starch, although if the amounts used are very small, the starch content may not be significant.

TABLE 7: Miscellaneous Foods and Fillers on the Advanced Diet

ALLOWED	BETTER TO AVOID	NOT ALLOWED
Cellulose	Ginger	Arrowroot
Gelatin	Mustard	Baking powder
Guar gum	Spices	Carrageenan
Gum arabic	Xanthan gum	Chicory
Hypromellose		Corn starch
Magnesium		Dextrose
stearate		Fructooligosaccharides
Pectin		Inulin
		Maize
		Maltodextrin
		Modified food starch
		Potato starch
		Tapioca starch

As for fillers in supplements such as vitamins and probiotics, the amount of starch present is often very small. Nevertheless, some people see better results by erring on the side of caution and avoiding supplements and medications that list starch or maltodextrin as ingredients. When shopping for alternative products, the best fillers for capsules are cellulose, methylcellulose, and lysine. Liquid-based and gel-cap formulations are also good options.

At the advanced level you may also decide to avoid probiotics that contain added *pre*biotics, such as fructooligosaccharides (FOS). At the time of writing, probiotics brands without starch, maltodextrin, or fructooligosaccharides include

- Pearls Digestion and Immunity
- BioGaia Protectis
- Renew Life
- GutPro

- BioK+ Capsules, dairy and soy versions
- Florastor

Dairy on the Advanced Low-Starch Diet

Like the intermediate level, the advanced level discourages dairy because of the prevalence of immune reactions to dairy proteins. The lactose in dairy can also promote the growth of undesirable gut microbes. If you do not appear to have an allergy or sensitivity to the proteins found in dairy and would like to include it in your diet, the best option is homemade yogurt that has been fermented for at least eight hours to reduce the lactose content.

A Ketogenic Version of the Low-Starch Diet

It is important to note that the advanced low-starch diet can be a ketogenic diet if you choose, but it does not need to be. A ketogenic diet involves drastically limiting carbohydrates and relying on the conversion of fat into ketones for fuel. In practice, this usually means having no fruit or other carbohydrate-rich foods and significantly increasing fat consumption.

When carbohydrate intake is kept very low for several days, the metabolism shifts from primarily carbohydrate-burning mode to primarily fat-burning mode. The liver begins converting fat to ketones, which can then be used for energy by most cells of the body. After several weeks of producing and using ketones as a primary energy source, the metabolism becomes very efficient at burning fat and one is said to be "fat adapted." To make this shift, people typically need to consistently keep net carbohydrate intake below 20 to 40 grams per day (excluding fiber) while significantly increasing fat intake. Most people following a ketogenic diet will obtain approximately 75 percent of calories from fat (approximately 100 to 150 grams) while also limiting protein intake in order to maximize ketone production.

The ketogenic diet was originally developed in the 1920s as a treatment for epilepsy. The goal was to mimic fasting, which was known to control seizures. It has since become a popular approach for weight loss and for treating a variety of other medical conditions involving the brain, such as multiple sclerosis, Alzheimer's, and Parkinson's disease. The ketogenic diet also shows some initial promise in the treatment of psoriasis and arthritis. As just one example, doctors in Italy reported that a ketogenic diet was able to completely clear psoriasis and psoriatic arthritis in a patient who had severe symptoms even after 12 months of treatment with Humira.[312]

Indeed, some people respond very well to a ketogenic diet and find that it eliminates carbohydrate cravings while providing steady energy levels throughout the day. Others do not fare as well and instead experience flu-like symptoms, particularly when first starting the ketogenic diet. These immediate side effects are typically caused by electrolyte imbalances. The kidneys function differently when you are in ketosis and excrete more water and sodium. If too much sodium is lost, the body will try to maintain the balance between sodium and potassium by also excreting more potassium. This loss of electrolytes, along with dehydration, can then lead to muscle cramps, fatigue, and feeling light-headed.

To circumvent this downward spiral, it is useful to consume at least half a teaspoon of salt per day, along with adequate water and perhaps a magnesium supplement. (You should also proceed with a low-carbohydrate diet only under medical supervision if you have a chronic condition such as diabetes or high blood pressure, because the dose of your medication may need to be adjusted.)

A ketogenic diet can also have more significant adverse effects over the longer term, with some people experiencing worsening fatigue, insomnia, or suppressed thyroid or adrenal function after following a ketogenic diet for several months. This likely happens because when insulin is kept very low, less of the active thyroid hormone (T3) is produced. The adrenal glands are also called upon to produce more cortisol, and it is thought that this can eventually become a stressor to the adrenals in some individuals.[313]

Additional demands on adrenal function may be particularly problematic for those with ankylosing spondylitis or psoriatic arthritis because it was recently discovered that these conditions are already associated with a greater risk of adrenal insufficiency.[314] Poorly functioning adrenal glands can manifest as fatigue, dizziness, low blood pressure, excess thirst, and worsening inflammation.

It may be possible to reap many of the benefits of a low-carbohydrate diet while minimizing these hormonal disruptions by keeping protein intake fairly high, reflecting an approach more like the Atkins diet. A true ketogenic diet limits protein intake because it triggers the release of insulin and glucagon, which temporarily inhibits ketosis. A reduction in ketone production may be suboptimal for endurance athletes or those with certain neurological diseases, but it is likely not a problem for those who simply want to rely primarily on fat and protein for fuel.

Humans can readily burn protein for energy. Indeed, most amino acids can be broken down and used directly in the energy-producing Krebs cycle. In addition, as long as carbohydrate intake is fairly low we can burn fat for fuel through fatty acid oxidation, even if we are not in ketosis.

This combination of higher protein, low carbohydrates, and moderate fat has actually been studied extensively in the context of epilepsy, where it is referred to as the modified Atkins diet. This diet was developed at Johns Hopkins Hospital as an attempt to create a more palatable and less restrictive treatment alternative to a ketogenic diet. It limits carbohydrates to 20 grams per day with no limits on protein. Typically, 30 percent of calories per day come from protein and 60 percent from fat. (A ketogenic diet typically has around 15 percent of calories from protein and 80 percent from fat). In more than 30 studies, the modified Atkins diet was found to be as effective as a ketogenic diet for controlling epilepsy, and much easier for patients to maintain long term.[315] As physicians at Johns Hopkins commented, "we suspect that the incidence of adverse effects, especially the long-term ones, may be less than with the ketogenic diet because of the inherently higher protein content."[316]

In short, for many people it is not necessary to follow the stringent ketogenic diet requirements of being very low carbohydrate, low-to-moderate protein, and very high fat. We can instead adopt a diet that is generally **low carbohydrate, high protein, and moderate fat**. This ratio will happen naturally on the advanced low-starch diet because the core of the diet is nonstarchy vegetables, lean animal proteins, and olive oil. If you would like confirmation that you are eating the right amounts, you can use a free carbohydrate tracking phone app, such as Carb Manager, to measure your intake over the course of the day. The app allows you to set a target for protein, fat, and carbohydrates and track your progress.

(You may, for example, aim for 50 grams of carbohydrates, 110 grams of fat, and 140 grams protein each day.)

Prioritizing higher protein intake over higher fat intake may be advantageous for many reasons. Additional protein not only prevents our hormonal systems from going into starvation mode but also provides more of the amino acids, vitamins, and minerals needed to build muscle and repair the skin and joints. Being able to obtain sufficient energy without an extremely high fat intake is also beneficial, given that diets very high in fat can increase intestinal permeability and dramatically increase the level of bacterial endotoxin (lipopolysaccharide) in the blood.[317]

As will be explained in chapter 6, the traditional sources of fat used by most people following a ketogenic diet, such as butter and coconut oil, are especially inflammatory. In any diet that keeps carbohydrate intake very low, moderate amounts of fat are useful to ensure adequate energy, but we can minimize inflammation by relying on the fats typically used in the Mediterranean diet, such as avocados, nuts, and olive oil.

A low-carbohydrate diet should also continue to emphasize high-fiber vegetables that can feed the microbiome. Good options include kale and cabbage, along with high-fiber seeds such as chia and flax.

Example daily meal: low carbohydrate, high protein, and moderate fat

Breakfast

- Smoothie with 2 scoops collagen peptides, 1/3 cup frozen blueberries, ½ cucumber, 1 tablespoon flax seeds, ice, and water

- Deli meat roll-up with ham, turkey, avocado, and lettuce

Lunch

- Salad with canned salmon, shredded cabbage, celery, scallions, parsley, baby spinach, olive oil, lemon juice

Dinner

- Grilled chicken breast
- Zucchini, kale, and mushrooms sautéed in olive oil
- ½ cup honeydew melon

CHAPTER 6

ANTI-INFLAMMATORY FATS AND OILS

Modifying our diet to include more of the foods that feed our beneficial microbes, and less of the foods that feed the harmful species, is just one piece of the puzzle. Another important way in which we can use food to calm the immune system is by choosing the right fats and oils. Specifically, the fats that are emphasized in the Mediterranean diet.

The Mediterranean diet has long been hailed as one of the healthiest diets by a variety of measures. It is correlated with a longer life expectancy and a lower risk of heart disease, cancer, and diabetes.[318] Most importantly for our purposes, the Mediterranean diet also lowers inflammation.[319] As a result, it can significantly reduce the severity of symptoms in people with psoriasis or arthritis.[320]

It appears that three specific components of the Mediterranean diet convey most of the anti-inflammatory effect: **fish**, **olive oil**, and **antioxidant-rich vegetables**. The importance of including vegetables with the highest antioxidant content was covered in chapter 4. This chapter focuses on how to get the most benefit from fish and olive oil, along with the specific problems with other fat sources.

The Power of Fish and Olive Oil

In those with psoriasis or rheumatoid arthritis, a higher consumption of fish and olive oil directly correlates with milder symptoms and lower levels of inflammatory markers.[321]

In one study illustrating this effect, Swedish researchers asked 50 patients with rheumatoid arthritis to follow a "Cretan Mediterranean" diet, which is rich in fish and olive oil. After only three months, the patients following the Mediterranean diet improved significantly compared to the control group.[322] This improvement was reflected in a wide variety of clinical measures, including a reduction in the number of tender and swollen joints and lower levels of inflammatory markers such as C-reactive protein (CRP). Notably, the patients who improved the most were the ones with the highest intake of omega-3 fats from fish.[323]

Similarly, a diet carefully designed to be high in omega-3 fatty acids was found to reduce the severity of psoriasis in three months.[324] An observational study performed in Italy also found that the more closely people with psoriasis followed the Mediterranean diet, the lower their psoriasis severity.[325] In that study, olive oil and fish consumption were the most important dietary factors.

These studies fit together with the immense body of research showing that the omega-3 fats found in fish can inhibit the production of inflammatory mediators. This effect is similar to the way in which nonsteroidal anti-inflammatory medications (NSAIDs) work, but the effect of omega-3 fats is in fact much broader, suppressing inflammation in a variety of ways.[326]

There is also a vast body of research showing that specific components in olive oil can protect against oxidative damage and inhibit the synthesis of inflammatory mediators.[327] After just a single meal including extra-virgin olive oil, a reduction in inflammatory markers and oxidative stress can be detected in the bloodstream.[328] When consumed regularly, this translates into improved symptoms of inflammatory diseases. In a double-blind, randomized study, olive oil significantly decreased symptoms of rheumatoid arthritis.[329]

Fish oil actually has even greater effects on inflammation than olive oil, but the two appear to work best together.[330] Studies have found that when a combination of fish oil and olive oil is compared to a fish oil supplement alone, the combination wins.[331] Omega-3 fats and olive oil yield a quicker and more significant drop in inflammation when used together than alone. The reduction in inflammation is greater still when omega-3 fats are added in the context of a diet low in omega-6 fats,[332] discussed further below.

To fight inflammation, the type of omega-3 fat is important. The two most useful forms are docosahexaenoic acid (DHA) and eicosapentaenoic acid (EPA), found in fish. The types of omega-3 fats found in plant sources (such as flax seed) have only limited anti-inflammatory effects, and humans cannot effectively convert these fats to EPA or DHA.[333]

Choosing the Best Fish

The following fish are the best choices to include in your daily diet because they are high in EPA and DHA but low in mercury:

- Salmon (farmed and wild)
- Sardines

- Farmed rainbow trout
- Atlantic mackerel
- Herring

These fish have five times more omega-3 fat than typical fish and should be eaten two or three times per week.

Cod is another fish that is usually very low in mercury, but it has too little omega-3 fat to combat inflammation. Sole is probably a better choice, with about one-third the omega-3 levels of salmon and low mercury levels. Many other fish that have substantial amounts of omega-3 fats, such as halibut, albacore tuna, king mackerel, and swordfish, are simply too high in mercury to eat regularly. A more detailed comparison of the omega-3 and mercury levels of some popular fish is set out in the table below.[334] A printable version is available online at www.keystonebook.com/resources.

THE BEST FISH: High omega-3, low mercury

Fish	DHA + EPA per 100 g (3.5 oz.)	Mercury (ppm)
Salmon, Atlantic, farmed	2.1	0.02
Salmon, Atlantic, wild	1.8	0.05
Herring	1.7	0.06
Salmon, pink	1.3	0.04
Salmon, sockeye	1.2	0.04
Mackerel, Atlantic	1.2	0.05
Farmed trout	1.2	0.03
Salmon, coho, wild	1.1	0.04
Sardines	1.0	0.08

GOOD FISH: moderate omega-3, low or moderate mercury

Fish	DHA + EPA per 100 g (3.5 oz.)	Mercury (ppm)
Mackerel, chub	1.8	0.1
Sablefish (black cod)	1.8	0.2
Halibut, from Greenland	1.2	0.2
Sole	0.5	0.09
Hake	0.5	0.2
Flounder	0.5	0.1
Tuna, yellowfin, canned	0.3	0.1
Tuna, light, canned	0.3	0.1
Snapper	0.3	0.2
Skipjack tuna	0.3	0.2
Perch	0.3	0.1
Haddock	0.2	0.2
Cod, Atlantic	0.12	0.03

MODERATE MERCURY (no more than 2 or 3 times per month)

Fish	Mercury (ppm)
Halibut, Pacific	0.3
Tuna, albacore, canned	0.3
Grouper	0.4
Mackerel, Spanish	0.4
Bass, Chilean	0.4
Orange roughy	0.5

AVOID: High in mercury

Fish	Mercury (ppm)
Marlin	1.5
Mackerel, king	1.1
Swordfish	0.9
Tuna, Bluefin	0.8

Choosing salmon over tuna is an important step to limit your mercury consumption if you eat fish regularly. A small can (3.5 oz.) of albacore tuna has approximately 75 percent of the weekly limit for mercury, while the mercury level in some types of tuna served at sushi restaurants (such as bigeye and bluefin) is higher still. Even the lowest-mercury tuna, such as canned chunk light, has 27 percent of the weekly limit of mercury in a small serving. By comparison, the same-sized serving of salmon has only 2 percent of the mercury limit. To look up mercury levels for other fish species, consult the Environmental Defense Fund Seafood Selector tool, available online at http://seafood.edf.org/.

Although wild-caught fish is generally preferable to farmed, the amount of omega-3 fat is similar in farmed and wild salmon. It is actually sometimes higher in farmed salmon due to the higher overall fat content.[335] Farmed salmon does pose some concern with respect to antibiotic use and potential environmental harm, but this can be minimized by only purchasing from sources such as WholeFoods, which impose strict standards on suppliers. Another cost-effective option is to buy frozen wild salmon in bulk.

If budget allows, grass-fed beef is also a relatively good

source of omega-3 fats, with levels approximately three times higher than conventional beef.[336]

Fish Oil Supplements

Can you just take a fish oil supplement instead of eating fish? There is some controversy on this point, but on balance the research suggests that fish oil supplements *are* effective in reducing inflammation and improving the symptoms of psoriasis and arthritis.

Numerous double-blind, placebo-controlled studies have found a consistent benefit of fish oil supplements, particularly at relatively high doses (3–4 grams per day) and when taken for several months.[337] This benefit is seen in psoriasis,[338] rheumatoid arthritis,[339] ankylosing spondylitis,[340] Crohn's disease,[341] and juvenile idiopathic arthritis.[342] Supplementing with additional fish oil has also been found to enhance the anti-inflammatory effect of a low-carbohydrate Mediterranean diet.[343]

Despite decades of positive results in clinical trials,[344] controversy has arisen in the past few years about whether supplements may do more harm than good on the basis that the omega-3 fats in fish oil are prone to oxidation.

Omega-3 fats are polyunsaturated, which means they are long-chain fats with many double bonds. These double bonds are inherently unstable. At each double bond, the fat molecule can be oxidized (by losing a hydrogen atom and ending up with a free radical), triggering chemical reactions that produce a variety of different compounds. Some of these compounds are inflammatory, theoretically undermining the anti-inflammatory effect of the fish oil.[345]

Oxidation is more prevalent in fish oil than fish itself because oxidation occurs during processing and storage of the isolated oil. Investigations of the extent of this problem have yielded conflicting results; depending on the study, anywhere between 10 percent and 75 percent of fish oil supplements exceed oxidation limits.[346]

Given the prevalence of oxidation in fish oil, experts conclude that "it is likely that the omega-3 supplements used in many clinical trials have also been significantly oxidized."[347] Yet the results of these trials are overwhelmingly positive, particularly when high doses are given.[348] Any oxidation that occurred to the fish oil supplements used in these studies therefore did not cancel out the therapeutic effects.

It is also worth noting that the average amount of oxidation products measured in fish oil supplements is comparable to that found in conventional cooking oils.[349] By eliminating these oils (discussed further below), it is possible to take fish oil supplements without adding to the overall burden of oxidized lipids. Indeed, studies adding a fish oil supplement in combination with a diet eliminating vegetable oils show the best results. In one such study, more than half of the patients had a moderate to excellent improvement in their psoriasis, while another 20 percent had a mild improvement.[350]

Fish oil supplements have been found to be helpful in the context of aggressive medical treatment of rheumatoid arthritis.[351] In a study at the Royal Adelaide Hospital in Australia, patients taking a high-dose fish oil (5 grams of EPA and DHA per day) were twice as likely as those taking a low dose (0.4 g) to achieve remission while on "triple DMARD therapy" (methotrexate, sulphasalazine, and hydroxychloroquine). Fish oil supplements can therefore effectively complement conventional medical approaches.

The major advantage of fish oil supplements over just

eating more fish is the ability to reach a high daily dose. It may take at least 3–4 grams per day of EPA and DHA to make a significant difference to psoriasis and arthritis,[352] which would require 5 to 6 ounces of high omega-3 fish every day. (In children with juvenile arthritis, a dose of 2 grams per day was effective.[353]) To meet the daily goal, it is probably easier in the long term to eat salmon, sardines, or mackerel a few times per week and **add a daily fish oil supplement of 2–4 grams (2000–4000 mg).**

We can also take steps to choose a fish oil supplement that is less likely to be oxidized. The most important factor seems to be the freshness of the supplement; in one study, almost all tested fish oil products that were more than 2½ years from expiration had low levels of oxidation.[354] Some other factors to consider when choosing a supplement:

- Light is a major contributor to oxidation during storage, so choose a product in a dark or opaque bottle.

- Krill oil has been found to have particularly high oxidation levels.[355]

- Soft gels have lower levels of oxidation than bulk oil.[356]

- Oils in triglyceride form are better absorbed than other forms.[357]

- If in doubt, cut open a capsule to smell and taste the oil. It should be only mildly fishy and not smell rancid.

- Look for a high concentration of EPA and DHA per capsule—at least 1000 mg.

One excellent choice is Nordic Naturals Ultimate Omega 2X. The company uses a proprietary oxygen-free manufacturing process to prevent oxidation and reports that the oxidation markers in their products are well below standard limits. Another good choice is Garden of Life Minami Platinum, which is produced using a carbon dioxide process to limit oxidation; the company also reports having independent lab verification of acceptable oxidation levels.

Like any supplement, check with your doctor before starting a fish oil supplement. There is some concern that it may increase bleeding risk in those taking blood-thinning medication, although this has not actually been observed in tests of moderate doses of fish oil in combination with warfarin.[358]

Buying Olive Oil

Like fish oil and other cooking oils, olive oil contains polyunsaturated fats that are prone to damage, although in a much lower concentration than seed and fish oils. Fortunately, olive oil also contains dozens of antioxidant compounds that help protect the oil from oxidation.

Extra-virgin olive oil has a higher level of these compounds than virgin or "light" olive oil. Many countries have strict guidelines for oil to meet the "extra virgin" description. Unfortunately, not all oil labeled as extra-virgin olive oil actually is. In 2010, researchers at the University of California found that the majority of olive oil samples tested did not meet U.S. or international standards for "extra virgin" status, usually because the oils were oxidized or poor quality.[359] Two brands that did meet the standards were California Olive Ranch and Costco's store brand, Kirkland Signature.

Beyond those two brands, the Australian and Californian

certifications for olive oil are good signifiers of quality, as is the presence of a harvest date printed on the bottle. Experts recommend only buying olive oil within 15 months of the harvest date. In addition, you can usually taste and smell whether olive oil is fresh and good quality. Good-quality extra-virgin olive oil will taste slightly bitter and peppery, be greenish in color, and have a fresh, grassy scent. Oxidized or poor-quality oil will smell musty, waxy, or rancid. To further minimize oxidation and preserve polyphenol content, buy olive oil in a dark glass bottle and store it in a cabinet, not next to the stove.

There is some controversy about whether cooking with olive oil is a good idea, but the current balance of the research suggests that olive oil is sufficiently stable to cook with, particularly at moderate temperatures. While it does contain polyunsaturated fats, olive oil also contains more than 20 different antioxidant compounds that limit oxidation during cooking.[360]

Avocado and Avocado Oil

Avocado is another good source of anti-inflammatory fat. As in olive oil, the predominant fat found in avocado is mostly the monounsaturated fat oleic acid. Processed avocado oil also has a level of oxidative stability during cooking similar to that of olive oil. It is, however, quite vulnerable to oxidation if exposed to light at room temperature for long periods of time, so it should be purchased in a dark bottle.[361] Fresh avocados are even better because they are particularly rich in antioxidants such as vitamin E.

Oils to Avoid

Using olive oil as the primary oil also makes it easier to side-step the two categories of fats that contribute most to inflammation: refined seed oils and saturated fat.

Seed Oils

Refined seed oils such as canola, soy, and sunflower contain significant amounts of polyunsaturated fats, which are quite unstable.[362] As a result, these oils readily oxidize when exposed to heat or light.[363] Consuming too many oxidized fats contributes to inflammation in a variety of ways, including by increasing oxidized LDL.[364]

In contrast, olive oil contains only around 10 percent polyunsaturated fats, along with a high concentration of antioxidant polyphenols that limit oxidation. Olive oil can therefore withstand some cooking without oxidizing significantly.[365]

The fats in seed oils are also problematic because they are more readily converted to trans fats, particularly after cooking at high heat.[366] Trans fats can increase inflammation throughout the body (reflected in higher levels of TNF, IL-6, and CRP, for example).[367] Olive oil is therefore clearly a better choice and oils such as canola and sunflower oil should only be used occasionally. If you find that you need to use seed oil regularly, high oleic safflower oil is the best choice, having a composition closer to olive oil.

Note that nut oils should also generally be avoided because they are readily oxidized.[368] Macadamia nut oil may be the exception because it is mostly monounsaturated fat, which is more stable.

Saturated Fats

To followers of health news, advising against saturated fat may seem antiquated. Saturated fat has long been vilified for playing a role in heart disease, resulting in a shift away from animal fats and toward refined vegetable oils from the 1960s to 1990s. Starting around 2007, the link between saturated fat and heart disease began to be seriously questioned, with high-profile studies over the subsequent decade finding no impact of saturated fat on the risk of dying from heart disease.[369] As that controversy continues, there has been a major shift toward using more saturated fats such as coconut oil, ghee, and palm oil, particularly among followers of the paleo diet.

While some of the authors who originally popularized the paleo diet have cautioned against excessive saturated fat (namely Loren Cordain, Robb Wolf, and Sarah Ballantyne), many other advocates for the paleo diet maintain that saturated fat is healthy and recommend coconut oil and ghee as primary cooking fats.

But saturated fat is definitely a problem for those with inflammatory diseases, as several groundbreaking studies have now revealed. In one study published in the journal *Metabolism* in 2016, a randomized crossover trial compared the effects of a high palmitic acid diet or high oleic acid diet in 12 young women for three weeks.[370] (Palmitic acid is a common saturated fatty acid, and oleic acid is the monounsaturated fat in olive oil.) The researchers looked at inflammatory mediators in the bloodstream and levels secreted by immune cells when stimulated with bacterial by-products. Even over this very short time period, the diet high in saturated fat resulted in higher levels of inflammatory mediators, including IL-6 and IL-1β, both of which are implicated in psoriasis and arthritis.

In a similar study published in the *Journal of Nutritional Biochemistry*, researchers found that when healthy adults reduced their normal consumption of palmitic acid for three weeks, their immune cells produced significantly lower levels of inflammatory mediators such as IL-1β and TNF. When the volunteers then increased their consumption of palmitic acid, TNF in the bloodstream increased.[371]

The findings from these human studies are consistent with what has recently been discovered at a molecular level: saturated fats can activate key receptors (called TLR-4 and NLRP3) and thereby trigger the release of inflammatory cytokines.[372] In this way, saturated fats stimulate inflammation in a range of different cell types, including various immune cells,[373] skeletal muscle,[374] the cells lining coronary arteries,[375] the placenta,[376] and brain cells.[377]

At a practical level, this research means that those with inflammatory diseases should definitely try to minimize saturated fat. The long-chain saturated fats found in palm oil and animal-based cooking fats are likely the worst.[378] The medium-chain saturated fatty acids found in coconut oil are still inflammatory, but to a lesser degree.[379]

Yet coconut oil may contribute to inflammation in another way—by facilitating the transport of bacterial by-products across the intestinal wall. As discussed earlier, endotoxin, also known as lipopolysaccharide, is a component of certain gut bacteria that can trigger systemic inflammation when it crosses into circulation. Even a small amount of endotoxin can trigger a widespread inflammatory response.

In a well-designed randomized study involving 20 healthy adults and published in 2016, researchers found that fish oil decreased the level of endotoxin in the bloodstream after a meal, whereas coconut oil significantly increased it. Olive oil and grapeseed oil had little effect.[380]

It appears that the fats in coconut oil have a somewhat unique ability to facilitate the transport of endotoxin across the gut barrier.[381] Animal and laboratory studies have found that the transport of endotoxin across the intestine was 60 percent higher in the presence of coconut oil, even without any observable harm to the integrity of the gut barrier.[382] Researchers now believe that the fatty acids in coconut oil help to form "lipid rafts" that transport endotoxin across the gut barrier.[383]

Taken together, the new research on saturated fats gives us good reason not to add additional saturated fats to our diet through coconut oil, butter, palm oil, or animal-based cooking fats. Avoiding these added fats allows room in the diet for the small amounts of saturated fat found in lean animal proteins. A chart setting forth the best choices for animal proteins is provided at the end of this chapter.

Omega-6 Fats

Another concern with animal-based fats is that they can be very high in a particular type of omega-6 fat called arachidonic acid (AA). Some forms of omega-6 fat, like the linoleic acid found in nuts and seeds, appear to have little impact on inflammation.[384] [385] Yet high levels of arachidonic acid—the type found in many animal foods—has been implicated in psoriasis and other inflammatory conditions.[386]

This is not sufficient reason to avoid animal-based proteins. Vegetarian and vegan diets are surprisingly not that effective for controlling psoriasis or arthritis. Arachidonic acid would be very low in a vegan diet, but the results of experiments involving vegan diets for arthritis have been disappointing.[387] In one of the few studies showing any significant benefit of a vegan diet, the researchers concluded that the reduction in arthritis symptoms was most likely due to the fact that the experimental diet was also gluten-free.[388] More recently, a diet carefully designed to be low in arachidonic acid showed just a 14 percent reduction in the number of painful joints in patients with rheumatoid arthritis.[389]

Strictly excluding arachidonic acid is therefore not worthwhile, but it may be wise to avoid the foods that contain extremely high levels of this fat.

- Fatty pork such as bacon
- Organ meat
- Walnut oil
- Farmed tilapia
- Wild rainbow trout

The true value in lowering your intake of arachidonic acid may actually be that doing so can help you get the best results from adding more fish and fish oil. That is because omega-3 fats are much better at suppressing inflammation in the context of a lower intake of arachidonic acid.[390]

Fats and Oils in Summary

The fats at the core of Mediterranean diet have an extraordinary ability to reduce inflammation. We should therefore try to obtain most of our fats from fish, olive oil, and avocado. Emphasizing these foods not only allows us to benefit from the anti-inflammatory powers of monounsaturated and omega-3 fats, it also allows us to avoid more harmful fats such as saturated fat and oxidized seed oils. In the end, choosing the right fats and oils is a powerful way to bring peace to the immune system.

TABLE 8: Preferred Proteins

BEST animal proteins	LIMIT (2 to 3 times per month)	AVOID
Chicken (skinless)	Chicken (with skin) [S, O6]	Fatty bacon [S, O6]
Pork tenderloin	Marbled beef [S]	Organ meats [O6]
Lean pork chop	Pork shoulder [S, O6]	Farmed tilapia [O6]
Pork loin	Pork ribs [S, O6]	Wild rainbow trout [O6]
Ham	Sausage [S, O6]	King mackerel [M]
Canadian bacon	Duck [S, O6]	Swordfish [M]
Turkey	Pacific halibut [M]	Bluefin tuna [M]
Lean beef	Grouper [M]	
Bison	Chilean sea bass [M]	
Lamb, trimmed of fat	Orange roughy [M]	
Salmon	Albacore tuna [M]	
Sardines	Spanish mackerel [M]	
Atlantic mackerel		
Cod		
Haddock		
Flounder		
Skipjack tuna		
Light canned tuna		
Yellowfin tuna		
Other low-mercury fish		

S: saturated fat. O6: omega-6 fat. M: mercury

TABLE 9: Anti-inflammatory Fats and Oils

BEST OILS	LIMIT (damaged polyunsaturated fats)	AVOID (saturated and/or omega-6)
Olive oil	Canola oil	Ghee
Avocado oil	Sunflower oil	Lard
	Safflower oil	Tallow
	Soybean oil	Palm oil
	Corn oil	Coconut oil
	Nut oils	Duck fat
	Other seed oils	

CHAPTER 7

TROUBLESHOOTING AND CUSTOMIZING THE KEYSTONE DIET

How to Find Your Own Trigger Foods

The Keystone Diet described so far provides the overall protocol for reducing inflammation, but it is not always enough. If you continue to have active inflammation, it may be worth doing further experimentation to determine whether you have any unique food sensitivities. To do so, you will systematically eliminate and then reintroduce foods that can trigger symptoms in some people with autoimmune disease, namely

- Common allergens (especially dairy, nuts, and eggs)
- Nightshades (tomatoes, peppers, potatoes, eggplants, certain spices)

These foods are not necessarily a problem for everyone. The only way to know how they affect you is to eliminate them for one or two months, then gradually reintroduce each food while carefully observing your response. The end goal is to develop your own personal maintenance diet that is tailored to your own particular sensitivities.

Identifying Food Allergies

Although most food allergies produce rapid and obvious symptoms, it is also possible for food allergies and sensitivities to contribute to autoimmune disease even in the absence of typical allergy symptoms.

For those affected by food allergy, identifying and removing the culprit can be enormously helpful—in rare cases even resulting in a complete resolution of joint pain. In the words of one doctor in the *British Medical Journal* in 1981, "No one would be foolish enough to claim that every case of rheumatoid arthritis is associated with a food allergy, but if only 1 in 20 is—and I suspect that it is considerably more—I question whether we have the right to withhold such a simple, safe, brief, and non-invasive investigation in a disease of such appalling chronicity."[391]

In the past two decades, there has been a stream of case reports in medical journals describing patients with severe rheumatoid arthritis who improved dramatically by eliminating a food allergen.[392] In each case, joint pain, swelling, and stiffness reduced or disappeared while on an "allergen-free" diet, followed by a clear exacerbation after repeated "blind" challenges. These blind challenges involved hiding the foods in capsules to ensure that both the patient and nurse assessing arthritis symptoms were unaware of the food being tested each time.

Food allergy has also been implicated in juvenile arthritis, with reports of some children making a complete recovery after eliminating an allergen, often milk.[393] One small study also found that a significant proportion of patients with "spondyloarthritis" (including ankylosing spondylitis and psoriatic arthritis) improved after eliminating dairy.[394] Pain severity decreased, morning stiffness improved, and joint and spine symptoms improved. Many of the patients in this study who had a good response were still following the dairy-free diet two years later, and some were able to discontinue all medications.

Researchers now estimate that food allergy impacts about 5 percent of rheumatoid arthritis cases.[395] We do not yet know how much of a role allergy plays in other autoimmune diseases, but anecdotal reports of reactions to dairy, nuts, and eggs are particularly common among those with psoriasis and various forms of autoimmune arthritis.

Detecting food allergies can be a laborious process. The only reliable method is to follow an allergy elimination diet and then systematically reintroduce foods one at a time. To that end, most allergy elimination diets focus on removing the set of foods that account for more than 90 percent of all serious food allergies. These foods are

- dairy
- eggs
- nuts
- wheat
- soy
- corn
- shellfish

It is also possible to have hidden allergies and sensitivities to many other foods. To identify which other foods you should consider eliminating, skin prick and blood tests can be helpful. These tests typically measure the antibody class associated with true allergies, called IgE antibodies. Blood tests are also available to look for the antibodies associated with delayed hypersensitivities, called IgG antibodies. IgG tests are less reliable than IgE tests, because they can produce many false positives and typically only reflect foods that have been eaten in the preceding few weeks. (There is also a subtype of IgG antibody, called IgG4, which can actually indicate tolerance to a food, rather than a sensitivity.)

Nevertheless, if we take the information with a healthy dose of skepticism, the results of allergy and sensitivity testing can be useful. The more information we have in guiding our elimination diet, the more likely we are to identify any culprits that are contributing to inflammation.

It is also important to note that if you do proceed with IgE and IgG testing and the results are negative for the common allergens listed above, it may still be worth eliminating some of these foods temporarily, particularly the worst offenders—nuts, eggs, and dairy. This is because the currently available tests are also prone to false negatives. That is, they fail to pick up true problems.

False negatives can happen if you have an IgG sensitivity and have not eaten the food for a while before the blood test, or if you have a local antibody response limited to the gut, not in the general circulation. Studies have actually found that some arthritis patients have antibodies against foods only in the intestines, not the general circulation, so these "allergies" would be missed by standard tests.[396]

Allergists and other doctors are often doubtful of the value of IgG food sensitivity testing, but if the results are used only to guide an elimination diet, it is clear these tests do have some value for those with autoimmune disease. As one example of an IgG hypersensitivity contributing to arthritis, a case report published in the journal *Arthritis and Rheumatism* described a patient who had suffered from rheumatoid arthritis for 11 years and believed her symptoms were exacerbated by foods.[397] Blood tests showed no allergy to milk as measured by IgE antibodies, but an increase in IgG antibodies to milk. After a month of hypoallergenic formula, her joint pain and stiffness had improved dramatically, and she was then given blind challenges with different foods or a placebo hidden in a capsule. She showed a major exacerbation from milk each time it was challenged, with an increase in swollen and painful joints peaking 24 to 48 hours after each challenge.

Practical Tips for the Allergy Elimination Diet

The most difficult aspect of eliminating dairy and eggs is developing a new breakfast routine. Good options include

- a smoothie made with collagen peptide powder, greens, and frozen berries
- meat patties or chicken sausage
- leftovers from dinner
- ham or turkey deli meat
- salmon

The adjustment becomes easier with time, particularly as you reframe breakfast as just another meal rather than one that involves typical "breakfast" foods.

Another hurdle that arises from eliminating dairy is ensuring sufficient calcium intake. Good nondairy calcium sources include leafy greens, such as kale or collards, and canned salmon or sardines with bones. Many people are surprised to learn that as much calcium can be absorbed from half a cup of cooked collard greens as from a glass of milk.[398] Calcium in broccoli, bok choy, and kale is also readily absorbed, but calcium in spinach is not. For children, a calcium supplement may be needed. Note that if you are taking a high dose vitamin D supplement, you will need very little calcium in your diet, because vitamin D facilitates calcium absorption.

If you end up eliminating dairy and eggs long term, it may be wise to begin supplementing with vitamin A (or ensure your multivitamin provides most of the recommended daily intake). Butter and eggs are often the main dietary sources of the active form of vitamin A (also called retinol). Many plant foods contain precursors to vitamin A (such as betacarotene), but some people may not perform this conversion process efficiently. Vitamin A is critical for immune regulation because it boosts regulatory T-cells and suppresses the inflammatory Th17 cells involved in autoimmunity.

Additional Tips

- It will be important to read labels to check for even small amounts of allergenic foods. If an allergy is present, occasional exposure to a very low dose can still perpetuate the immune response and obscure the results of the elimination diet.

- The trace amounts of dairy in probiotic supplements may be too trivial to cause a reaction, but you can also err on the side of caution with a dairy-free probiotic such as GutPro Infant Powder, Jarrow Allergen Free, or Renew Life.

- Eliminate the common allergens for at least one month, or longer if the results are not clear.

- When you are ready to perform a challenge, start with a small amount of a particular food, then gradually increase the amount each day over the course of a week or until you observe a reaction.

- A positive reaction may include symptoms other than your usual skin or joint symptoms. If a food causes abdominal pain, for example, it may contribute to arthritis symptoms over the longer term.

- Wait at least a week between each challenge or until symptoms return to normal after a positive challenge.

- Test the foods in "pure" form so that other ingredients do not interfere with the results (for example, using plain yogurt to test dairy).

- Do not perform challenges if you have a history of anaphylactic reactions.

- The most allergenic proteins in eggs are found in the white, so if you react to whole eggs, it may be worth testing egg yolk separately.

- Reintroduce different nuts individually because some people react to all nuts, while others only react to certain varieties.

- If you find that you react to cow's milk dairy, it may be worth testing goat and sheep milk products. Some people with cow's milk allergy will cross-react to the similar proteins in these other forms of dairy, but others will be able to tolerate them without any problem.[399]

An Allergy Impersonator: Food Chemical Sensitivity

If you notice reactions to a large number of foods, and these reactions are inconsistent and unpredictable, bear in mind that this may not reflect a true allergy or IgG-based sensitivity. Rather, it is possible to be intolerant to natural chemicals found in foods, such as histamine and salicylates. It is not yet clear the extent to which these reactions impact psoriasis or arthritis, so investigating sensitivity to these foods should be a lower priority for most people. If, however, you have other symptoms that are typical of food chemical intolerance, such as headaches, flushing, and dizziness after eating certain foods, or if you have noticed reactions to the specific foods that are highest in amines or salicylates, it is worth exploring this possibility.

The most common symptoms of intolerance to amines and/or salicylates include the following:[400]

- chronic hives
- flushing, itching, or burning skin, particularly on the face
- eczema
- asthma
- nasal congestion
- headaches
- stomach pain or diarrhea
- low blood pressure/dizziness
- fatigue or irritability
- joint pain
- muscle pain

Foods high in salicylates include berries, nuts, tea, watermelon, tomatoes, avocado, and spices.[401] Aspirin is another major source of salicylates.

Foods high in amines include cheese, chocolate, aged or processed meats, and fermented foods such as wine, soy sauce, and sauerkraut. (Amines include histamine, tyramine, and several other similar chemicals that form when protein breaks down.)

When considering whether you may have a food chemical intolerance, it is worth noting that this intolerance often presents very differently from allergies; reactions are more unpredictable, and a wider variety of foods seem to be involved. This is because the chemicals are found in a broad array of foods but will only trigger symptoms once the cumulative dose exceeds the amount the body can break down or excrete.[402]

Depending on your threshold for reacting, a small amount of a particular food may have no noticeable effect, yet when consumed in a larger amount or in combination with other problematic foods over the course of the day, the level of amines or salicylates can build up, triggering symptoms. This is quite different from an allergy, where even a small amount of an allergenic food predictably causes symptoms every time.

Investigating sensitivity to these food chemicals is now part of the conventional medical treatment of hives, asthma, eczema, and chronic headache. This is particularly true in Australia, where allergists at major teaching hospitals have led research in this area for the past 30 years.[403] As a result of this research, salicylate sensitivity has now been found to trigger attacks in at least 20 percent of asthmatics, while amine sensitivity has been linked to chronic headache and irritable bowel syndrome.[404]

It is likely that amines and salicylates can contribute to

joint pain and psoriasis in the same way they cause these other symptoms, but only in those with a sensitivity. The Royal Prince Alfred Hospital's Allergy Unit notes joint pain as a common symptom of amine and salicylate intolerance.[405] There are also numerous anecdotal reports of joint pain and psoriasis resolving after eliminating amines and/or salicylates.[406] One small study found that when a group of rheumatoid arthritis patients followed a low-chemical diet (eliminating additives, preservatives, fruit, red meat, herbs, and dairy products), a small subset of the patients showed a dramatic improvement and chose to stay on the diet long term.[407]

If you have reason to suspect amine or salicylate intolerance, it may be worth reducing your intake of the foods with the highest concentration of these chemicals. (For more extensive lists of high amine and salicylate foods, see www.keystonebook. com/foodchemical.) If you find that you do have a food chemical sensitivity, your focus should then shift to addressing the underlying cause, rather than restricting these foods indefinitely.

Although the precise causes may differ for different individuals, experts in this field strongly suspect that small intestinal bacterial overgrowth (SIBO) is a major factor in histamine and salicylate intolerance. This is based on clinical observations on the overlap between patients experiencing food chemical intolerance and SIBO symptoms, and the frequent improvement in food chemical intolerance when SIBO is addressed.

The detailed mechanisms for food chemical sensitivity are still poorly understood but appear to involve hyper-responsive mast cells. An overgrowth of bacteria, yeast, or parasites in the gut may contribute to this process by increasing the numbers and activation of mast cells. This is effectively a form of "mast cell activation syndrome." When there are too many mast cells and they are in an active state, this then sets the stage for overreactions to salicylates and other chemicals from foods.[408] (Note that mast cells are also key players in the inflammatory process in psoriasis and arthritis.[409])

In addition, we know that many of the bacteria that can cause SIBO or dysbiosis in the large intestine can produce large amounts of histamine, overwhelming the body's natural histamine-breakdown mechanisms. You can find out if this may be a factor for you through comprehensive stool testing, such as the GI-Map. Histamine-producing bacteria include *E. coli*, *Citrobacter*, and *Morganella morganii*.[410] *Candida* yeast and various parasites may also trigger substantial histamine production. Addressing these overgrowths using the strategies described in chapter 3, along with a diet that is lower in sugar and starch, can therefore significantly improve food chemical intolerance.

There can also be other contributing factors, such as genetics and hormones (particularly disrupted thyroid and adrenal hormones). Celiac disease can also play a role in some cases, because when the gut lining is damaged, there is a reduction in the enzyme that breaks down histamine (Diamine oxidase). For most people, however, the best place to start in addressing food chemical intolerance is reducing pathogen overgrowth, using the approaches discussed in previous chapters.

Supplementing with high-dose vitamin C is another way to reduce histamine sensitivity. A dose of 2 grams per day has been found to significantly reduce blood histamine levels and the biological effects of histamine.[411] Fish oil supplementation may also be useful for those with salicylate sensitivity. A small study found that supplementing with 10 grams per day of fish oil for six to eight weeks produced a complete or virtually complete resolution of symptoms in three patients with severe salicylate sensitivity.[412] This is an excessive dose of fish oil, but it is possible that a longer-term intake of a more reasonable dose (such as 2 grams per day) could also help reduce salicylate sensitivity.

Nightshades

The final category of foods that some people can have a particular sensitivity to is fruits, vegetables, and spices in the nightshade plant family. Nightshades have long been implicated in arthritis, starting with the work of a horticulturalist named Norman Childers, who, in the 1970s, suspected that his own arthritis was triggered by potatoes, tomatoes, and eggplant.[413] He understood that these were all members of the Solanaceae plant family—historically known as nightshades because this family includes the deadly nightshade used by the Romans to poison enemies. There are actually thousands of plants in the nightshade family, many of which are toxic or inedible, such as tobacco. The edible nightshades include

- tomatoes
- potatoes (but not sweet potatoes or yams)
- bell peppers/capsicum/sweet peppers
- chili peppers (and derivative spices such as cayenne, paprika, and chipotle)
- eggplant
- tomatillos
- goji berries
- ashwaganda (often found in herbal thyroid supplements)

After eliminating all foods from this plant family, Dr. Childers's symptoms rapidly improved. He shared this finding in a book published in the 1970s, and in the decades since, thousands of people have reported that they too have reduced the severity of their arthritis by eliminating night-shades. A recent study also found that 52 percent of psoriasis patients reported improvement in their symptoms after elim-inating nightshades.[414] Yet there have never been any rigorous scientific studies supporting the link between nightshades and inflammation; all we have to rely on is a plausible bio-chemical explanation.

This biochemical explanation is based on two potentially toxic components found in nightshades: glycoalkaloids and lectins. Glycoalkaloids are chemicals produced by plants to defend against insects. The best-studied glycoalkaloids are solanine and chaconin, found in potato; tomatine, found in tomato; and a group of similar chemicals found in peppers.

There is no doubt that these chemicals are extremely toxic in high doses, with reports throughout history of "solanine poisoning" from green potatoes. Potatoes produce much larger amounts of glycoalkaloids when stored improperly (conditions which also cause them to turn green), but even fresh pota-toes contain a significant amount.[415] The critical question is what happens when we are exposed to low doses over the long term. There is some limited evidence that even in low doses, these chemicals can damage cell membranes and contribute to increased intestinal permeability.[416] In theory, this would allow bacterial by-products and other molecules to cross the gut barrier and activate the immune system, spurring further inflammation.

In laboratory and animal studies, potato glycoalkaloids

were found to disrupt the intestinal barrier.[417] In another laboratory experiment, a glycoalkaloid found in sweet peppers increased the permeability of human intestinal cells.[418] Capsaicin, the chemical responsible for the heat of hot peppers, also appears to disrupt the gut barrier.[419]

The second plausible biochemical explanation for a link between nightshades and arthritis comes down to lectins, and here, too, we have limited but intriguing evidence. We know that the lectins in potato and tomato survive cooking and digestion and can cross the gut barrier and enter the circulatory system.[420] Once in circulation, the "stickiness" of these proteins allows them to bind to molecules on the surface of mast cells, sending a signal to activate and release histamine and other inflammatory mediators. Researchers have shown that potato lectin activates human mast cells and triggers histamine release.[421] Tomato lectin is expected to behave in the same way because it has the same binding properties.[422] Because mast cells are the source of many inflammatory mediators involved in psoriasis and arthritis, we should be wary of anything suspected of increasing mast cell activation.

There is no definitive answer as to whether the glycoalkaloids or lectins are the reason nightshades appear to worsen arthritis symptoms in many people. But even without definitive proof, we have sufficient reason to avoid these foods on a short-term trial basis. Some people may find that they have less joint pain when avoiding tomatoes, potatoes, and nightshade-based spices, but they can tolerate sweet peppers or eggplant, for example. It is also possible to tolerate these foods in small amounts when eaten occasionally, but to react if they are consumed too often.

Practical Tips for Eliminating Nightshades

- Nightshades are the basis of many commonly used spices such as paprika, cayenne pepper, chili powder, chipotle, and red pepper flakes.

- Paprika and chili powder are often used in spice blends in processed foods and may not be specifically listed as an ingredient. For this reason, it is best to avoid any foods that contain the catchall term "spices."

- Black pepper comes from an unrelated plant family, but it should be used sparingly because it contains a chemical called piperine, which appears to have similar biological effects to capsaicin, causing a similar increase in intestinal permeability.[423] In two recent animal studies, piperine increased the ability of other compounds to cross the intestinal barrier two- to fourfold.[424]

- Lectins and glycoalkaloids are typically concentrated in the skin and seeds, so some people may be able to tolerate small amounts of tomatoes and bell peppers that have been peeled and deseeded.

- Ripe tomatoes also have a much lower lectin concentration than green tomatoes.

- In the end, sensitivity to nightshades may vary widely between people. The only way to determine how you are affected is through trial and error.

The Keystone Diet at a Glance

General Principles

- Support your microbiome and antioxidant defenses by eating more high-fiber and brightly colored fruit and vegetables.

- Eat more fish, especially salmon, sardines, and Atlantic mackerel.

- Consider supplementing with 2–4 grams of fish oil per day.

- Use olive oil and avocado oil as the primary added fats.

- Choose leaner proteins such as chicken, fish, and lean pork.

- Trim visible fats from meat before cooking.

Level 1: Basic low-starch plan

- Eliminate gluten-containing grains.

- Avoid gut-damaging grains and legumes (soy, corn, potato, peanut).

- Limit other starchy foods to two servings per day, preferably in the form of starchy root vegetables such as parsnip or sweet potato.

- Cut back on sugar.

Level 2: Intermediate low-starch plan

- Eliminate grains, legumes, and very starchy vegetables.

- Minimize added sugars.

- Limit fruit to two or three small servings per day.
- Avoid dairy, other than homemade yogurt if tolerated.
- Avoid the highest-starch nuts and seeds, such as cashews.

Level 3: Advanced low-starch plan

In addition to the steps listed above for level 2:

- Choose vegetables with the lowest starch content.
- Limit fruit to one or two small servings per day.
- Use only the lowest-starch nuts and seeds, such as flax and macadamias.
- Try to avoid maltodextrin and other starchy fillers in supplements.
- Increase fat and protein to compensate for the reduction in carbohydrates. If you emphasize fat this will become a ketogenic diet. Some people may feel better long term by emphasizing protein instead in order to prevent hormonal disturbances.
- You may need to increase salt to prevent the electrolyte imbalances that can result from a very low carbohydrate diet.

Troubleshooting and Customizing the Keystone Diet

Consider eliminating the following for at least 30 days to determine if you have a sensitivity:

- Common allergens: nuts, eggs, dairy, soy, corn, shellfish
- Nightshades: tomatoes, potatoes, peppers, chili spices, eggplant

If you have symptoms of food chemical intolerance and react to a wide range of foods that are high in histamines or salicylates, you may be able to reduce this sensitivity by addressing SIBO and pathogen overgrowth. Other alternative strategies include testing for thyroid and adrenal hormones and adding a high-dose vitamin C supplement to reduce histamine levels.

Part 3

Beyond Food

CHAPTER 8

ANTI-INFLAMMATORY SUPPLEMENTS

Our primary focus throughout this book is targeting the underlying causes of autoimmunity through diet and other strategies that aim to heal the gut and rebalance the microbiome. For even further help, there are additional supplements that can help fine-tune the immune system. These supplements may only make an incremental difference to the severity of symptoms, but they are worth considering as optional extras to your own personalized program.

Vitamin D

Vitamin D performs many important functions, including regulating immunity and calcium absorption. When vitamin D levels are low, bone density suffers and the immune system becomes unbalanced, with a weaker defense against infections and greater autoimmune activity and inflammation.[425]

Vitamin D is obtained primarily from sun exposure, and most people simply do not get enough sunlight to produce an adequate amount. A substantial length of time outdoors is required even on sunny days, and in winter in most climates the sunlight is simply too weak to generate any vitamin D. As a result, serious deficiencies are widespread.[426]

More than one-third of otherwise healthy young adults in the United States have low levels of vitamin D. This figure may be even higher in those with autoimmune disease, with studies finding that more than half of those with rheumatoid arthritis, ankylosing spondylitis, psoriasis, and juvenile arthritis are deficient.[427] In each of these conditions, vitamin D deficiency is also correlated with disease activity: those with the lowest levels have the most severe symptoms.[428]

For many with psoriasis, adding a vitamin D supplement can make an extraordinary difference. Although most clinical studies in this area have been open label (not blinded or placebo controlled), they have consistently found a benefit when high doses are given for three to six months. Five separate studies have reported a moderate or greater improvement in psoriasis in at least 50 percent of patients.[429] Some patients taking high doses even show complete resolution of their psoriasis.[430] Vitamin D is in fact so effective in psoriasis that topical vitamin D–based prescription creams, such as calcipotriene, are now used as first-line therapy.[431]

Vitamin D supplements also appear to improve joint symptoms in psoriatic and rheumatoid arthritis, with several open-label studies finding that most patients taking a high-dose supplement for three to six months had a significant reduction in pain.[432] It is unclear whether this approach can also reduce pain in other forms of arthritis such as juvenile arthritis or ankylosing spondylitis. Yet even with these conditions, vitamin D is worth supplementing for another reason.

Aside from potential pain reduction, supplementing

with vitamin D is useful for preserving bone strength.[433] Inflammatory arthritis is typically associated with a significant loss of bone minerals, causing bones to become more prone to fracture. This is especially pronounced in juvenile arthritis and ankylosing spondylitis as well as in those using steroids such as prednisone.[434] Vitamin D limits this loss of bone density because it facilitates calcium absorption. The American College of Rheumatology in fact recommends vitamin D supplementation for all patients using steroids such as prednisone.[435] (To further support bone density, supplementing with calcium, magnesium, and vitamin K2 may also be useful, particularly if you do not include kale or collards in your daily diet.)

More broadly, a panel of 25 experts from 15 countries recently recommended that all people with autoimmune disease or musculoskeletal health problems should have their vitamin D level tested.[436] The panel established clinical practice recommendations stating that in this group, the optimum level is 30 ng/mL, higher than typically considered sufficient for the general population. The panel also recommended that even without testing for a deficiency, people with autoimmune disease should take a low-dose supplement (800 IU) each day. In the winter or for those not often exposed to sunlight, a significantly higher dose may be needed to maintain an adequate vitamin D level.[437] In one study, more than 60 percent of rheumatoid arthritis patients taking 800 IU of vitamin D were still below the preferred level of 30 ng/mL.[438]

For those with a known deficiency, the expert panel recommends a short-term treatment of approximately 7000 IU per day (as 50,000 IU once per week) for eight weeks, followed by a maintenance dose of 800 IU per day, with regular monitoring to ensure that this low-maintenance dose is sufficient.

An alternative approach, if regular testing is not feasible, is to start with 5000 IU each day for one to two months, then continue at 2000 IU per day as a maintenance dose. The clinical practice recommendations state that "international authorities consider a vitamin D intake of 2000 IU daily as absolutely safe, although a recent review found that even doses of up to 10,000 IU per day supplemented over several months did not lead to any adverse events."[439]

For children, the U.S. government's recommended daily intake for vitamin D is 600 IU per day. Clinical trials of vitamin D to prevent other childhood diseases often use 1200–2000 IU per day.[440]

To maximize absorption, the preferred form of vitamin D supplement is vitamin D3 (cholecalciferol) as a liquid softgel (or liquid drops) rather than a solid tablet. Good-quality brands (such as Doctor's Best, Jarrow, and Seeking Health) often use extra-virgin olive oil as the carrier oil rather than soy or corn oil.

Glucosamine and Chondroitin

Glucosamine and chondroitin are among the most commonly used supplements to treat joint pain, with a long track record of safety and minimal side effects. Both are components needed to make cartilage and the fluid that cushions joints. They have also been studied in clinical trials for decades, although largely in the context of osteoarthritis.

In osteoarthritis, it is clear from several large, double-blind, placebo-controlled studies that glucosamine can help limit cartilage destruction.[441] In one of the best-known studies, published in the *Lancet* in 2001, those patients taking

1500 mg of glucosamine sulfate per day had significantly less pain and cartilage loss after three years.[442]

Although most glucosamine products contain a combination of glucosamine and chondroitin, it may be that this combination adds no further benefit. One large study funded by the National Institutes of Health (at a cost of $12.5 million) compared glucosamine and chondroitin alone or in combination in 500 patients with knee osteoarthritis. The patients with the least cartilage loss after two years were those taking glucosamine alone. Those taking the combination of glucosamine and chondroitin actually fared no better than those taking the placebo. This could have been a random aberration, but it led the authors to suggest that the two compounds may interfere with one another when used in combination.[443]

The question for those with autoimmune forms of arthritis is whether the cartilage-sparing effect of glucosamine is limited to osteoarthritis or applies more generally. There is little research in this area, but what is known so far does point to a likely benefit for long-term cartilage protection in rheumatoid, psoriatic, and juvenile arthritis.

Osteoarthritis is driven by a different process than autoimmune forms of arthritis, but they share similarities, including degradation of cartilage by the same enzymes (called matrix metalloproteinases).[444] In one of the only trials of glucosamine in rheumatoid arthritis, there was a modest reduction in pain after 12 weeks, but most interestingly, there was also a decrease in the level of matrix metalloproteinase-3 (MMP-3) in the bloodstream.[445] This enzyme is activated by inflammation and causes much of the destruction to cartilage in both rheumatoid arthritis and osteoarthritis.[446] MMP-3 is also elevated in psoriatic and juvenile arthritis and correlates with greater disease severity.[447]

The finding that glucosamine reduces MMP-3 in patients with rheumatoid arthritis suggests that this supplement not only provides a building block for new cartilage and joint fluid but also lessens the attack on existing cartilage. This finding is also supported by numerous animal and laboratory studies showing that glucosamine does indeed reduce the production of MMP-3.[448]

When we put together the pieces of the puzzle, it is reasonable to expect that glucosamine can limit long-term cartilage damage in all these forms of arthritis, not just osteoarthritis. It may therefore be worth adding a glucosamine supplement, particularly since this compound has been studied extensively for safety and side effects. The two common forms of glucosamine supplements, sulfate and hydrochloride, are roughly equivalent. The typical dose is 1000 to 1500 milligrams per day.

Many glucosamine and chondroitin products now also include a compound called MSM, which stands for methylsulfonylmethane. This is included because it provides a source of sulfur, which is needed to make connective tissue. A small number of studies have found that MSM produces a mild benefit in osteoarthritis, but side effects such as gastrointestinal symptoms, insomnia, and headaches have been reported.[449] Unlike glucosamine and chondroitin, there have not been any large studies establishing the safety of MSM supplements. As a result, it may be preferable to choose a glucosamine supplement that does not contain MSM. (An alternative source for the sulfur needed to make and repair connective tissue is sulfur-rich vegetables, particularly those in the cabbage family and mushrooms.)

Gamma-Linolenic Acid (GLA) as Borage or Evening Primrose Oil

Borage oil and evening primrose oil are mildly anti-inflammatory because they contain a specific omega-6 fatty acid called gamma-linolenic acid (GLA). This fatty acid can inhibit the production of one particular inflammatory mediator called leukotriene B4 (LTB4).[450] LTB4 attracts immune cells to the site of inflammation and helps orchestrate the immune attack.[451] LTB4 plays a particularly key role in psoriasis because it is also involved in the proliferation of skin cells to produce plaques.[452] GLA helps block the conversion of arachidonic acid to LTB4. This mechanism explains the anecdotal reports that borage or evening primrose oil supplements can significantly reduce psoriasis, although this has not been established in clinical trials.

In the rheumatoid arthritis context, there have been some human studies, although the results have been mixed. Studies involving low doses or short time periods often find little to no benefit,[453] while very high doses have been found to reduce the number of tender and swollen joints.[454] The successful high-dose studies have given doses of 1.4 or 2.8 grams per day of GLA. Since borage oil is only about 20 percent GLA, this would translate to five to 10 large capsules. Evening primrose oil is only 10 percent GLA, so 10 or 20 capsules would be required. There is no data supporting the long-term safety of these high doses. A middle-ground dose of 500 milligrams (0.5 grams) per day of borage oil (typically two capsules) would be a more reasonable approach and may be sufficient to noticeably reduce inflammation in the context of an anti-inflammatory diet.[455]

One of the concerns with GLA supplements is that they can increase the level of arachidonic acid in the bloodstream.[456] This could in theory worsen inflammation in the long term and increase the risk of blood clotting. One study indicated that it is possible to prevent the increase in arachidonic acid after taking GLA supplement by adding an omega-3 supplement.[457] As a result, if you are using a borage or evening primrose oil supplement, it is particularly important to take at least 2 grams of fish oil per day. This combination does appear to reduce inflammation more than fish oil alone.[458]

Vitamin E

Vitamin E is widely known as a powerful antioxidant. This vitamin is actually a group of eight similar compounds (four tocopherols and four trienols), usually present as a mixture in different plant oils, nuts, and seeds. Although vitamin E compounds are typically known for their antioxidant properties, some forms have entirely separate anti-inflammatory effects because they directly suppress the enzymes that produce inflammatory mediators.[459]

Several clinical studies have found vitamin E supplements useful for rheumatoid arthritis, producing an equivalent pain reduction as the NSAID diclofenac.[460] A double-blind, placebo-controlled clinical study also found that a combination of vitamin E, selenium, and CoQ10 significantly decreased the severity of psoriasis and joint pain.[461]

Yet the Mediterranean diet is naturally high in vitamin E, so a supplement is probably unnecessary in the context of the diet outlined in this book. In a clinical trial of rheumatoid arthritis patients following the Mediterranean diet, all patients exceeded the minimum recommended vitamin E intake.[462] It is also preferable to obtain vitamin E from food (such as avocado and olive oil) because foods contain a mixture of the different tocopherols and trienols, whereas supplements often contain only alpha-tocopherol. Studies suggest that a mixture of different forms of vitamin E produces a greater anti-inflammatory effect than alpha-tocopherol alone.[463]

Turmeric / Curcumin

Turmeric is a spice from the ginger family that has been used for thousands of years in Indian cuisine and traditional medicine. Curcumin is one of the many compounds found in turmeric and is widely regarded as having powerful anti-inflammatory effects, based on thousands of laboratory studies.

Yet the ability of curcumin to calm inflammation is limited by its poor absorption and stability.[464] As a result, the real-world effects of curcumin are less impressive than lab studies would suggest. Many human clinical studies of standard curcumin supplements have produced underwhelming results, particularly in the context of autoimmune disease.[465]

There are, however, some new formulations of turmeric that are better absorbed and much more effective.[466] Among these new formulations, Meriva® is supported by the most clinical research, particularly in the context of joint pain and psoriasis.

Meriva contains all three curcuminoids found in turmeric, rather than just curcumin. These curcuminoids are combined with phosphatidylcholine (a component of our cell membranes) to make the curcuminoids more soluble and stable. Meriva is sold by various good-quality supplement brands, including Doctor's Best, Thorne, Jarrow, and Pure Encapsulations.

There is convincing evidence that Meriva can improve joint inflammation and pain, at least in the context of nonautoimmune arthritis. In a placebo-controlled clinical study of osteoarthritis, patients taking Meriva saw a significant improvement in pain, swelling, and stiffness, along with a drop in all measured inflammatory markers.[467] The patients taking Meriva were also able to reduce their NSAIDs usage by 63 percent and as a result had fewer gastrointestinal complaints.

Although this study was done in the context of osteoarthritis, not autoimmune arthritis, it does support the view that the Meriva form of curcumin can reduce joint pain and inflammation. By contrast, similar studies using other formulations of curcumin, such as BCM-95 (in CuraMed) produced very little reduction in joint pain and no improvement in inflammatory markers.[468]

In addition to reducing some aspects of inflammation, Meriva also reduces perception of pain in the short term, in a similar way to acetaminophen. (Acetaminophen is the active ingredient in Tylenol, also known as paracetamol.) A dose of 2 grams of Meriva was found to produce a short-term reduction in pain equivalent to a full dose of acetaminophen.[469] In this study, the pain-relieving effects started about two hours after it was taken and lasted about four hours. Note that pain relief was barely noticeable at a lower dose. A relatively large dose of 2 grams is required, which is typically four capsules.

Although the main value of Meriva is likely pain reduction, it does also show promise in directly controlling some autoimmune diseases. For example, one study found that Meriva can reduce the relapse rate in chronic anterior uveitis.[470] This is an autoimmune eye condition that is closely linked to psoriatic arthritis and ankylosing spondylitis. Another clinical study found that Meriva is helpful for maintenance of remission in ulcerative colitis.[471] Finally, in the context of psoriasis, Meriva significantly reduced the severity of psoriasis after 12 weeks, along with a reduction in one of the main inflammatory mediators that drives psoriasis (IL-22).[472] This lies in sharp contrast to the disappointing results seen with other versions of curcumin, which produced no benefit in psoriasis.[473]

It may be that Meriva is so much more effective than standard curcumin supplements because this formulation specifically improves the absorption of other related compounds found in turmeric, not just curcumin. In fact, the major curcuminoid present in plasma after taking Meriva is not actually curcumin, but demethoxycurcumin, a related compound that may have even more potent anti-inflammatory effects.[474]

An area of research to watch when it comes to curcumin is the effect on the microbiome. Initial studies published in 2017 and 2018 suggest that curcumin may have beneficial effects on the microbiome, such as increasing the abundance of beneficial butyrate-producing microbes and thereby boosting regulatory T cells.[475]

New studies also hint at a possible role for curcumin in improving the gut barrier.[476] This is at odds with the old idea that the gut barrier was an obstacle that needed to be overcome in order for curcumin to work. Older formulations of curcumin actually used an ingredient called piperine to improve the absorption of curcumin by increasing intestinal permeability.[477] This is counterproductive because it also helps other molecules cross the gut barrier too, including bacterial toxins that may increase immune activation.

If you decide to add curcumin to your supplement regime, the best option is to choose one of the many Meriva supplements available, such as Thorne Meriva 500-SF, Jarrow Curcumin Phytosome, or Pure Encapsulations Curcumasorb.

Clinical trials showing beneficial effect in autoimmune disease and joint pain use either 1 or 2 grams per day, which is typically two to four capsules.

Approaching Supplements with Caution

Apart from the thoroughly investigated supplements discussed above, it is prudent to consider other "anti-inflammatory" supplements with great skepticism, given the lack of regulation and oversight of the supplement industry. It is important to keep in mind that supplement manufacturers are not required to test for safety or effectiveness. As a result, most supplements have not been studied in clinical trials, and it is difficult to know their true impact on inflammation. Contamination of supplements with lead and other toxins is also a major concern. "Not only are the advertised ingredients of some supplements potentially dangerous," says Pieter Cohen, MD, Assistant Professor of Medicine at Harvard Medical School, "but because of the way they're regulated, you often have no idea what you're actually ingesting."[478]

Supplements can also obscure the results of dietary changes, as explained by Dr. Suskind of Seattle Children's Hospital: "Caution should be used when considering additional herbal supplements or other alternative therapies . . . I have met families where the SCD did not seem to be working effectively, but when other adjunct therapies were removed, the SCD worked."[479] For this reason, it is useful to keep other supplements to a bare minimum while experimenting with dietary changes.

Summary of Anti-inflammatory Supplements
Supported by Clinical Studies

Supplement	Priority	Example products	Typical Dose
Probiotic	High	· Culturelle · Jarrow Allergen Free · BioK+ · Florastor	10 billion CFU per day (varies greatly depending on strain)
Fish oil	High	· Nordic Naturals Ultimate Omega 2x · Garden of Life Omega 3 Minami Platinum	2000–4000 mg (2–4 grams) per day EPA + DHA
Vitamin D	High	· Doctor's Best Vitamin D3 Softgels	2000 IU per day
Glucosamine	Medium	· Jarrow Glucosamine HCL Mega · NOW Glucosamine 1000	1000–1500 mg per day
Meriva	Medium	· Pure Encapsulations Curcumasorb · Jarrow Curcumin Phytosome · Thorne Meriva 500-SF	1000–2000 mg per day
Borage oil	Low	· Nature's Way EFA Gold Borage · Jarrow Formulas Borage GLA	500 mg GLA per day (~2500 mg borage oil)

CHAPTER 9

THE SCIENCE OF LOW-DOSE NALTREXONE

Naltrexone is a pharmaceutical that has been used for decades to treat opioid addiction, but more recently it has shown great promise as a medication for various inflammatory diseases. When taken in very low doses, naltrexone can regulate the immune system and reduce pain.[480]

In one of the earliest studies on low-dose naltrexone (LDN), researchers found that it could reduce muscle spasms associated with multiple sclerosis (MS).[481] In 2010, a placebo-controlled study at the University of California, San Francisco, also found that LDN significantly reduced pain and improved quality of life in MS patients.[482]

Low-dose naltrexone has also been found to significantly reduce pain in some people with fibromyalgia.[483] The treatment does not work for everyone, but a small double-blind trial at Stanford University reported that the majority of fibromyalgia patients taking LDN had at least a 30 percent reduction in pain.[484]

Aside from these pain-relieving effects, LDN may actually

be able to reduce underlying inflammation, particularly in the gut. There is good evidence for this from double-blind, placebo-controlled trials in Crohn's disease.[485] In one such study, when patients were examined by endoscopy after taking naltrexone for three months, 78 percent showed significant intestinal healing, compared to just 28 percent of those taking a placebo.[486] Even more starkly, one-third of the patients taking naltrexone achieved remission, compared to 8 percent of those on the placebo. These extraordinary effects suggest that naltrexone can actually disrupt the inflammatory process in the gut.

Although most of the controlled trials in Crohn's disease have so far originated from a single research institution, other gastroenterologists have also reported success in some patients.[487] A case report from the Cleveland Clinic, for example, describes a 14-year-old girl who had suffered from abdominal pain for three years and had intestinal damage consistent with Crohn's disease. After four weeks of LDN treatment, her symptoms were significantly reduced, and by three months an endoscopy showed complete healing of the damaged intestinal lining.[488] A 2018 study found that LDN induced clinical improvement in three-quarters of patients with inflammatory bowel disease and induced remission in one-quarter of patients.[489] Physicians in Australia also reported that LDN was successful in treating five out of 14 Crohn's patients, and four of those patients also showed gut healing on an endoscopy.[490]

It was initially suggested that naltrexone has this powerful anti-inflammatory effect because it boosts natural endorphins and it is these endorphins that regulate the immune system.[491] More recently, another mechanism has come to light, one that is particularly relevant to psoriasis and various forms of inflammatory arthritis.

This newly discovered mechanism is entirely separate from the opioid/endorphin system. It is instead based on the fact that naltrexone can directly interfere with the activation of immune cells by bacterial toxins such as lipopolysaccharide.[492]

Naltrexone does this by binding to and blocking a receptor called TLR4.[493] This receptor is normally how "first-responder" immune cells (such as mast cells) can detect the presence of lipopolysaccharide and other bacterial by-products. When lipopolysaccharide binds to TLR4 on the surface of cells, this triggers the release of inflammatory mediators. In effect, TLR4 receptors are the eyes that allow a variety of different immune cells to see bacterial by-products in the intestines and in the bloodstream. Naltrexone blindfolds these cells and stops them from overreacting to the presence of bacteria.

The TLR4 mechanism suggests that the extraordinary effects seen in Crohn's disease could also apply in several other autoimmune diseases. This is particularly true in those conditions where TLR4 clearly plays a role, including psoriasis, psoriatic arthritis, rheumatoid arthritis, and ankylosing spondylitis. In each of these conditions, mutations in the TLR4 genes are more common than in the rest of the population,[494] and there is a higher than normal level of TLR4 receptors on immune cells.[495] When bacterial by-products bind to TLR4 receptors, this also triggers the production of the precise inflammatory mediators that are the hallmarks of psoriasis and inflammatory arthritis.[496] Naltrexone could disrupt this process and thereby calm the immune system.

Interestingly, in the fibromyalgia clinical study, the patients with the greatest drop in pain on LDN treatment were those who started out with the highest level of inflammation, shown by erythrocyte sedimentation rate (ESR). According to the researchers performing the study, this suggested "that the clinical effect of LDN may be physiologically associated with the reduction of inflammation."[497] The researchers further commented that "the observed relationship between ESR and LDN response raises the intriguing possibility that other chronic conditions characterized by high ESR may also benefit from LDN therapy." Psoriasis and inflammatory arthritis are unquestionably conditions characterized by high ESR levels, and ESR is in fact used by rheumatologists to monitor disease severity. The pain-reducing and anti-inflammatory effects of low-dose naltrexone thus hold great promise for those with these conditions.

In the United States, naltrexone is already approved by the FDA to treat addiction, so physicians are allowed to prescribe it "off-label" for other uses. When used to treat inflammatory diseases, the dose is far lower than that used for addiction (1.5–4.5 mg compared to 50–100 mg). As a result, the prescription must be filled at a specialist compounding pharmacy that can prepare capsules containing low doses. The dose is often titrated, meaning one starts at a dose of 1.5 mg or 2 mg and then increases to 3 mg after several weeks. The dose is only increased further if necessary.

The side effects of LDN reported in the clinical studies so far are headache, difficulty sleeping, and vivid dreams, but it has also been reported that these side effects can be minimized by keeping the dose at or below 3 mg per day.[498] LDN cannot be used in conjunction with opioids, because it causes withdrawal symptoms, but rheumatologists have been prescribing LDN in combination with methotrexate and biologics. At the time of writing, several clinical trials are underway to determine the efficacy of LDN in treating conditions such as rheumatoid and psoriatic arthritis.

LDN is not yet an FDA-approved treatment option for autoimmune disease, but as explained by Stanford researchers, "Our replicated observation that low-dose naltrexone affects levels of pain, together with the low cost and tolerable nature of low-dose naltrexone, makes it a promising target for future investigation."[499]

CHAPTER 10

PUTTING IT ALL TOGETHER

The Basic Plan

If you suffer from any form of autoimmune disease, there is a small set of fundamental dietary changes and supplements that can produce an immense payoff when it comes to calming inflammation. These basic steps are the most critical for shifting the balancing of species in the microbiome, healing the gut barrier, and giving the immune system the healthy fats it needs to return to a normal equilibrium.

Diet

- Start by focusing on what you should be eating more of: **high-fiber and antioxidant-rich vegetables, fish, poultry, lean meat, and olive oil.** These foods should be the foundation of most meals.

- Adopt the **Level 1 low-starch diet** by removing gluten-containing grains, corn, soy, peanuts, quinoa, and potatoes. Limit other starches to two servings per day (preferably rice, legumes, or starchy vegetables).

- Cut back on added sugar.
- Try to space meals four hours apart with no snacking, to allow time for the digestive system to perform its important cleaning cycle.

Supplements

- To help support the levels of other anti-inflammatory resident microbes, suppress harmful bacteria, and heal the gut, start taking a **Level 1 probiotic** with breakfast each day. Look for a product that includes *L. rhamnosus GG* (e.g., Culturelle) or *B. infantis*, *B. breve*, or *B. longum* (e.g., Jarro-dophilus Allergen-Free, Klaire Ther-Biotic Metabolic Formula). Take the probiotic with breakfast each day.
- Consider adding a vitamin D supplement containing at least 2000 IU of vitamin D3 (cholecalciferol) in an oil-based liquid or soft-gel. You may need a short-term treatment with a higher dose, such as 5000 IU per day, if you are deficient.
- On days that you do not eat oily fish such as salmon, sardines, or mackerel, add a fish oil supplement containing at least 2 grams of DHA and EPA.

Beyond the Basics

To go further and address more specific root causes of autoimmunity, it is helpful to tailor the approach to your particular autoimmune condition. To that end, intermediate and advanced diet and supplement plans are provided below for psoriasis, psoriatic arthritis, rheumatoid arthritis, and ankylosing spondylitis.

If budget permits, it may also be useful to pursue laboratory testing to guide the next steps in your personalized program. The most helpful tests are (in order of priority)

- a stool test to detect overgrowth of specific pathogens
- a breath test to detect SIBO
- a blood test for IgE-based food allergy and IgG-based food sensitivity

Depending on where you live, you may be able to order these tests yourself, or you may need the assistance of a functional medicine physician. (See www.keystonebook.com/testing.)

Laboratory testing is not always reliable, however, and it is certainly not required. We can instead look to the factors that are most likely to be at play in a given autoimmune disease to guide our plan of attack. In doing so, we are effectively relying on the body of scientific research to identify the most likely root causes.

Psoriasis and PsA—Intermediate and Advanced Plans

If you have psoriasis or psoriatic arthritis (PsA), the basic plan above will provide the most important groundwork for healing, but there are additional steps you can take that focus on the unique issues and contributing factors that are more likely to play a role in psoriasis than other autoimmune conditions. These potential contributing factors include small intestinal bacterial overgrowth (SIBO), *Candida* yeast, and

Streptococcus bacteria, whether in the gastrointestinal tract or in the form of chronic low-level throat infection.

Note that individuals with psoriatic arthritis that impacts the spine and sacroiliac joints may benefit the most from reducing or eliminating starch, because this form is closely related to ankylosing spondylitis and has a clearer link to the harmful bacteria that thrive on starch.

Psoriasis/PsA Diet—Intermediate

- The foundation of your diet should be high-fiber and antioxidant-rich vegetables, fish, poultry, lean meat, and olive oil.

- To combat SIBO and *Streptococcus* overgrowth, adopt the **level 2 low-starch diet**, which eliminates grains, legumes, and very starchy vegetables. Minimize high-fructose fruits, added sugars, dairy, and very starchy nuts and seeds.

Psoriasis/PsA Diet—Advanced

- Experiment with the **level 3 low-starch diet** for at least three months and then try to gradually return to the intermediate low-starch diet to determine your tolerance for starches. If psoriatic arthritis impacts your spine or sacroiliac joints, you may benefit from keeping starch very low for an even longer period of time.

- For at least one month, eliminate **nightshades, nuts, eggs, dairy**, and any other foods that test positive for an allergy or IgG-based sensitivity. Systematically reintroduce these foods one at a time to find out how they affect you.

- For further troubleshooting, another possible culprit to investigate is fruit. Some individuals may feel better avoiding fruit entirely and following a very low-carbohydrate diet. This diet can be ketogenic but does not need to be if protein intake is increased to meet energy demands.

Psoriasis/PsA Supplements—Intermediate

In addition to the vitamin D and fish oil recommended for the basic level above, consider adding the following supplements:

- A **Level 2 probiotic** such as a high potency *Bifidobacteria* combination containing multiple strains and including *B. bifidum* (e.g., Jarrow Bifidus Balance, GutPro, Renew Life 50 Plus).

- If you are prone to throat infections or tonsillitis, add a probiotic lozenge containing *S. salivarius K12*, such as HyperBiotics ProDental.

- If you suspect SIBO, consider adding further supplements to support the digestion and cleansing cycle. This may include bile and a combination of betaine HCL, pepsin, and pancreatin with larger meals and Iberogast between meals.

Psoriasis/PsA Supplements—Advanced

- To reduce excess *Candida, Streptococcus*, and other harmful bacteria in the small intestine, follow a short-term pathogen-fighting protocol for 30 days. This includes a **Level 3 probiotic** (BioK+, Mutaflor, *S. boulardii*), taken before bed each day, along with **lactoferrin**, **allicin,** and **berberine** half an hour before meals.

- To combat SIBO, consider adding supplements to support the digestion and cleansing cycle. This may include bile and a combination of betaine HCL, pepsin, and pancreatin with larger meals and Iberogast between meals.

- For additional long-term anti-inflammatory maintenance, consider supplementing with **Borage oil** or curcumin in the form of **Meriva**.

Rheumatoid Arthritis—Intermediate and Advanced Plans

If you have rheumatoid arthritis (RA), it is particularly helpful to adopt the core tenets of the Mediterranean diet. Clinical studies show that RA often responds quite well to dietary changes such as increasing the consumption of fish, olive oil, and antioxidant-rich vegetables. From that point you can begin to explore whether your inflammation may be influenced by food allergy, an overgrowth of bacteria such as *Proteus mirabilis,* or a combination of factors.

Rheumatoid Arthritis Diet—Intermediate

- Start by focusing on what you should be eating more of: **high-fiber and antioxidant-rich vegetables, fish, poultry, lean meat, and olive oil**. These foods should be the foundation of most meals.

- Adopt the **level 1 low-starch diet by** removing gluten-containing grains, corn, soy, peanuts, quinoa, and potatoes. Limit other starches to two servings per day (preferably rice, legumes, or starchy vegetables).

- Avoid sugar.

- Try to space meals four hours apart with no snacking, to allow time for the digestive system to perform its important cleaning cycle.

Rheumatoid Arthritis Diet—Advanced

- For at least one month, eliminate **nightshades**, **nuts**, **eggs**, **dairy**, and any other foods that test positive for an allergy or IgG-based sensitivity. Systematically reintroduce these foods one at a time to find out how they affect you.

- Consider experimenting with the **level 2 low-starch diet** for three months, to determine whether you may be sensitive to starch and other carbohydrates.

Rheumatoid Arthritis Supplements—Intermediate

In addition to the vitamin D and fish oil recommended for the basic level above, consider adding the following supplements:

- **Level 2 probiotic** such as a more potent *Bifidobacteria* combination containing multiple strains and including *B. bifidum* (e.g., Jarrow Bifidus Balance, GutPro, Renew Life 50 Plus).

- If you suspect SIBO, further supplements to support the digestion and cleansing cycle may be helpful. This can include bile and a combination

of Betaine HCL, pepsin, and pancreatin with
larger meals and Iberogast between meals.

Rheumatoid Arthritis Supplements—Advanced

- Consider following a short-term pathogen-
  fighting protocol for one month to target pathogens implicated in RA, such as *Proteus mirabilis*.
  This includes a **Level 3 probiotic** (BioK+,
  Mutaflor, *S. boulardii*), taken before bed each
  day, along with **lactoferrin**, **allicin**, and **berberine** half an hour before meals.

- When additional pain relief is needed, consider
  supplementing with turmeric in the form of
  Meriva.

- A **glucosamine** supplement may help prevent
  further cartilage deterioration in the long term.

Ankylosing Spondylitis—
Intermediate and Advanced Plans

If you have ankylosing spondylitis (AS), you have the most
to gain from a stricter approach to starch and sugars. The
low-starch diet has a long history of successfully treating
many patients with AS, and there is substantial evidence that
this condition is driven by the immune response to starch-
loving bacteria, such as *Klebsiella* and adherent-invasive *E.
coli*. Because overgrowths of these bacteria often occur in
the form of SIBO, you may also benefit from strategies that
reduce the overall bacterial population in the small intestine.

AS Diet—Intermediate

- The foundation of your diet should be **high-fiber and antioxidant-rich vegetables, fish, poultry, lean meat, and olive oil.**

- Start with the **level 3 low-starch diet** for several months to find out how starch impacts your symptoms. If you experience a significant reduction in inflammation, at that point you can gradually introduce additional fruits and vegetables from the intermediate level to determine your tolerance.

- If you continue to have active inflammation even on the advanced low-starch diet, it may just be that more time is required to see a benefit. Dr. Ebringer reports that from his three decades of experience treating AS with a low-starch diet, "it normally takes around six to eight months for the diet to show its effects."[500]

AS Diet—Advanced

- Continued inflammation on the advanced low-starch diet may also be due to a food sensitivity. For at least one month, eliminate **nightshades, nuts, eggs,** and **dairy** and then reintroduce each food individually to gauge your reaction.

- For further troubleshooting, another possible culprit to investigate is fruit. Some individuals with AS feel better avoiding fruit entirely and following a very low carbohydrate diet. This diet can be ketogenic but does not need to be if protein intake is increased to meet energy demands.

AS Supplements—Intermediate

- Consider a **Level 2 probiotic** such as a more potent *Bifidobacteria* combination containing multiple strains and including *B. bifidum* (e.g., Jarrow Bifidus Balance, GutPro, Renew Life 50 Plus).

- Given that *Klebsiella* and *E. coli* overgrowths can take the form of SIBO, consider adding further supplements to support the digestion and cleansing cycle. This may include bile and a combination of Betaine HCL, pepsin, and pancreatin with larger meals and Iberogast between meals.

AS Supplements—Advanced

- To combat *E. coli* and *Klebsiella,* follow a short-term pathogen-fighting protocol for one or two months. This consists of a **Level 3 probiotic** (Mutaflor is the preferred option for AS) taken before bed each day, along with **lactoferrin, berberine**, and **allicin** taken half an hour before meals. Mutaflor can also be continued longer term if needed.

- For additional anti-inflammatory maintenance or pain relief, consider supplementing with curcumin in the form of **Meriva**.

Part 4

In the Kitchen

CHAPTER 11

PLANNING AHEAD AND OTHER KITCHEN TIPS

Adapting to a new diet is challenging enough, but if you are also battling joint pain or chronic illness, it is particularly important to minimize the stress and effort involved in preparing healthy meals. The best way to do this is by keeping meals simple, planning ahead, and taking every shortcut available to you. To that end, this provides basic tips to make low-starch, allergen-free food preparation quicker and easier.

General Tips

Keep it simple. Rather than trying to alter recipes for favorite foods by substituting with "safe" ingredients, start with a clean slate and focus on simple meals built around vegetables and protein.

Double recipes. Whenever you cook something that will store well, double or triple the recipe then save a portion for breakfast or lunch the next day and freeze the leftovers. This strategy will dramatically cut down on meal preparation time.

Batch cook. Every two to four weeks, spend a couple of

hours batch cooking foods to have on hand in the freezer. Good freezer staples include chicken soup, stews, and breakfast sausage patties (specific recipes are provided in chapter 12).

Order supplies online. Items such as collagen peptides and good-quality canned salmon are useful to have on hand and are often cheaper if you order online, particularly if you buy in bulk or through programs such as Amazon's Subscribe and Save.

Rely on meals, not snacks. Snacking halts the natural process that sweeps the small intestine clear of food debris and pathogens between meals. Separating meals by four hours is therefore a useful tool to treat and prevent bacterial overgrowth and to allow the digestive system time to enter into cleaning and repair mode. To avoid snacking, it is important to eat meals that are substantial enough to hold you over until the next meal, with a good amount of protein and fiber at each meal. If you do need to snack, the best options are fruit, additive-free deli meat, and raw vegetables with guacamole.

Take shortcuts. If joint pain makes chopping vegetables difficult for you, cook them whole, use a food processor, microwave briefly to soften before cutting, or buy precut vegetables. It is also worth investing in a very sharp knife and vegetable peeler.

Freeze herbs. To save fresh herbs such as basil, parsley, or cilantro, simply blend with olive oil and then pour the mixture into ice cube trays to freeze. When frozen, the herb cubes can be transferred to a zip-top bag until you need them. Fresh ginger also freezes well. If you have excess thyme or rosemary, allow the leaves to dry thoroughly in the sun or a low oven (200°F) then combine with sea salt in a small jar.

Stock your freezer with proteins. Freeze uncooked

hamburger patties, chicken pieces, and fish fillets so you are never caught without an easy dinner option. To thaw, the best method is a warm-water bath. Place the food in a zip-top bag then submerge in a pot or large bowl filled with warm water. (Partially immerse the bag in the water before sealing, to force the air out.) Individual portions will typically take 10 to 30 minutes to thaw. To speed up thawing, replace the water with more warm water after 10 minutes. Larger items such as a whole chicken may take over an hour to thaw, so the container must be refrigerated during thawing.

Rely on add-ons for family members. Instead of cooking entirely different meals for children or other family members who are not following such a restrictive diet, an easier approach is to prepare a protein and one or two vegetables, then round out meals for other family members with an easy-to-prepare carbohydrate such as rice or gluten-free pasta.

Breakfast Strategies

Breakfast is usually the meal that changes the most when people begin an anti-inflammatory elimination diet because typical Western breakfast foods heavily emphasize starch, dairy, and eggs. Yet a protein-rich breakfast without these problematic ingredients does not have to be complicated or time consuming. By stocking your freezer in advance, breakfast can be as simple as heating one or two chicken sausage patties and then adding fresh berries or melon. You can also make a quick roll-up with turkey or ham deli meat, avocado, and lettuce. Another good option is to make a smoothie with frozen berries and hydrolyzed collagen protein powder.

Collagen powder has the added bonus of including the specific amino acids needed to repair skin and joints. The optimal form of collagen for this purpose is marine collagen, but hydrolyzed beef collagen is also a good choice for most people. (The main advantage of marine collagen is that it is much lower in glutamate, which can cause insomnia or mood disturbances in some individuals.) Note that most collagen supplements are a combination of type 1 and type 3 collagen, which provide the amino acids needed to repair collagen throughout the body. Specialized type 2 collagen powders are also available to target cartilage repair, but these are typically taken in small doses as a supplement, rather than a dietary protein source.

Lunch Strategies

Salads are the best default for quick and easy lunches. A good way to streamline weekday lunches is to wash and slice enough salad vegetables for several days then store each prepared vegetable in its own individual container in the fridge. You will then be able to assemble a salad in a few minutes on busy weekday mornings. Vegetables that store well preprepared include sliced radishes, shredded carrots, shredded cabbage, sliced mushrooms, and raw or very lightly steamed broccoli florets, green beans, and snap peas. All of these vegetables will typically stay fresh for at least three days. You can also preroast a large batch of vegetables to add to salads, including carrots, zucchini, Brussels sprouts, and fennel.

For a complete meal, just assemble the salad with a basic dressing, then add a preprepared protein such as good-quality deli meats, canned salmon, or leftover roast or grilled chicken. (The next chapter includes a simple recipe for brining chicken, which allows cooked chicken to freeze well without drying out.)

Another simple strategy for lunches is to make a large batch of chicken soup and freeze individual portions. You can then either microwave the soup at work if you have that option, or heat the soup at home and take it in a thermos container.

Dinner Strategies

There are three basic approaches for preparing quick and easy dinners in the context of the Keystone Diet:

1. **Sheet-pan dinners.** Add a protein with one or two vegetables and roast together on a single sheet pan. The entire meal typically takes 20 to 30 minutes to prepare and is almost entirely hands-off (see specific tips below).

2. **Simply grilled, stir-fried, steamed.** By pan-frying fish, chicken, or steak while steaming or stir-frying a mix of vegetables, you can make a complete meal in 10 minutes.

3. **Pressure-cooker stews.** By investing in an Instant Pot, you can combine inexpensive cuts of meat (such as lean beef stew or bone-in chicken thighs) with herbs and vegetables, then cook for 20 to 40 minutes to make a large batch of fork-tender meat that freezes well.

Tips for Sheet-Pan Dinners

Sheet-pan dinners are a perfect way to make a quick meal with very little cleanup. For best results, use a rimmed metal sheet pans and take care not to overcrowd the sheet. When there is not enough space around chicken and other meats for juices to evaporate, they can steam and become tough. (If needed, use two separate sheet pans.)

There are endless combinations of ingredients to use for sheet-pan dinners, but the process is even simpler if you pair proteins with vegetables that take approximately the same time to cook. Examples include

- Chicken drumsticks with Brussels sprouts and carrots (35 to 40 minutes)
- Chicken breasts with mushrooms and zucchini (20 minutes)
- Salmon with green beans (15 minutes)

You can also use whatever combination you have on hand by adding components to the sheet pan in stages, giving ingredients that require longer cooking times a head start. Before roasting, lightly coat everything with olive oil and add flavorings such as dried herbs. Herbs that work well include thyme, rosemary, sage, and oregano. You can also finish dishes with fresh basil, parsley, cilantro, or chives.

Precise cooking times will depend on sizes, spacing on the sheet pan, and taste preferences, but a rough guide is provided below (for a preheated 400°F oven).

Chicken drumsticks	40 minutes
Bone-in chicken thighs	35 minutes
Boneless chicken thighs	25 minutes
Chicken breasts	20 minutes
Lamb chops	17 minutes
Salmon	15 minutes
Meatballs	15 minutes

Shrimp	8 minutes
Brussels sprouts, halved	35 minutes
Carrots	35 minutes
Fennel	35 minutes
Baby carrots	25 minutes
Cauliflower	25 minutes
Mushrooms, sliced	20 minutes
Zucchini	20 minutes
Broccoli	20 minutes
Summer squash	15 minutes
Green beans	15 minutes

Perfectly Steamed Vegetables

For maximum antioxidants (and flavor), it is important to steam vegetables for only a very short time, until they are just tender but still crisp. The exact time will vary depending on your setup and how much you are cooking at once, but approximate times are given below.

Asparagus	3 to 5 minutes
Broccoli	2 to 3 minutes
Cabbage	2 to 3 minutes
Carrots	5 to 7 minutes
Cauliflower	4 to 5 minutes
Green beans	3 to 5 minutes
Sugar snap peas	2 to 3 minutes
Summer squash	3 to 4 minutes
Zucchini	3 to 4 minutes

Basic Steaming Method

Place a large metal steamer basket (OXO is a good brand) in a pot with 1 inch of boiling water. Vegetables will cook more evenly if the pot is large enough for the metal basket to remain fully open. Chop vegetables into large chunks (1 to 2 inches). Distribute the vegetables evenly in the steamer basket, ideally in a single layer. Cover the pan and set a timer for 2 or 3 minutes. Check whether the vegetables have become slightly tender and continue cooking a few minutes longer if needed. Immediately transfer to a plate to serve. If using a mixture of different vegetables, add longer-cooking vegetables, such as carrots or cauliflower, a couple of minutes before adding quicker-cooking vegetables, such as broccoli and zucchini.

Leftover steamed vegetables can be stored in the refrigerator for several days. They can then be added to salads or used as crudité with guacamole. For these uses, it is particularly important to remove the vegetables from the heat when still slightly crunchy.

Adding flavor

After steaming, you can drizzle the vegetables with olive oil and flavorings. Examples include

- 2 tablespoons olive oil and juice of ½ lemon with ½ teaspoon salt
- 2 tablespoons olive oil and 1 tablespoon rice syrup (works best for carrots)
- 2 tablespoons olive oil and 5 to 10 fresh basil leaves, sliced

CHAPTER 12

THE RECIPES

All the recipes in this section are suitable for the basic, intermediate, and advanced low-starch plans, although minor modifications may be noted for the advanced plan. The recipes are also suitable for those eliminating nightshades, dairy, nuts, and eggs.

To avoid the fructans in garlic and onion, the recipes use garlic-infused oil and the green part of scallions (spring onions) instead of red or white onions. If you do not notice any benefit from limiting fructans, you can modify recipes to simply use crushed garlic and red or white onion if you prefer.

For the recipes that contain mayonnaise, an olive oil– or avocado oil–based mayonnaise is the best choice for those that tolerate egg. If you are eliminating egg, there are egg-free brands available (such as Hellman's vegan), but these should be used sparingly because they typically contain a small amount of corn or potato starch and undesirable oils.

Most recipes include a small amount of added salt, but this can be omitted or reduced if you prefer. There is some evidence that a high-salt diet is inflammatory,[501] but more than 75 percent of the salt Americans consume comes from packaged, processed, and restaurant foods. Once these foods are eliminated, you can add salt to meals and still maintain a relatively low-sodium diet. A very low carbohydrate diet also requires additional sodium to maintain proper electrolyte balance.

BREAKFAST

Green Juice

(serves 1)

> 1 small bunch kale or collard greens (or ½ large bunch)
> 4 celery stalks
> ½ cup cubed honeydew melon
> ½ cucumber, peeled
> ½ cup parsley (optional)
> 5 to 10 mint or basil leaves (optional)
> Juice of ½ lemon

Juice all the ingredients except the lemon in an electric juicer or high-speed blender. Squeeze the lemon juice into a glass then add ice and the green juice. Stir to combine.

Blueberry Smoothie

(serves 1)

> 2 to 3 scoops collagen peptide powder
> ½ cup water
> ½ cup frozen blueberries
> ½ banana (omit for advanced low-starch)
> ½ cup crushed ice
> 1 tablespoon olive or avocado oil

Mix the collagen powder and water in a glass. Add to the blender with the other ingredients and blend until smooth.

Keto Green Smoothie
(serves 1)

> 2 to 3 scoops collagen peptide powder
> ¾ cup water
> 3 to 5 kale leaves or a handful of spinach
> ½ avocado
> ½ cup crushed ice
> Juice of ½ lime
> Handful parsley, basil, mint, or a combination

Mix the collagen powder and water in a glass. Add to the blender with the remaining ingredients and blend until smooth.

Apple and Sage Chicken Sausage
(serves 6)

> 2 pounds ground chicken (preferably made from a mix of skinless thighs and breast)
> 2 peeled apples, finely diced (optional)
> 5 fresh sage leaves, finely chopped, or 1 teaspoon dried sage
> 1 teaspoon sea salt
> 2 tablespoons olive oil
> 1 to 2 teaspoons honey or brown rice syrup (optional)

Preheat the oven to 425°F. In a large bowl, mix together all the ingredients and then shape into patties about 2 inches wide. Bake on a foil-lined baking sheet for 12 to 15 minutes. Alternatively, for additional flavor (but more effort), pan-fry the patties in olive oil.

To freeze, allow the patties to cool then place in small zip-top freezer bags or wrap in plastic wrap and store in freezer-safe containers.

American Breakfast Sausage

(serves 6)

> 2 pounds lean ground beef
> 1 tablespoon olive oil
> 1 scallion/spring onion, green portion, chopped
> 1 teaspoon sea salt
> 1 teaspoon dried sage
> ¼ teaspoon dried marjoram
> 1 tablespoon brown rice syrup (optional)

Preheat the oven to 425°F. In a large bowl, mix together all the ingredients and then shape into patties about 2 inches wide. Bake on a foil-lined baking sheet for 12 to 15 minutes.

To freeze, allow the patties to cool then place in small zip-top freezer bags or wrap in plastic wrap and store in freezer-safe containers.

Chia Protein Pudding

(serves 1)

> 2 scoops collagen peptide powder
> ½ cup water (or any form of milk)
> 2 tablespoons chia seeds
> 1 tablespoon nut butter or sunflower butter (optional)
> Fresh, frozen, or dried berries (optional)
> ½ tablespoon avocado oil (optional)
> 2 tablespoons unsweetened shredded coconut (optional)

Put the collagen peptides in a small bowl or cup then pour the water and stir to combine. Add the chia seeds, stir, then refrigerate overnight. When ready to eat, top with your choice of nut butter or sunflower butter, berries, avocado oil, or dried coconut.

Flax Porridge

(serves 1)

> 2 tablespoons freshly ground flax seeds
> ½ cup boiling water
> 2 tablespoons hemp hearts
> 2 tablespoons unsweetened shredded coconut
> 2 tablespoons collagen peptide powder
> ¼ teaspoon ground cinnamon
> 1 teaspoon brown rice syrup (optional)
> ½ tablespoon avocado oil (optional)
> Fresh, frozen, or dried berries (optional)

Combine the ground flax seeds and boiling water in a bowl. Add the remaining ingredients and stir until well combined. Add additional water or a milk of your choice if needed and any toppings you choose, such as berries or chopped nuts. If you prefer, hemp hearts can also be substituted with chia seeds that have been soaked in water or a milk of your choice.

Chicken and Kale Hash

(serves 1)

> 3 large kale leaves
> 1 leftover cooked chicken breast
> 2 tablespoons avocado oil
> ¼ teaspoon salt
> 1 pinch poultry seasoning
> ¼ cup water
> ¼ cup chopped parsley

Remove the center ribs from the kale and chop the leaves. Slice the chicken into cubes and fry in the avocado oil until lightly browned. Transfer the chicken to a plate. Add the kale to the pan with the salt, poultry seasoning, and water. At this stage you can also add any other leftover cooked vegetables. Cover and cook for 3 minutes. Return the chicken to the pan, along with the parsley, and toss to combine.

SALADS

Perfect Brined Roast Chicken Breasts for Salads

(serves 6)

>   2 tablespoons salt
>   1 tablespoon fresh rosemary
>   1 teaspoon dried thyme
>   ½ cup boiling water
>   2 cups ice water
>   3 large chicken breasts
>   Olive oil

Brining chicken allows it to retain its flavor and moisture when stored in the refrigerator or freezer. To prepare the brine, dissolve the salt, rosemary, and thyme in the boiling water. In a large glass bowl or zip-top bag, mix the salt solution with the ice water. Add the chicken breasts then cover and refrigerate for 2 to 12 hours. (If brining for more than 3 or 4 hours, only use 1½ tablespoons of salt.) When ready to cook the chicken, preheat the oven to 425°F. Rinse then dry the chicken with paper towels. Coat lightly with olive oil and then roast for 17 to 20 minutes until cooked through. (Alternatively, grill or broil until cooked through.)

Store in the refrigerator for 2 to 3 days or in the freezer for 1 month. If freezing, allow to cool completely, wrap individual portions tightly in plastic wrap, then combine portions in a labeled zip-top bag. Thaw briefly in the microwave then add to salads or other dishes.

This approach also works well with a whole chicken. Simply double the brine recipe then roast the chicken at 425°F for 1 hour, 15 minutes or until the juices run clear.

Californian Chicken Salad

(serves 2)

2 to 3 tablespoons mayonnaise

1 tablespoon olive oil

1 tablespoon freshly squeezed lemon juice

2 roast chicken breasts, cubed

½ cup black or red grapes, halved

2 celery stalks, sliced

5 basil leaves, sliced into ribbons

½ avocado, diced (optional)

In a large bowl, combine the mayonnaise, oil, and lemon juice and whisk. Add the chicken, grapes, and celery, and stir to combine. Add the basil and avocado. Stir gently to combine again.

Ranch Chicken Wrap

(serves 2)

> 2 to 3 tablespoons mayonnaise
>
> 1 tablespoon olive oil
>
> 1 tablespoon freshly squeezed lemon juice
>
> 1 tablespoon each chopped fresh dill, parsley, basil, chives (or any combination)
>
> ½ teaspoon onion powder (optional)
>
> ½ teaspoon mustard (optional)
>
> ½ avocado, mashed
>
> 1 scallion/spring onion
>
> 1 celery stalk, finely chopped
>
> 2 roast chicken breasts, cubed
>
> Lettuce, collards, or kale for serving

Whisk together the mayonnaise, oil, lemon juice, herbs, onion powder, and mustard. Add the avocado, chopped scallion, and celery, then stir in the chicken. Serve in lettuce cups or wrap in a collard or kale leaf with the rib removed.

Arugula Chicken Salad

(serves 2)

> Juice of 1 lemon (3 tablespoons)
>
> 1 teaspoon brown rice syrup
>
> 2 tablespoons extra-virgin olive oil
>
> ½ teaspoon salt
>
> 1 package arugula/rocket (or baby kale or spinach)
>
> 1 roast chicken breast, shredded

In a small bowl, whisk together the lemon juice, brown rice syrup, olive oil, and salt. Pour the dressing over the arugula, add the chicken, and toss to combine.

Salmon Salad Wrap

(serves 1)

¼ or ½ avocado, mashed

1 tablespoon mayonnaise

½ scallion/spring onion, white and green parts

Squeeze of lemon juice

1 teaspoon olive oil

1 can salmon, drained

½ celery stalk, chopped

In a small bowl, combine the avocado, mayonnaise, scallion, lemon juice, and olive oil. Lightly mash the salmon and add to the dressing along with the chopped celery. Mix to combine.

Enjoy as is, wrap in a sturdy green leaf (collard, kale, lettuce), or use as a dip for sliced cucumber or celery sticks. To use as a dip, omit the celery from the salmon mixture. If you prepare the salad in advance to take to work, omit the avocado.

Kale Salad

(serves 2 to 4)

> 1 garlic clove, crushed
> 2 tablespoons olive oil
> 1 bunch kale, rinsed
> Juice of 1 lemon
> ½ teaspoon salt

Crush or chop the garlic and add it to the olive oil in a small pan. Heat gently for 5 minutes. Meanwhile, cut each kale leaf lengthwise to remove the tough rib, then stack the leaves and slice into small ribbons. Transfer the kale to a large bowl and add the lemon juice and salt. Scrunch and release handfuls of kale to massage the juice into the leaves to soften them. Drizzle over the olive oil (remove and discard the garlic) and toss to combine. Allow to sit for at least 15 minutes before serving.

MAIN DISHES

FISH

Simple Crispy Salmon
(serves 4)

> 4 fresh salmon fillets (about 6 ounces each)
> 1 tablespoon olive oil
> Salt

For a crispy flesh side: Preheat the oven to 400°F. Set an oven-safe pan over medium-high heat. While the pan heats, thoroughly dry the salmon with paper towels and lightly coat with the olive oil and a sprinkle of salt. Place the salmon in the pan, flesh-side down, and cook for 5 minutes or until it releases easily from the pan. Flip the salmon to skin-side down and immediately transfer the pan to the oven. Bake for 5 to 10 minutes until cooked.

For a crispy skin: Heat a pan over medium-high heat. Dry the salmon with paper towels and coat with the olive oil and a sprinkle of salt. Lower the heat to medium-low. Place the salmon skin-side down in the pan and continuously push down on the fillets with a spatula for several minutes to keep the skin in contact with the pan. (For multiple fillets, push down using a metal pot lid smaller than the skillet.) After the first few minutes, push down occasionally until the skin is browned and crispy, about 6 minutes. Flip the salmon to flesh-side down and cook another 1 to 2 minutes.

Tartare Sauce

2 teaspoons fresh chives
2 teaspoons fresh dill
2 teaspoons fresh parsley
2 scallions/spring onions
1 teaspoon capers
4 tablespoons mayonnaise
¼ teaspoon Dijon mustard
Juice of ½ lemon

Finely chop the herbs, scallions, and capers, then combine with the mayonnaise, mustard, and lemon juice. Allow the flavors to combine before serving, preferably for at least an hour. Store in the refrigerator for up to 2 days.

Cuban Salmon

(serves 4)

 4 salmon fillets
 Zest of 1 lime
 1 teaspoon orange zest
 ¼ cup finely chopped fresh cilantro
 1 tablespoon chopped fresh rosemary
 ¼ cup olive oil
 ½ teaspoon turmeric
 ½ teaspoon salt
 1 teaspoon brown rice syrup (optional)
 Juice of ½ lemon

Remove the skin from the salmon. To prepare the marinade, combine the lime and orange zest, cilantro, rosemary, oil, turmeric, salt, and brown rice syrup. Marinate the salmon for 2 to 6 hours. Remove from the refrigerator 30 minutes before cooking and add the lemon juice. When ready to cook, lightly pat the salmon dry, then grill, broil, or panfry until cooked through.

Parisian Fish

(serves 4)

3 shallots

2 teaspoons capers, drained

3 tablespoons mayonnaise

1 tablespoon Dijon mustard

1 tablespoon olive oil

1 tablespoon freshly squeezed lemon juice

1 teaspoon grated lemon zest

4 fish fillets (any flaky white fish)

Chives or parsley (optional)

Preheat the oven to 425°F. Finely chop the shallots, then combine with the capers, mayonnaise, mustard, olive oil, lemon juice, and zest. Place the fish fillets skin-side down in a shallow baking dish. Spread the sauce over the top of each fillet, then bake for 10 to 15 minutes until the fish flakes easily with a fork. Serve garnished with finely chopped chives or parsley.

Ginger Lime Fish Parcels
(serves 4)

4 fish portions (salmon or any flaky white fish)
1 tablespoon olive oil
Zest and juice of 1 or 2 limes
2-inch piece of fresh ginger, thinly sliced
3 scallions/spring onions, sliced
½ teaspoon salt

Preheat the oven to 400°F. Place each piece of fish on a large square of parchment paper. Brush the fish lightly with the oil, then top with the lime zest, ginger, scallions, and a sprinkle of salt. Bring the edges of the parchment paper together and fold over several times to close into a parcel. Bake for 12 to 16 minutes, depending on the thickness of the fish. When cooked through, remove the fish from the parcel, discard the ginger pieces, and sprinkle with the lime juice.

Peruvian Ceviche
(serves 2 to 4)

1 pound very fresh white fish (such as halibut), skin removed
½ cup freshly squeezed lime juice
2 scallions/spring onions (green part only), finely sliced
1 tablespoon chopped fresh cilantro or parsley
1 teaspoon salt

Using a large, very sharp knife, slice the fish into 1½-inch cubes. Place the cubes in a bowl of chilled water. Drain the fish and combine with the lime juice, scallions, cilantro, and salt. Cover and refrigerate for 30 minutes before serving.

Panfried Fish with Greek Herb Sauce

(serves 2)

> 2 to 4 fillets of any flaky white fish
> 1 garlic clove
> ½ cup olive oil
> ¼ cup fresh oregano, chopped
> ¼ cup fresh parsley, chopped
> 2 to 3 tablespoons freshly squeezed lemon juice
> ½ teaspoon salt

To prevent sticking, rest the fish at room temperature between layers of paper towel for 20 minutes before cooking. To prepare the sauce, slice the garlic and add to the olive oil in a small pan. Heat gently for 5 minutes. Discard the garlic and blend the garlic-infused oil with the oregano, parsley, lemon juice, and salt in a blender or small food processor.

When ready to cook the fish, heat the olive oil in a large pan over medium-high heat. Place the fish in the pan, skin-side down. Cook until the skin is crisp and releases from the pan, 3 to 4 minutes. Flip the fish and finish cooking 1 to 2 minutes longer. Serve with the herb sauce.

Sardine Salad

(serves 1)

 1 can sardines in water, drained
 1 scallion/spring onion, finely chopped
 2 tablespoons chopped fresh parsley and/or chives
 2 tablespoons freshly squeezed lemon juice
 1 tablespoon olive oil
 1 teaspoon capers
 Bib lettuce

Drain and lightly mash the sardines. Combine the sardines with the remaining ingredients and serve in lettuce cups.

CHICKEN

Chicken and Vegetable Soup
(serves 8)

> 3 to 4 pounds bone-in chicken pieces or whole chicken,
>   cut into pieces
> 2 teaspoons salt
> 4 large carrots (omit for advanced low-starch), divided
> 4 celery stalks, divided
> 2 teaspoons dried thyme (or 2 fresh sprigs)
> 1 teaspoon dried sage (or 5 fresh leaves)
> 2 bay leaves
> 2 zucchini (or summer squash)
> ½ cup broccoli florets
> 2 tablespoons chopped fresh parsley
> 2 tablespoons chopped fresh dill

Remove the skin from the chicken pieces. Place the chicken in a large soup pot and cover with water. Add the salt, 2 carrots, 2 celery stalks, thyme, sage, and bay leaves. Simmer for approximately 1½ hours, occasionally skimming the foam that appears on the surface. Use tongs to transfer the chicken pieces to a plate to cool. Strain the broth into another pot, discarding the solids. Dice the remaining carrots and celery, zucchini, and broccoli then add to the broth and simmer for 5 minutes. Meanwhile, pull the chicken meat from the bones and chop into small pieces. Return the chicken to the pot, along with the parsley and dill.

(Alternatively, if you prefer chicken breast, you can add two skinless chicken breasts after the first hour of simmering the broth, then discard the dark-meat chicken on the bones.)

Lemon-Herb Roast Chicken

(serves 4)

> 1 lemon, zested and then quartered
> 1 to 2 tablespoons fresh thyme (or 2 teaspoons dried)
> 1 teaspoon dried sage or dried mixed herbs
> 2 tablespoons olive oil
> 1 teaspoon sea salt
> 1 whole (4- to 5-pound) chicken
> 6 garlic cloves

Preheat the oven to 425°F. To prepare the herb rub, combine the lemon zest in a small bowl with the thyme, sage, olive oil (substitute garlic-infused oil for additional flavor), and salt. Remove any giblets from the chicken cavity and dry the outside with paper towels. Gently separate the skin from the chicken breasts and add spoonfuls of the herb rub to the space underneath the skin. Cover with the skin again and rub the outside to evenly distribute the herb mixture. Rub any leftover mixture (or a drizzle of olive oil and salt) over the outside of the bird.

Stuff the chicken cavity with the lemon quarters and whole garlic cloves. Roast for 1 hour, 15 minutes until juices run clear when a knife is inserted near the thigh.

(To serve with roasted vegetables, add carrots and Brussels sprouts on a rimmed baking sheet after the first 45 minutes of cooking time.)

Chicken Souvlaki

(serves 4)

> 2 garlic cloves, sliced
> ¼ cup chopped fresh oregano (or 2 tablespoons dried)
> 1 teaspoon dried marjoram, rosemary, or mixed herbs
> ¼ cup olive oil
> Zest and juice of ½ lemon (2 to 3 tablespoons)
> 1 teaspoon sea salt
> 3 large chicken breasts, cut into quarters

Warm the garlic, oregano, and marjoram in the olive oil over low to medium heat for 5 minutes. Allow the oil to cool then discard the garlic. Pour the infused oil into a bowl or zip-top bag, reserving 1 tablespoon for the sauce. Add the lemon zest, lemon juice, salt, and chicken breasts. Marinate the chicken for 30 minutes at room temperature. Place the chicken on a rimmed baking sheet lined with foil and broil under high heat until cooked through, 5 to 10 minutes (or grill).

To serve with a Greek tzatziki-style sauce, combine 1 avocado, 1 grated cucumber, 1 tablespoon garlic-infused oil, the juice of ½ lemon, ½ teaspoon salt, and 1 tablespoon chopped fresh dill.

Grilled Italian Lemon Chicken

(serves 2)

- 2 chicken breasts
- 3 tablespoons olive oil
- 2 tablespoons freshly squeezed lemon juice
- 1 tablespoon finely chopped fresh rosemary
- 2 garlic cloves, sliced
- 1 teaspoon grated lemon zest

Place the chicken breasts in a plastic bag and pound to an even thickness. Transfer the chicken to a glass bowl or baking dish, add the remaining ingredients, and marinate for 30 minutes at room temperature or several hours refrigerated. Remove the garlic slices. Grill or panfry the chicken until cooked through, 3 to 5 minutes on each side.

Chicken Florentine

(serves 2)

> 1 (8-ounce) package mushrooms, such as chanterelle, crimini, or button
> 1 shallot
> 2 garlic cloves
> 2 boneless skinless chicken breasts
> 1 teaspoon dried thyme (or Italian seasoning)
> ½ teaspoon salt, plus more to taste
> 4 tablespoons olive oil, divided
> 1 (6- to 8-ounce) package baby spinach

Quarter the mushrooms and finely slice the shallot and garlic. Place each chicken breast between two layers of plastic wrap and pound lightly to flatten to an even thickness. Sprinkle the chicken with the thyme and salt. Set a cast-iron skillet over medium heat and add the olive oil. Add the chicken and cook until lightly brown, about 5 minutes on each side. Meanwhile, in a separate pan, heat the remaining 2 tablespoons of olive oil over medium heat. Add the mushrooms, garlic, and shallot and sauté 5 minutes. Remove the garlic and add the spinach. Cover the pan and cook until the spinach wilts. Stir well and add salt to taste. To serve, top each chicken breast with the spinach and mushroom mixture.

Chicken Stir-Fry with Ginger and Garlic

(serves 4)

8 boneless chicken thighs

3 tablespoons olive oil, divided

3 garlic cloves

1 to 2 cups sliced red cabbage

1 zucchini, sliced

1 cup mushrooms

2 tablespoons grated ginger

2 scallions/spring onions (green parts), sliced

1 teaspoon salt

½ teaspoon white pepper

¼ cup water

Panfry the chicken thighs in 1½ tablespoons of olive oil over high heat, 3 to 5 minutes per side. Meanwhile, in a separate large pan, heat the remaining 1½ tablespoons of olive oil over medium heat. Add the garlic and cook for 2 minutes then remove and discard the garlic. Add the cabbage, zucchini, mushrooms, grated ginger, scallions, salt, and pepper. Add the water. Cover the pan and steam the vegetables for 2 minutes. Slice the chicken thighs then add to the pan with the vegetables. Toss to combine.

Chicken with Mushrooms and Sage (Instant Pot)

(serves 4)

- 2 tablespoons olive oil
- 4 garlic cloves, sliced
- 8 boneless chicken thighs, skin removed
- 2 cups mushrooms, halved
- 8 fresh sage leaves, chopped
- ½ cup water
- ½ teaspoon dried thyme
- ½ teaspoon sea salt
- 2 tablespoons chopped fresh basil

Set the Instant Pot to sauté. Combine the olive oil and garlic in the pot and lightly brown the chicken thighs. Remove and discard the garlic. Add the mushrooms, sage, water, thyme, and salt. Close the lid and cook at high pressure for 15 minutes (or 25 minutes if the chicken is frozen). Quick release the pressure. Serve topped with the fresh basil.

Alternate cooking method: Brown the chicken in an oven-safe cast-iron pan. Add the remaining ingredients and braise in a 325°F oven for 30 to 40 minutes.

BEEF

Steak with Argentinian Chimichurri
(serves 2)

    2 steaks
    ½ teaspoon salt
    ¾ cup extra-virgin olive oil, plus 1 tablespoon
    2 garlic cloves, sliced
    1 bunch flat-leaf parsley
    Zest and juice of 1 lemon
    1 tablespoon diced onion

Take the steaks out of the refrigerator 30 minutes before cooking and sprinkle lightly with the salt. Warm ¾ cup of olive oil with the garlic for 5 minutes. Allow the oil to cool then discard the garlic. To prepare the chimichurri sauce, process the garlic-infused oil with the parsley, lemon zest and juice, and onion in a blender or food processor.

To prepare the steaks, preheat the oven to 325°F. Dry the steaks thoroughly with a paper towel then coat with the remaining tablespoon of olive oil. Heat an ovenproof cast-iron pan over medium-high heat. Briefly sear the steaks on one side (2 to 3 minutes). Flip the steaks and transfer the pan to the oven to finish cooking, about 5 minutes for rare, 10 minutes for well done. (Use caution removing the pan from the oven, as the handle will be hot.) Allow to rest for 5 minutes before serving with the chimichurri.

Burger Salad

(serves 4)

>   2 pounds lean ground beef
>   Salt
>   1 tablespoon olive oil
>   1 cup mushrooms
>   2 radishes
>   2 small cucumbers
>   1 scallion (green parts)
>   1 head lettuce
>   1 avocado, pitted and sliced

Dressing

>   ¼ cup olive oil
>   2 tablespoons Dijon mustard
>   ½ teaspoon brown rice syrup (optional)
>   Juice of ½ lemon

Shape the ground beef into four large patties. Heat a grill pan over medium-high heat. Lightly coat the burger patties with salt and olive oil. Grill for 3 to 5 minutes on each side until cooked through. In a small bowl, whisk together the dressing ingredients. Slice the mushrooms, radishes, cucumber, and scallion, then combine with the lettuce in a large bowl. Dress the salad and toss to combine. Serve to individual plates, then top with the burger patties and sliced avocado.

Beef and Cabbage Stir-Fry

(serves 4)

 2 pounds ground beef
 2 tablespoons olive oil
 ½ red cabbage, shredded
 2 garlic cloves, sliced
 ½ teaspoon powdered ginger or 1 teaspoon fresh ginger
 1 teaspoon salt
 2 scallions/spring onions (green parts), chopped
 3 small bunches baby bok choy
 1 tablespoon freshly squeezed lemon or lime juice

Sauté the beef in the olive oil until cooked through. Transfer the beef to a bowl, then in the same pan sauté the cabbage with the garlic, ginger, and salt until the cabbage is tender, approximately 5 minutes. Remove and discard the garlic. Add the scallions, bok choy, cooked beef, and lemon juice. Cook for 1 to 2 minutes more, then serve.

Turkish Beef Kebabs

(serves 4)

- ¼ cup minced fresh parsley
- 2 teaspoons finely chopped fresh rosemary
- 1 teaspoon dried oregano
- 1 scallion/spring onion (green part), finely chopped
- 1 teaspoon salt
- 1 pinch saffron (optional)
- 2 pounds lean ground beef

In a large mixing bowl, combine the parsley, rosemary, oregano, scallion, salt, saffron, and ground beef. Shape into sausages and place on skewers to grill (3 to 5 minutes on each side) or on a foil-lined rimmed baking sheet to bake or broil. (Bake at 425°F for 10 to 15 minutes.)

PORK

Pork tenderloin
(Serves 2 to 4)

- 1 garlic clove, sliced
- 1 tablespoon chopped fresh rosemary
- 1 tablespoon chopped fresh thyme
- 2 tablespoons olive oil
- 1 pork tenderloin
- 1 teaspoon salt

Warm the garlic, rosemary, and thyme in the olive oil over low to medium heat for 5 minutes. Allow to cool then remove and discard the garlic solids. Rub the garlic-infused oil over the pork tenderloin, sprinkle with the salt, then refrigerate for at least 2 hours or overnight. Take out of the refrigerator 30 minutes before cooking. Preheat the oven to 425°F degrees. Roast for 18 to 20 minutes or until a thermometer shows an internal temperature of 145°F. (Additional time may be needed if the tenderloin is larger than 1 pound.) This recipe can also be made with boneless pork loin by doubling the amount of herbs, garlic, and oil, and roasting at 350°F for 1 to 1½ hours.

TURKEY

Turkey Burgers
(serves 2 to 4)

> 1 medium zucchini
> 1 carrot (omit for advanced low-starch)
> 1 pound lean ground turkey
> 3 scallions/spring onions (green parts), finely chopped
> 1 teaspoon salt
> 2 tablespoons olive oil or avocado oil

Grate the zucchini then wrap in a clean kitchen towel and squeeze out as much moisture as possible. Grate the carrot and combine with the zucchini and remaining ingredients. Form into patties and refrigerate for at least 2 hours or overnight. Separate the patties with plastic wrap or parchment paper if needed to stop them sticking together. Grill or panfry over medium-high heat for about 4 minutes each side until cooked through.

Turkey Meatball Soup

3 carrots (omit for advanced low-starch)

3 celery stalks

3 cups low-sodium chicken broth

1 pound lean ground turkey

1 tablespoon olive or avocado oil

1 teaspoon salt

1 to 2 cups chopped kale or spinach

Place the carrots, celery, and broth in a pot over medium-high heat. Bring to a boil then reduce the heat to low and simmer for 5 minutes. While the vegetables are cooking, prepare the meatballs. Combine the turkey, oil, and salt in a bowl and form into one-inch meatballs. Add the meatballs to the broth and simmer over low heat for 10 to 15 minutes or until cooked through. In the last 5 minutes of cooking, add the kale, spinach, or any other leafy greens.

LAMB

Roast Leg of Lamb
(serves 8 to 10)

> 10 garlic cloves, halved or quartered into long slivers
> ¼ cup olive oil
> ½ cup fresh rosemary leaves
> ½ tablespoon salt
> 1 (5 pound) boneless leg of lamb, tied with netting

Preheat the oven to 425°F. Prepare the garlic-infused oil by warming the sliced garlic in the olive oil. Allow to cool, then remove and discard the garlic. Combine the garlic-infused oil, rosemary, and salt then rub over the lamb to coat. (If it is tied with stretchy netting, remove the netting, unroll the lamb and coat the inner surface with the flavored oil before rolling back up and re-covering with the netting.)

Place the lamb in a roasting pan and transfer to the oven. After 15 minutes, turn the oven down to 325°F and continue roasting for another 1½ to 2 hours (add or subtract 20 minutes per pound for larger or smaller roasts) until a meat thermometer reads 120°F for rare, 130°F for medium-rare, or 140°F for well done. Cover tightly with foil and let rest for 20 minutes before carving.

Cut leftovers into thick steaks, wrap tightly with plastic wrap, and place slices together in a labeled zip-top bag. Freeze. When ready to use, thaw slightly in the microwave then slice thinly and fry in olive oil.

Lamb Shawarma Salad

(serves 2)

12 ounces leftover roast lamb

2 tablespoons olive oil

2 teaspoons chopped fresh rosemary (or ½ teaspoon dried)

1 teaspoon dried oregano

½ teaspoon salt

½ head lettuce

Tzatziki dressing

1 cucumber, grated

1 avocado, mashed

1 tablespoon olive oil

2 tablespoons freshly squeezed lemon juice

2 teaspoons chopped fresh dill

1 to 2 tablespoons water (if needed)

Combine the ingredients for the tzatziki dressing and set aside. Thinly slice the leftover roast lamb (this is even easier if the lamb is still slightly frozen). Fry the lamb in the olive oil with the rosemary, oregano, and salt, until warmed through and slightly browned. Serve over lettuce, topped with the tzatziki dressing.

Moroccan Lamb Stew (Instant Pot)

(serves 4)

- 2 pounds lamb stew meat
- 1 tablespoon olive oil
- 3 carrots, chopped
- 2-inch piece fresh ginger
- 1 teaspoon dried rosemary
- Zest and juice of 1 orange
- 1 tablespoon brown rice syrup
- 1 teaspoon salt
- 1 cup water
- 2 zucchini, chopped
- 2 tablespoons chopped fresh parsley or cilantro

With the Instant Pot set to sauté, lightly brown the lamb in the olive oil. Add the carrots, ginger, rosemary, orange zest and juce, brown rice syrup, salt, and water. Close the lid and cook at high pressure for 35 minutes. Manually release the pressure, then add the zucchini and cilantro and set to sauté for 5 minutes until the zucchini softens and the sauce reduces.

(Alternatively, lightly brown the lamb in a large Dutch oven. Add the remaining ingredients then simmer over low heat for 1½ hours, adding the zucchini in the last 5 minutes.)

SIDE DISHES

Kale Slaw

(serves 4)

> ½ head red cabbage
>
> 4 large kale leaves
>
> 3 carrots (omit for advanced low-starch)

Dressing

> ¼ cup olive oil
>
> ¼ cup freshly squeezed lemon juice
>
> 2 tablespoons finely chopped fresh parsley
>
> 1 tablespoon chopped fresh basil
>
> 1 scallion/spring onion, finely chopped
>
> 1 teaspoon brown rice syrup
>
> ½ teaspoon salt

Shred the cabbage in a food processor or finely slice. Remove the ribs from the kale and finely chop the leaves. Grate the carrots. Combine the remaining ingredients to make the dressing and pour over the vegetables, tossing to coat.

Fennel Slaw

(serves 4)

1 fennel bulb

½ head cabbage, shredded

2 scallions/spring onions, finely chopped

Dressing

2 tablespoons egg-free mayonnaise

1 tablespoon olive oil

Juice of ½ lemon

1 teaspoon honey

1 teaspoon sea salt

1 tablespoon chopped fresh parsley

2 tablespoons roughly chopped fennel fronds

Quarter the fennel bulb, remove the core, and then slice thinly. Reserve some of the fennel fronds for the dressing. Combine the sliced fennel with the shredded cabbage and scallions. Combine the dressing ingredients in a small bowl and whisk. Pour the dressing over the vegetables and toss to coat.

Garden Salad with Citrus Dressing
(serves 2 to 4)

1 yellow squash
½ head lettuce
2 cups baby spinach or other salad greens
3 radishes
½ cup white mushrooms

Dressing
2 tablespoons orange juice
2 teaspoons freshly squeezed lime juice
2 teaspoons freshly squeezed lemon juice
6 tablespoons olive oil
½ teaspoon salt

Slice the squash into thin ribbons with a vegetable peeler. Chop the remaining vegetables. In a small bowl, whisk together the dressing ingredients. Pour the dressing over the salad and toss to combine.

Kale Chips

(serves 2 to 4)

> 1 bunch kale
> 1 tablespoon olive oil
> ½ teaspoon sea salt

Preheat the oven to 275°F. Wash the kale and dry thoroughly using paper towels (or wash well in advance and allow to dry). Remove the center ribs and tear or cut the kale leaves into large pieces. Pile the leaves on a large baking tray and lightly coat with the olive oil and salt. Mix with your hands then spread the kale out evenly across the tray. If the leaves are overlapping, it may be necessary to split into two batches or use two trays. Bake until crisp, about 20 minutes.

Celery Fennel Salad

(serves 4)

> 1 large fennel bulb
> 4 celery stalks
> 3 tablespoons olive oil
> 2 tablespoons freshly squeezed lemon juice
> ¼ teaspoon salt
> ¼ cup fresh basil leaves

Remove the stems and core from the fennel bulb. Slice the fennel as thinly as possible (or use a mandolin). Cut the celery diagonally into thin slices. Combine the fennel and celery with the olive oil, lemon juice, and salt and toss to coat. Stack the basil leaves on top of each other then roll up and slice into thin ribbons. Sprinkle the basil over the salad and serve immediately.

Sautéed Kale
(serves 2 to 4)

    1 bunch kale
    2 garlic cloves, sliced
    2 tablespoons olive oil
    ¼ cup water
    ½ teaspoon sea salt
    Juice of ½ lemon

Rinse the kale leaves then remove the ribs and chop the leaves into large pieces. In a deep pan, cook the garlic in the olive oil over medium heat for 2 to 5 minutes. Remove and discard the garlic then add the kale, water, and salt. Cover the pan for 3 minutes. Uncover and continue cooking for another few minutes. Squeeze the lemon juice over the kale and serve.

Marinated Mushrooms
(serves 4)

    1 pound small mushrooms
    2 tablespoons freshly squeezed lemon juice
    ½ teaspoon salt
    ½ teaspoon dried thyme
    ¼ cup chopped fresh parsley

Bring a pot of water to the boil. Remove the stems from the mushrooms and add the caps to the pot. After 5 minutes, drain the mushrooms and transfer to a bowl with the lemon juice, salt, thyme, and parsley. Allow to marinate overnight. Serve at room temperature.

Fried Cabbage with Ham
(serves 4)

>   3 slices ham (or lean Canadian bacon)
>   3 tablespoons olive oil
>   1 head cabbage, chopped
>   ½ teaspoon salt
>   ¼ cup water

Dice the ham and fry in the olive oil until lightly browned.
Add the cabbage, salt, and water. Cover the pan and cook
over medium heat for 3 to 5 minutes. Remove the lid and
continue cooking until the cabbage is tender.

DESSERTS

Blueberry Mint Jelly
(serves 4)

>   2 tablespoons gelatin
>   ½ cup pomegranate juice
>   1 cup frozen blueberries
>   1 cup boiling water
>   6 mint leaves, roughly chopped

Combine the gelatin and pomegranate juice. Microwave the
blueberries for 1 to 2 minutes until they release some juices.
Pour the boiling water over the gelatin and stir well until dissolved. Mix in the blueberries and mint. Pour into a muffin
tray or a large baking dish and refrigerate until set.

Berry Compote

(serves 2 to 4)

1 ripe pear, grated or finely chopped
½ teaspoon vanilla extract
1 cup frozen blueberries, divided
1 cup frozen blackberries, divided
1 tablespoon freshly squeezed lemon juice

Place the pear, vanilla, half the blueberries, and half the blackberries in a microwave-safe bowl. Microwave for 5 minutes. Stir in the remaining berries and lemon juice and microwave for an additional minute. The compote will thicken slightly as it cools. For an even thicker consistency, add 1 tablespoon of gelatin mixed with ¼ cup of water to the berries before microwaving.

Pomegranate Jelly

(serves 8)

2 tablespoons gelatin
1½ cups pomegranate juice, divided
1 cup boiling water

Bloom the gelatin in ½ cup of pomegranate juice. Add the boiling water and stir to combine. When the gelatin is fully dissolved, stir in the remaining 1 cup of pomegranate juice. Pour into a rectangular baking dish, silicon molds, or a muffin tray. Refrigerate until set (1 to 2 hours).

Melon Mint Salad

(serves 2 to 4)

- 1 to 2 tablespoons freshly squeezed lime juice
- 1 tablespoon olive oil
- 2 cups cubed honeydew melon
- 2 tablespoons chopped fresh mint
- 1 teaspoon grated lime zest

Pour the lime juice and olive oil over the melon, add the mint and lime zest, then toss to combine.

AUTHOR'S NOTE

There is something uniquely unsettling about having a chronic health condition in which the body essentially turns upon itself. Many of us are told that autoimmune disease will be a permanent fixture in our lives and that medication to suppress the immune system is the only answer. This perspective is not only disheartening, it is also just plain wrong.

The latest science shows that we are not helpless. There is so much we can do to address the underlying causes of autoimmunity. It may take a great deal of effort and persistence, but we can work to reset our microbiome, heal our gut, and recalibrate our immune system. By doing so we can directly tackle the autoimmune process, rather than merely subduing the symptoms.

Until the medical establishment catches up with this new paradigm, it is up to all of us to learn as much as possible and make the best use we can of the latest research. When we use this research to guide our everyday choices, the cumulative effect can be extraordinarily powerful.

THE KEYSTONE DIET
AT A GLANCE

General Principles:

- Support your microbiome and antioxidant defenses by eating more high-fiber and brightly colored fruit and vegetables.

- Eat more fish, especially salmon, sardines, and Atlantic mackerel.

- Consider supplementing with 2–4 grams of fish oil per day.

- Use olive oil and avocado oil as the primary added fats.

- Choose leaner proteins such as chicken, fish, and lean pork.

- Trim visible fats from meat before cooking.

Level 1: Basic low-starch plan

- Eliminate gluten-containing grains.

- Avoid gut-damaging grains and legumes (soy, corn, potato, peanut).
- Limit other starchy foods to two servings per day, preferably in the form of starchy root vegetables such as parsnip or sweet potato.
- Cut back on sugar.

Level 2: Intermediate low-starch plan

- Eliminate grains, legumes, and very starchy vegetables.
- Minimize added sugars.
- Limit fruit to two or three small servings per day.
- Avoid dairy, other than homemade yogurt if tolerated.
- Avoid the highest-starch nuts and seeds, such as cashews.

Level 3: Advanced low-starch plan

In addition to the steps listed above for level 2:

- Choose vegetables with the lowest starch content.
- Limit fruit to one or two small servings per day.
- Use only the lowest-starch nuts and seeds, such as flax and macadamias.
- Try to avoid maltodextrin and other starchy fillers in supplements.
- Increase fat and protein to compensate for the reduction in carbohydrates. If you emphasize fat this will become a ketogenic diet. Some

people may feel better long term by emphasizing protein instead in order to prevent hormonal disturbances.

- You may need to increase salt to prevent the electrolyte imbalances that can result from a very low carbohydrate diet.

Troubleshooting and Customizing the Keystone Diet

Consider eliminating the following for at least 30 days to determine if you have a sensitivity:

- Common allergens: nuts, eggs, dairy, soy, corn, shellfish
- Nightshades: tomatoes, potatoes, peppers, chili spices, eggplant

If you have symptoms of food chemical intolerance and react to a wide range of foods that are high in histamines or salicylates, you may be able to reduce this sensitivity by addressing SIBO and pathogen overgrowth. Other alternative strategies include testing for thyroid and adrenal hormones and adding a high-dose vitamin C supplement to reduce histamine levels.

REFERENCES

Scientific publications are available from the
National Institutes of Health database at www.
ncbi.nlm.nih.gov/pubmed

Chapter 1. Understanding the Root Causes of Autoimmunity

1   Cypers, H., Varkas, G., Beeckman, S., Debusschere, K., Vogl, T., Roth, J.,...& De Vos, M. (2015). Elevated calprotectin levels reveal bowel inflammation in spondyloarthritis. Annals of the rheumatic diseases, Dec. 23 2015;
Stebbings, S., Jenks, K., Treharne, G. J., García, J. A., Schultz, M., Highton, J., & Dudley-Brown, S. (2011). Validation of the Dudley Inflammatory Bowel Symptom Questionnaire for the assessment of bowel symptoms in axial SpA: prevalence of clinically relevant bowel symptoms and association with disease activity. Rheumatology, ker359;
Stoll, M. L., Punaro, M., & Patel, A. S. (2011). Fecal calprotectin in children with the enthesitis-related arthritis subtype of juvenile idiopathic arthritis. The Journal of rheumatology, 38(10), 2274-2275;
Bjarnason, I., Helgason, K. O., Geirsson, Á. J., Sigthorsson, G., Reynisdottir, I., Gudbjartsson, D.,...& Thjodleifsson, B. (2003). Subclinical intestinal inflammation and sacroiliac changes in relatives of patients with ankylosing spondylitis. Gastroenterology, 125(6), 1598-1605.
Klingberg, E., Strid, H., Ståhl, A., Deminger, A., Carlsten, H., Öhman, L., & Forsblad-d'Elia, H. (2017). A longitudinal study of fecal calprotectin and the development of inflammatory bowel disease in ankylosing spondylitis. Arthritis research & therapy, 19(1), 21.
Tayel, M., Megid, M. A., Nouh, H. H., & Rofaeil, B. (2014). AB0340 Fecal Calprotectin in Rheumatoid Disease, and Its Relation to Disease State. Annals of the Rheumatic Diseases, 73(Suppl 2), 917-917.

2   Van Praet, L., Van den Bosch, F. E., Jacques, P., Carron, P., Jans, L., Colman, R.,...& Cuvelier, C. (2013). Microscopic gut inflammation in axial spondyloarthritis: a multiparametric predictive model. Annals of the rheumatic diseases, 72(3), 414-417.
Van Praet, L., Jans, L., Carron, P., Jacques, P., Glorieus, E., Colman, R.,...& Van den Bosch, F. (2014). Degree of bone marrow oedema in sacroiliac joints of patients with axial spondyloarthritis is linked to gut inflammation and male sex: results from the GIANT cohort. Annals of the rheumatic diseases, 73(6), 1186-1189.
Duran, A., Kobak, S., Sen, N., Aktakka, S., Atabay, T., & Orman, M. (2016). Fecal calprotectin is associated with disease activity in pa-

tients with ankylosing spondylitis. Bosnian Journal of Basic Medical Sciences, 16(1), 71.

Tayel, M., Megid, M. A., Nouh, H. H., & Rofaeil, B. (2014). AB0340 Fecal Calprotectin in Rheumatoid Disease, and Its Relation to Disease State. Annals of the Rheumatic Diseases, 73(Suppl 2), 917-917.

Stebbings, S., Jenks, K., Treharne, G. J., García, J. A., Schultz, M., Highton, J., & Dudley-Brown, S. (2011). Validation of the Dudley Inflammatory Bowel Symptom Questionnaire for the assessment of bowel symptoms in axial SpA: prevalence of clinically relevant bowel symptoms and association with disease activity. Rheumatology, ker359;

3   Viladomiu, M., Kivolowitz, C., Abdulhamid, A., Dogan, B., Victorio, D., Castellanos, J. G., ... & Chai, C. (2017). IgA-coated E. coli enriched in Crohn's disease spondyloarthritis promote TH17-dependent inflammation. Science Translational Medicine, 9(376), eaaf9655; Eppinga, H., Weiland, C. J. S., Thio, H. B., van der Woude, C. J., Nijsten, T. E., Peppelenbosch, M. P., & Konstantinov, S. R. (2016). Similar depletion of protective Faecalibacterium prausnitzii in psoriasis and inflammatory bowel disease, but not in Hidradenitis suppurativa. Journal of Crohn's and Colitis, 10(9), 1067-1075; Scher, J. U., Sczesnak, A., Longman, R. S., Segata, N., Ubeda, C., Bielski, C., ... Littman, D. R. (2013). Expansion of intestinal Prevotella copri correlates with enhanced susceptibility to arthritis. eLife, 2, e01202.

Maeda, Y., Kurakawa, T., Umemoto, E., Motooka, D., Ito, Y., Gotoh, K., ... & Sakaguchi, N. (2016). Dysbiosis contributes to arthritis development via activation of autoreactive T cells in the intestine. Arthritis & Rheumatology, 68(11), 2646-2661.

Chen, J., Wright, K., Davis, J. M., Jeraldo, P., Marietta, E. V., Murray, J., ... & Taneja, V. (2016). An expansion of rare lineage intestinal microbes characterizes rheumatoid arthritis. Genome medicine, 8(1), 43.

Scher, J. U., Ubeda, C., Artacho, A., Attur, M., Isaac, S., Reddy, S. M., ... & Manasson, J. (2015). Decreased bacterial diversity characterizes the altered gut microbiota in patients with psoriatic arthritis, resembling dysbiosis in inflammatory bowel disease. Arthritis & rheumatology, 67(1), 128-139.

4   Mathew, J. L., Singh, S., & Sankar, J. (2015). Is antibiotic exposure associated with newly diagnosed juvenile idiopathic arthritis?. Indian pediatrics, 52(10), 883-888.

5   Kohn, D (2015, January 12). Joint Pain, from the Gut. *The Atlantic*

6   Ghouri, Y. A., Richards, D. M., Rahimi, E. F., Krill, J. T., Jelinek, K. A., & DuPont, A. W. (2014). Systematic review of randomized controlled trials of probiotics, prebiotics, and synbiotics in inflammatory bowel disease. Clinical and experimental gastroenterology, 7, 473.

7   Skoldstam, L., Hagfors, L., & Johansson, G. (2003). An experimental

study of a Mediterranean diet intervention for patients with rheumatoid arthritis. Annals of the Rheumatic Diseases, 62(3), 208–214; Abendroth, A., Michalsen, A., Luedtke, R., Rueffer, A., Musial, F., Dobos, G. J., & Langhorst, J. (2010). Changes of intestinal microflora in patients with rheumatoid arthritis during fasting or a Mediterranean diet. Forschende Komplementärmedizin/Research in Complementary Medicine, 17(6), 307-313;

McKellar, G., Morrison, E., McEntegart, A., Hampson, R., Tierney, A., Mackle, G., ... & Capell, H. A. (2007). A pilot study of a Mediterranean-type diet intervention in female patients with rheumatoid arthritis living in areas of social deprivation in Glasgow. Annals of the rheumatic diseases, 66(9), 1239-1243.

Preedy, V. R., & Watson, R. R. (Eds.). (2014). The Mediterranean Diet: An Evidence-Based Approach. Academic press.

Barrea, L., Balato, N., Di Somma, C., Macchia, P. E., Napolitano, M., Savanelli, M. C., ... & Savastano, S. (2015). Nutrition and psoriasis: is there any association between the severity of the disease and adherence to the Mediterranean diet?. Journal of translational medicine, 13(1), 18.

Di Giuseppe, D., Crippa, A., Orsini, N., & Wolk, A. (2014). Fish consumption and risk of rheumatoid arthritis: a dose-response meta-analysis. Arthritis research & therapy, 16(5), 1.

8   Dumas, J. A., Bunn, J. Y., Nickerson, J., Crain, K. I., Ebenstein, D. B., Tarleton, E. K., ... & Kien, C. L. (2016). Dietary saturated fat and monounsaturated fat have reversible effects on brain function and the secretion of pro-inflammatory cytokines in young women. Metabolism, 65(10), 1582-1588.

Kien, C. L., Bunn, J. Y., Fukagawa, N. K., Anathy, V., Matthews, D. E., Crain, K. I., ... & Poynter, M. E. (2015). Lipidomic evidence that lowering the typical dietary palmitate to oleate ratio in humans decreases the leukocyte production of proinflammatory cytokines and muscle expression of redox-sensitive genes. The Journal of nutritional biochemistry, 26(12), 1599-1606.

9   Rocha, D. M., Caldas, A. P., Oliveira, L. L., Bressan, J., & Hermsdorff, H. H. (2016). Saturated fatty acids trigger TLR4-mediated inflammatory response. Atherosclerosis, 244, 211-215.

Reynolds, C. M., McGillicuddy, F. C., Harford, K. A., Finucane, O. M., Mills, K. H., & Roche, H. M. (2012). Dietary saturated fatty acids prime the NLRP3 inflammasome via TLR4 in dendritic cells—implications for diet-induced insulin resistance. Molecular nutrition & food research, 56(8), 1212-1222.

Snodgrass, R. G., Huang, S., Choi, I. W., Rutledge, J. C., & Hwang, D. H. (2013). Inflammasome-mediated secretion of IL-1β in human monocytes through TLR2 activation; modulation by dietary fatty acids. The Journal of Immunology, 191(8), 4337-4347.

10   Morris, Z. S., Wooding, S., & Grant, J. (2011). The answer is 17
      years, what is the question: understanding time lags in translational
      research. Journal of the Royal Society of Medicine, 104(12), 510-520.

11   Proudman, S. M., James, M. J., Spargo, L. D., Metcalf, R. G., Sullivan,
      T. R., Rischmueller, M., ... & Cleland, L. G. (2013). Fish oil in recent
      onset rheumatoid arthritis: a randomised, double-blind controlled
      trial within algorithm-based drug use. Annals of the rheumatic
      diseases, annrheumdis-2013.

12   Meadows, S. (2013, February 1). The Boy with the Thorn in his
      Joints. The New York Times, Magazine.

13   Mielants, H., De Vos, M., Goemaere, S., Schelstraete, K., Cuvelier,
      C., Goethals, K., ... & Veys, E. M. (1991). Intestinal mucosal perme-
      ability in inflammatory rheumatic diseases. II. Role of disease. The
      Journal of rheumatology, 18(3), 394-400.
      Martínez-González O1, Cantero-Hinojosa J, Paule-Sastre P, Gómez-
      Magán JC, Salvatierra-Ríos D, Br J Rheumatol. 1994 Jul;33(7):644-7.
      Intestinal permeability in patients with ankylosing spondylitis and
      their healthy relatives
      Picco, P., Gattorno, M., Marchese, N., Vignola, S., Sormani, M. P.,
      Barabino, A., & Buoncompagni, A. (2000). Increased gut perme-
      ability in juvenile chronic arthritides. A multivariate analysis of the
      diagnostic parameters. Clinical and experimental rheumatology,
      18(6), 773-778.
      Humbert P, Bidet A, Treffel P, Drobacheff C, Agache P. Intestinal
      permeability in patients with psoriasis. J Dermatol Sci. 1991;2:324–
      6.

14   Merga, Y., Campbell, B. J., & Rhodes, J. M. (2014). Mucosal barrier,
      bacteria and inflammatory bowel disease: possibilities for therapy.
      Digestive diseases, 32(4), 475-483.

15   Ciccia, F., Guggino, G., Rizzo, A., Saieva, L., Peralta, S., Giardina,
      A., ... & Triolo, G. (2015). Type 3 innate lymphoid cells producing
      IL-17 and IL-22 are expanded in the gut, in the peripheral blood,
      synovial fluid and bone marrow of patients with ankylosing spondy-
      litis. Annals of the rheumatic diseases, annrheumdis-2014
      May, E., Märker–Hermann, E., Wittig, B. M., Zeitz, M., Zum
      Büschenfelde, K. H. M., & Duchmann, R. (2000). Identical T-cell
      expansions in the colon mucosa and the synovium of a patient with
      enterogenic spondyloarthropathy. Gastroenterology, 119(6), 1745-
      1755.
      Fantini, M. C., Pallone, F., & Monteleone, G. (2009). Common im-
      munologic mechanisms in inflammatory bowel disease and spondy-
      larthropathies. World J Gastroenterol, 15(20), 2472-2478;
      Suurmond, J., Rivellese, F., Dorjee, A. L., Bakker, A. M., Rombouts,
      Y. J. P. C., Rispens, T., ... & Toes, R. E. M. (2015). Toll-like receptor

triggering augments activation of human mast cells by anti-citrullinated protein antibodies. Annals of the rheumatic diseases, 74(10), 1915-1923

16   Cypers, H., Varkas, G., Beeckman, S., Debusschere, K., Vogl, T., Roth, J., ... & De Vos, M. (2015). Elevated calprotectin levels reveal bowel inflammation in spondyloarthritis. Annals of the rheumatic diseases, Dec. 23 2015;

Stebbings, S., Jenks, K., Treharne, G. J., García, J. A., Schultz, M., Highton, J., & Dudley-Brown, S. (2011). Validation of the Dudley Inflammatory Bowel Symptom Questionnaire for the assessment of bowel symptoms in axial SpA: prevalence of clinically relevant bowel symptoms and association with disease activity. Rheumatology, ker359;

Stoll, M. L., Punaro, M., & Patel, A. S. (2011). Fecal calprotectin in children with the enthesitis-related arthritis subtype of juvenile idiopathic arthritis. The Journal of rheumatology, 38(10), 2274-2275;

Bjarnason, I., Helgason, K. O., Geirsson, Á. J., Sigthorsson, G., Reynisdottir, I., Gudbjartsson, D., ... & Thjodleifsson, B. (2003). Subclinical intestinal inflammation and sacroiliac changes in relatives of patients with ankylosing spondylitis. Gastroenterology, 125(6), 1598-1605.

Klingberg, E., Strid, H., Ståhl, A., Deminger, A., Carlsten, H., Öhman, L., & Forsblad-d'Elia, H. (2017). A longitudinal study of fecal calprotectin and the development of inflammatory bowel disease in ankylosing spondylitis. Arthritis research & therapy, 19(1), 21.

Tayel, M., Megid, M. A., Nouh, H. H., & Rofaeil, B. (2014). AB0340 Fecal Calprotectin in Rheumatoid Disease, and Its Relation to Disease State. Annals of the Rheumatic Diseases, 73(Suppl 2), 917-917.

17   Mielants, H., Veys, E. M., Cuvelier, C., & De Vos, M. (1988). Ileocolonoscopic findings in seronegative spondylarthropathies. Rheumatology, 27(suppl 2), 95-105.

18   Van Praet, L., Van den Bosch, F. E., Jacques, P., Carron, P., Jans, L., Colman, R., ... & Cuvelier, C. (2013). Microscopic gut inflammation in axial spondyloarthritis: a multiparametric predictive model. Annals of the rheumatic diseases, 72(3), 414-417.

Cypers, H., Varkas, G., Beeckman, S., Debusschere, K., Vogl, T., Roth, J., ... & De Vos, M. (2015). Elevated calprotectin levels reveal bowel inflammation in spondyloarthritis. Annals of the rheumatic diseases, Dec. 23 2015;

Leirisalo-Repo, M., Turunen, U., Stenman, S., Helenius, P., & Seppälä, K. (1994). High frequency of silent inflammatory bowel disease in spondylarthropathy. Arthritis & Rheumatology, 37(1), 23-31.

Scarpa R, Manguso F, D'Arienzo A, D'Armiento FP, Astarita C, Mazzacca G, et al. Microscopic inflammatory changes in colon of

patients with both active psoriasis and psoriatic arthritis without
bowel symptoms. J Rheumatol. 2000;27:1241–6.

19   Li, W. Q., Han, J. L., Chan, A. T., & Qureshi, A. A. (2012). Psoriasis,
psoriatic arthritis and increased risk of incident Crohn's disease in
US women. Annals of the rheumatic diseases, annrheumdis-2012.

20   De Vos, Mielants, Cuvelier, C., Elewaut, A., & Veys, E. R. I. C.
(1996). Long-term evolution of gut inflammation in patients with
spondyloarthropathy. Gastroenterology, 110(6), 1696-1703.

21   Lucaciu, L., Ilies, M., Iuga, C., & Seicean, A. (2018). P136 Serum
IL-17 and IL-23 levels can distinguish between severe and non-
severe inflammatory bowel disease. *Journal of Crohn's and Colitis, 12*(supplement_1), S163-S163.
Kuwabara, T., Ishikawa, F., Kondo, M., & Kakiuchi, T. (2017). The
role of IL-17 and related cytokines in inflammatory autoimmune
diseases. *Mediators of inflammation, 2017.*
Krueger, J. G., & Brunner, P. M. (2018). Interleukin-17 alters the
biology of many cell types involved in the genesis of psoriasis,
systemic inflammation and associated comorbidities. *Experimental
dermatology, 27*(2), 115-123.
Sakkas, L. I., & Bogdanos, D. P. (2017). Are psoriasis and psoriatic
arthritis the same disease? The IL-23/IL-17 axis data. *Autoimmunity
reviews, 16*(1), 10-15.
Poddubnyy, D., & Sieper, J. (2017). What is the best treatment target
in axial spondyloarthritis: tumour necrosis factor α, interleukin 17,
or both?. *Rheumatology.*
Suurmond, J., Rivellese, F., Dorjee, A. L., Bakker, A. M., Rombouts,
Y. J. P. C., Rispens, T., . . . & Toes, R. E. M. (2015). Toll-like receptor
triggering augments activation of human mast cells by anti-citrullinated protein antibodies. Annals of the rheumatic diseases, 74(10),
1915-1923.
Baricza, E., Marton, N., Királyhidi, P., Kovács, O. T., Kovácsné
Székely, I., Lajkó, E., . . . & Nagy, G. (2018). Distinct In Vitro T-helper
17 Differentiation capacity of Peripheral naive T cells in rheumatoid
and Psoriatic arthritis. *Frontiers in immunology, 9*, 606.
Bazzazi, H., Aghaei, M., Memarian, A., Asgarian-Omran, H.,
Behnampour, N., & Yazdani, Y. (2018). Th1-Th17 Ratio as a New Insight in Rheumatoid Arthritis Disease. *Iranian Journal of Allergy,
Asthma and Immunology, 17*(1), 68-77.

22   Park, J. H., Jeong, S. Y., Choi, A. J., & Kim, S. J. (2015). Lipopolysaccharide directly stimulates Th17 differentiation in vitro modulating
phosphorylation of RelB and NF-κB1. *Immunology letters, 165*(1),
10-19.
McAleer, J. P., Liu, B., Li, Z., Ngoi, S. M., Dai, J., Oft, M., & Vella,
A. T. (2010). Potent intestinal Th17 priming through peripheral

lipopolysaccharide-based immunization. *Journal of leukocyte biology*, *88*(1), 21-31.

Dekita, M., Wu, Z., Ni, J., Zhang, X., Liu, Y., Yan, X., ... & Takahashi, I. (2017). Cathepsin S Is Involved in Th17 Differentiation Through the Upregulation of IL-6 by Activating PAR-2 after Systemic Exposure to Lipopolysaccharide from Porphyromonas gingivalis. *Frontiers in pharmacology*, *8*, 470.

Chovanova, L., Vlcek, M., Krskova, K., Penesova, A., Radikova, Z., Rovensky, J., ... & Imrich, R. (2013). Increased production of IL-6 and IL-17 in lipopolysaccharide-stimulated peripheral mononuclears from patients with rheumatoid arthritis. *Gen Physiol Biophys*, *32*(3), 395-404.

Supajatura, V., Ushio, H., Nakao, A., Okumura, K., Ra, C., & Ogawa, H. (2001). Protective roles of mast cells against enterobacterial infection are mediated by Toll-like receptor 4. The Journal of Immunology, 167(4), 2250-2256.

Abraham, S. N., & John, A. L. S. (2010). Mast cell-orchestrated immunity to pathogens. Nature Reviews Immunology, 10(6), 440-452.

Suurmond, J., Rivellese, F., Dorjee, A. L., Bakker, A. M., Rombouts, Y. J. P. C., Rispens, T., ... & Toes, R. E. M. (2015). Toll-like receptor triggering augments activation of human mast cells by anti-citrullinated protein antibodies. Annals of the rheumatic diseases, 74(10), 1915-1923.

Lee, G. R. (2018). The Balance of Th17 versus Treg Cells in Autoimmunity. *International journal of molecular sciences*, *19*(3), 730.

Lucaciu, L., Ilies, M., Iuga, C., & Seicean, A. (2018). P136 Serum IL-17 and IL-23 levels can distinguish between severe and nonsevere inflammatory bowel disease. *Journal of Crohn's and Colitis*, *12*(supplement_1), S163-S163.

Kuwabara, T., Ishikawa, F., Kondo, M., & Kakiuchi, T. (2017). The role of IL-17 and related cytokines in inflammatory autoimmune diseases. *Mediators of inflammation*, *2017*.

Krueger, J. G., & Brunner, P. M. (2018). Interleukin-17 alters the biology of many cell types involved in the genesis of psoriasis, systemic inflammation and associated comorbidities. *Experimental dermatology*, *27*(2), 115-123.

Sakkas, L. I., & Bogdanos, D. P. (2017). Are psoriasis and psoriatic arthritis the same disease? The IL-23/IL-17 axis data. *Autoimmunity reviews*, *16*(1), 10-15.

Poddubnyy, D., & Sieper, J. (2017). What is the best treatment target in axial spondyloarthritis: tumour necrosis factor α, interleukin 17, or both?. *Rheumatology*.

Suurmond, J., Rivellese, F., Dorjee, A. L., Bakker, A. M., Rombouts, Y. J. P. C., Rispens, T., ... & Toes, R. E. M. (2015). Toll-like receptor triggering augments activation of human mast cells by anti-citrulli-

23

nated protein antibodies. Annals of the rheumatic diseases, 74(10), 1915-1923.

Baricza, E., Marton, N., Királyhidi, P., Kovács, O. T., Kovácsné Székely, I., Lajkó, E.,... & Nagy, G. (2018). Distinct In Vitro T-helper 17 Differentiation capacity of Peripheral naive T cells in rheumatoid and Psoriatic arthritis. *Frontiers in immunology*, 9, 606.

Bazzazi, H., Aghaei, M., Memarian, A., Asgarian-Omran, H., Behnampour, N., & Yazdani, Y. (2018). Th1-Th17 Ratio as a New Insight in Rheumatoid Arthritis Disease. *Iranian Journal of Allergy, Asthma and Immunology*, 17(1), 68-77.

Suurmond, J., Rivellese, F., Dorjee, A. L., Bakker, A. M., Rombouts, Y. J. P. C., Rispens, T.,... & Toes, R. E. M. (2015). Toll-like receptor triggering augments activation of human mast cells by anti-citrullinated protein antibodies. Annals of the rheumatic diseases, 74(10), 1915-1923.

Fotis, L., Shaikh, N., Baszis, K. W., Samson, C. M., Lev-Tzion, R., French, A. R., & Tarr, P. I. (2017). Serologic evidence of gut-driven systemic inflammation in juvenile idiopathic arthritis. *The Journal of rheumatology*, 44(11), 1624-1631

24   Atarashi, K., Tanoue, T., Shima, T., Imaoka, A., Kuwahara, T., Momose, Y.,... & Taniguchi, T. (2011). Induction of colonic regulatory T cells by indigenous Clostridium species. Science, 331(6015), 337-341;

Frank, D. N., Amand, A. L. S., Feldman, R. A., Boedeker, E. C., Harpaz, N., & Pace, N. R. (2007). Molecular-phylogenetic characterization of microbial community imbalances in human inflammatory bowel diseases. Proceedings of the National Academy of Sciences, 104(34), 13780-13785.

Gevers, D., Kugathasan, S., Denson, L. A., Vázquez-Baeza, Y., Van Treuren, W., Ren, B.,... & Morgan, X. C. (2014). The treatment-naive microbiome in new-onset Crohn's disease. Cell host & microbe, 15(3), 382-392.

Kang, S., Denman, S. E., Morrison, M., Yu, Z., Dore, J., Leclerc, M., & McSweeney, C. S. (2010). Dysbiosis of fecal microbiota in Crohn's disease patients as revealed by a custom phylogenetic microarray. Inflammatory bowel diseases, 16(12), 2034-2042.

25   Kolho, K. L., Korpela, K., Jaakkola, T., Pichai, M. V., Zoetendal, E. G., Salonen, A., & De Vos, W. M. (2015). Fecal microbiota in pediatric inflammatory bowel disease and its relation to inflammation. The American journal of gastroenterology, 110(6), 921-930.

26   Geirnaert, A., Calatayud, M., Grootaert, C., Laukens, D., Devriese, S., Smagghe, G.,... & Van de Wiele, T. (2017). Butyrate-producing bacteria supplemented in vitro to Crohn's disease patient microbiota increased butyrate production and enhanced intestinal epithelial

barrier integrity. Scientific Reports, 7(1), 11450.

27   Scher, J. U., Ubeda, C., Artacho, A., Attur, M., Isaac, S., Reddy, S.
     M.,...& Manasson, J. (2015). Decreased bacterial diversity charac-
     terizes the altered gut microbiota in patients with psoriatic arthritis,
     resembling dysbiosis in inflammatory bowel disease. Arthritis &
     rheumatology, 67(1), 128-139.
     Casellas, F., Borruel, N., Manichanh, C., Varela, E., Antolín, M., Tor-
     rejón, A.,...& MetaHIT Consortium. (2014). OP022 Low microbial
     gene diversity and depletion of Akkermansia muciniphila is associ-
     ated with a relapsing course of ulcerative colitis. Journal of Crohn's
     and Colitis, 8(Supplement 1), S12-S13.

28   Vaahtovuo, J., Munukka, E., KORKEAMÄKI, M., Luukkainen, R., &
     Toivanen, P. (2008). Fecal microbiota in early rheumatoid arthritis.
     The Journal of rheumatology, 35(8), 1500-1505.
     Di Paola, M., Cavalieri, D., Albanese, D., Sordo, M., Pindo, M.,
     Donati, C.,...& Lionetti, P. (2016). Alteration of Fecal Microbiota
     Profiles in Juvenile Idiopathic Arthritis. Associations with HLA-B27
     Allele and Disease Status. Frontiers in Microbiology, 7.
     Eppinga, H., Weiland, C. J. S., Thio, H. B., van der Woude, C. J.,
     Nijsten, T. E., Peppelenbosch, M. P., & Konstantinov, S. R. (2016).
     Similar depletion of protective Faecalibacterium prausnitzii in
     psoriasis and inflammatory bowel disease, but not in Hidradenitis
     suppurativa. Journal of Crohn's and Colitis, 10(9), 1067-1075.
     Stoll, M. L., Kumar, R., Morrow, C. D., Lefkowitz, E. J., Cui, X.,
     Genin, A.,...& Elson, C. O. (2014). Altered microbiota associated
     with abnormal humoral immune responses to commensal organisms
     in enthesitis-related arthritis. Arthritis research & therapy, 16(6), 486.

29   Gevers, D., Kugathasan, S., Denson, L. A., Vázquez-Baeza, Y., Van
     Treuren, W., Ren, B.,...& Morgan, X. C. (2014). The treatment-naive
     microbiome in new-onset Crohn's disease. Cell host & microbe,
     15(3), 382-392.
     Scher, J. U., Ubeda, C., Artacho, A., Attur, M., Isaac, S., Reddy, S.
     M.,...& Manasson, J. (2015). Decreased bacterial diversity charac-
     terizes the altered gut microbiota in patients with psoriatic arthritis,
     resembling dysbiosis in inflammatory bowel disease. Arthritis &
     rheumatology, 67(1), 128-139.

30   Stoll, M. L., Kumar, R., Morrow, C. D., Lefkowitz, E. J., Cui, X.,
     Genin, A.,...& Elson, C. O. (2014). Altered microbiota associated
     with abnormal humoral immune responses to commensal organ-
     isms in enthesitis-related arthritis. Arthritis research & therapy,
     16(6), 486.

31   Di Paola, M., Cavalieri, D., Albanese, D., Sordo, M., Pindo, M.,
     Donati, C.,...& Lionetti, P. (2016). Alteration of Fecal Microbiota
     Profiles in Juvenile Idiopathic Arthritis. Associations with HLA-B27

Allele and Disease Status. Frontiers in microbiology, 7.

32   Vaahtovuo, J., Munukka, E., KORKEAMÄKI, M., Luukkainen, R., & Toivanen, P. (2008). Fecal microbiota in early rheumatoid arthritis. The Journal of rheumatology, 35(8), 1500-1505

33   Reunanan (2015) Akkermansia muciniphila Adheres to Enterocytes and Strengthens the Integrity of the Epithelial Cell Layer; Atarashi, K., Tanoue, T., Shima, T., Imaoka, A., Kuwahara, T., Momose, Y.,…& Taniguchi, T. (2011). Induction of colonic regulatory T cells by indigenous Clostridium species. Science, 331(6015), 337-341.

34   Atarashi, K., Tanoue, T., Shima, T., Imaoka, A., Kuwahara, T., Momose, Y.,…& Taniguchi, T. (2011). Induction of colonic regulatory T cells by indigenous Clostridium species. Science, 331(6015), 337-341

35   Gri, G., Piconese, S., Frossi, B., Manfroi, V., Merluzzi, S., Tripodo, C.,…& Pucillo, C. E. (2008). CD4+ CD25+ regulatory T cells suppress mast cell degranulation and allergic responses through OX40-OX40L interaction. Immunity, 29(5), 771-781; Frossi, B., D'Incà, F., Crivellato, E., Sibilano, R., Gri, G., Mongillo, M.,…& Pucillo, C. E. (2011). Single-cell dynamics of mast cell–CD4+ CD25+ regulatory T cell interactions. European journal of immunology, 41(7), 1872-1882.

36   Smith, P. M., Howitt, M. R., Panikov, N., Michaud, M., Gallini, C. A., Bohlooly-y, M.,…& Garrett, W. S. (2013). The microbial metabolites, short-chain fatty acids, regulate colonic Treg cell homeostasis. Science, 341(6145), 569-573.

37   Keijsers, R. R. M. C., van der Velden, H. M. J., van Erp, P. E. J., de Boer-van Huizen, R. T., Joosten, I., Koenen, H. J. P. M., & van de Kerkhof, P. C. M. (2013). Balance of Treg vs. T-helper cells in the transition from symptomless to lesional psoriatic skin. British Journal of Dermatology, 168(6), 1294-1302.

38   Furusawa, Y., Obata, Y., Fukuda, S., Endo, T. A., Nakato, G., Takahashi, D.,…& Takahashi, M. (2013). Commensal microbe-derived butyrate induces the differentiation of colonic regulatory T cells. Nature, 504(7480), 446-450. Arpaia, N., Campbell, C., Fan, X., Dikiy, S., van der Veeken, J., Liu, H.,…& Rudensky, A. Y. (2013). Metabolites produced by commensal bacteria promote peripheral regulatory T-cell generation. Nature, 504(7480), 451-455. Smith, P. M., Howitt, M. R., Panikov, N., Michaud, M., Gallini, C. A., Bohlooly-y, M.,…& Garrett, W. S. (2013). The microbial metabolites, short-chain fatty acids, regulate colonic Treg cell homeostasis. Science, 341(6145), 569-573.

39 Sarrabayrouse, G., Bossard, C., Chauvin, J. M., Jarry, A., Meurette, G., Quévrain, E., ... & Altare, F. (2014). CD4CD8αα lymphocytes, a novel human regulatory T cell subset induced by colonic bacteria and deficient in patients with inflammatory bowel disease. PLoS Biol, 12(4), e1001833.
Omenetti, S., & Pizarro, T. T. (2015). The Treg/Th17 axis: a dynamic balance regulated by the gut microbiome. *Frontiers in immunology*, 6, 639.

40 Viladomiu, M., Kivolowitz, C., Abdulhamid, A., Dogan, B., Victorio, D., Castellanos, J. G., ... & Chai, C. (2017). IgA-coated E. coli enriched in Crohn's disease spondyloarthritis promote TH17-dependent inflammation. Science Translational Medicine, 9(376), eaaf9655;
Eppinga, H., Weiland, C. J. S., Thio, H. B., van der Woude, C. J., Nijsten, T. E., Peppelenbosch, M. P., & Konstantinov, S. R. (2016). Similar depletion of protective Faecalibacterium prausnitzii in psoriasis and inflammatory bowel disease, but not in Hidradenitis suppurativa. Journal of Crohn's and Colitis, 10(9), 1067-1075;
Scher, J. U., Sczesnak, A., Longman, R. S., Segata, N., Ubeda, C., Bielski, C., ... Littman, D. R. (2013). Expansion of intestinal Prevotella copri correlates with enhanced susceptibility to arthritis. eLife, 2, e01202.
Maeda, Y., Kurakawa, T., Umemoto, E., Motooka, D., Ito, Y., Gotoh, K., ... & Sakaguchi, N. (2016). Dysbiosis contributes to arthritis development via activation of autoreactive T cells in the intestine. Arthritis & Rheumatology, 68(11), 2646-2661.
Chen, J., Wright, K., Davis, J. M., Jeraldo, P., Marietta, E. V., Murray, J., ... & Taneja, V. (2016). An expansion of rare lineage intestinal microbes characterizes rheumatoid arthritis. Genome medicine, 8(1), 43.
Blankenberg-Sprenkels, S. H., Fielder, M., Feltkamp, T. E., Tiwana, H., Wilson, C., & Ebringer, A. (1998). Antibodies to Klebsiella pneumoniae in Dutch patients with ankylosing spondylitis and acute anterior uveitis and to Proteus mirabilis in rheumatoid arthritis. The Journal of rheumatology, 25(4), 743-747.
Ramírez-Boscá, A., Navarro-López, V., Martínez-Andrés, A., Such, J., Francés, R., de la Parte, J. H., & Asín-Llorca, M. (2015). Identification of bacterial DNA in the peripheral blood of patients with active psoriasis. JAMA dermatology, 151(6), 670-671.

41 Maeda, Y., Kurakawa, T., Umemoto, E., Motooka, D., Ito, Y., Gotoh, K., ... & Sakaguchi, N. (2016). Dysbiosis contributes to arthritis development via activation of autoreactive T cells in the intestine. Arthritis & Rheumatology, 68(11), 2646-2661;
Viladomiu, M., Kivolowitz, C., Abdulhamid, A., Dogan, B., Vic-

torio, D., Castellanos, J. G.,...& Chai, C. (2017). IgA-coated E. coli enriched in Crohn's disease spondyloarthritis promote TH17-dependent inflammation. Science Translational Medicine, 9(376), eaaf9655;

Shawki, A., & McCole, D. F. (2017). Mechanisms of Intestinal Epithelial Barrier Dysfunction by Adherent-Invasive Escherichia coli. CMGH Cellular and Molecular Gastroenterology and Hepatology, 3(1), 41-50.

Kivolowitz, C., Abdulhamid, A., Victorio, D., Castellanos, J., Simpson, K., Scherl, E., & Longman, R. (2016). O-006 Expansion of Immunologically-Relevant E. Coli in the Intestinal Microbiota of Patients with IBD-Associated Spondyloarthritis Promotes Mucosal RORgt-Dependent Immunity. Inflammatory bowel diseases, 22, S3.

Cosorich, I., Dalla-Costa, G., Sorini, C., Ferrarese, R., Messina, M. J., Dolpady, J.,...& Comi, G. (2017). High frequency of intestinal TH17 cells correlates with microbiota alterations and disease activity in multiple sclerosis. Science Advances, 3(7), e1700492.

42 Agus, A., Massier, S., Darfeuille-Michaud, A., Billard, E., & Barnich, N. (2014). Understanding host-adherent-invasive Escherichia coli interaction in Crohn's disease: opening up new therapeutic strategies. BioMed research international, 2014.

43 Martinez-Medina, M., Aldeguer, X., Lopez-Siles, M., González-Huix, F., López-Oliu, C., Dahbi, G.,...& Darfeuille-Michaud, A. (2009). Molecular diversity of Escherichia coli in the human gut: new ecological evidence supporting the role of adherent-invasive E. coli (AIEC) in Crohn's disease. Inflammatory bowel diseases, 15(6), 872-882.

Baumgart, M., Dogan, B., Rishniw, M., Weitzman, G., Bosworth, B., Yantiss, R.,...& Berg, D. (2007). Culture independent analysis of ileal mucosa reveals a selective increase in invasive Escherichia coli of novel phylogeny relative to depletion of Clostridiales in Crohn's disease involving the ileum. The ISME journal, 1(5), 403-418.

Eaves-Pyles, T., Allen, C. A., Taormina, J., Swidsinski, A., Tutt, C. B., Jezek, G. E.,...& Torres, A. G. (2008). Escherichia coli isolated from a Crohn's disease patient adheres, invades, and induces inflammatory responses in polarized intestinal epithelial cells. International Journal of Medical Microbiology, 298(5), 397-409.

Kotlowski, R., Bernstein, C. N., Sepehri, S., & Krause, D. O. (2007). High prevalence of Escherichia coli belonging to the B2+ D phylogenetic group in inflammatory bowel disease. Gut, 56(5), 669-675.

Conte, M. P., Schippa, S., Zamboni, I., Penta, M., Chiarini, F., Seganti, L.,...& Cucchiara, S. (2006). Gut-associated bacterial microbiota in paediatric patients with inflammatory bowel disease. Gut, 55(12), 1760-1767.

44 Viladomiu, M., Kivolowitz, C., Abdulhamid, A., Dogan, B., Victorio, D., Castellanos, J. G., ... & Chai, C. (2017). IgA-coated E. coli enriched in Crohn's disease spondyloarthritis promote TH17-dependent inflammation. Science Translational Medicine, 9(376), eaaf9655.
Kivolowitz, C., Abdulhamid, A., Victorio, D., Castellanos, J., Simpson, K., Scherl, E., & Longman, R. (2016). O-006 Expansion of Immunologically-Relevant E. Coli in the Intestinal Microbiota of Patients with IBD-Associated Spondyloarthritis Promotes Mucosal RORgt-Dependent Immunity. Inflammatory bowel diseases, 22, S3.

45 Viladomiu, M., Kivolowitz, C., Abdulhamid, A., Dogan, B., Victorio, D., Castellanos, J. G., ... & Chai, C. (2017). IgA-coated E. coli enriched in Crohn's disease spondyloarthritis promote TH17-dependent inflammation. Science Translational Medicine, 9(376), eaaf9655.
Kivolowitz, C., Abdulhamid, A., Victorio, D., Castellanos, J., Simpson, K., Scherl, E., & Longman, R. (2016). O-006 Expansion of Immunologically-Relevant E. Coli in the Intestinal Microbiota of Patients with IBD-Associated Spondyloarthritis Promotes Mucosal RORgt-Dependent Immunity. Inflammatory bowel diseases, 22, S3.

46 Rashid, T., & Ebringer, A. (2007). Ankylosing spondylitis is linked to Klebsiella—the evidence. Clinical rheumatology, 26(6), 858-864.

47 Tani, Y., Tiwana, H., Hukuda, S., Nishioka, J., Fielder, M., Wilson, C., ... & Ebringer, A. (1997). Antibodies to Klebsiella, Proteus, and HLA-B27 peptides in Japanese patients with ankylosing spondylitis and rheumatoid arthritis. The Journal of rheumatology, 24(1), 109-114.

48 Blankenberg-Sprenkels, S. H., Fielder, M., Feltkamp, T. E., Tiwana, H., Wilson, C., & Ebringer, A. (1998). Antibodies to Klebsiella pneumoniae in Dutch patients with ankylosing spondylitis and acute anterior uveitis and to Proteus mirabilis in rheumatoid arthritis. The Journal of rheumatology, 25(4), 743-747.

49 Tiwana, H., Wilson, C., Walmsley, R. S., Wakefield, A. J., Smith, M. S. N., Cox, N. L., ... & Ebringer, A. (1997). Antibody responses to gut bacteria in ankylosing spondylitis, rheumatoid arthritis, Crohn's disease and ulcerative colitis. Rheumatology international, 17(1), 11-16.

50 Puccetti, A., Dolcino, M., Tinazzi, E., Moretta, F., D'Angelo, S., Olivieri, I., & Lunardi, C. (2017). Antibodies Directed against a Peptide Epitope of a Klebsiella pneumoniae-Derived Protein Are Present in Ankylosing Spondylitis. PloS one, 12(1), e0171073.

51 Puccetti, A., Dolcino, M., Tinazzi, E., Moretta, F., D'Angelo, S., Olivieri, I., & Lunardi, C. (2017). Antibodies Directed against a Peptide Epitope of a Klebsiella pneumoniae-Derived Protein Are Present in Ankylosing Spondylitis. PloS one, 12(1), e0171073.

52   Christopoulos, G., Christopoulou, V., Routsias, J. G., Babionitakis,
        A., Antoniadis, C., & Vaiopoulos, G. (2017). Greek rheumatoid
        arthritis patients have elevated levels of antibodies against antigens
        from Proteus mirabilis. Clinical rheumatology, 36(3), 527-535.
        Rashid, T., Jayakumar, K. S., Binder, A., Ellis, S., Cunningham, P., &
        Ebringer, A. (2007). Rheumatoid arthritis patients have elevated anti-
        bodies to cross-reactive and non cross-reactive antigens from Proteus
        microbes. Clinical and experimental rheumatology, 25(2), 259.
        Tani, Y., Tiwana, H., Hukuda, S., Nishioka, J., Fielder, M., Wilson,
        C.,...& Ebringer, A. (1997). Antibodies to Klebsiella, Proteus, and
        HLA-B27 peptides in Japanese patients with ankylosing spondylitis
        and rheumatoid arthritis. The Journal of rheumatology, 24(1), 109-114.
        Newkirk, M. M., Goldbach-Mansky, R., Senior, B. W., Klippel, J.,
        Schumacher Jr, H. R., & El-Gabalawy, H. S. (2005). Elevated levels
        of IgM and IgA antibodies to Proteus mirabilis and IgM antibodies
        to Escherichia coli are associated with early rheumatoid factor (RF)-
        positive rheumatoid arthritis. Rheumatology, 44(11), 1433-1441.

53   Pyleris, E., Giamarellos-Bourboulis, E. J., Tzivras, D., Koussoulas, V.,
        Barbatzas, C., & Pimentel, M. (2012). The prevalence of overgrowth
        by aerobic bacteria in the small intestine by small bowel culture:
        relationship with irritable bowel syndrome. Digestive diseases and
        sciences, 57(5), 1321-1329;
        Dukowicz, A. C., Lacy, B. E., & Levine, G. M. (2007). Small intesti-
        nal bacterial overgrowth: a comprehensive review. Gastroenterology
        & hepatology, 3(2), 112.

54   Ely, P. H. (1980). The bowel bypass syndrome: A response to bacte-
        rial peptidoglycanss. Journal of the American Academy of Derma-
        tology, 2(6), 473-487.
        Zhao, H., Zhao, L., Shi, W., Luo, H., Duan, L., You, Y.,...& Zuo, X.
        (2016). Is it bowel-associated dermatosis-arthritis syndrome induced
        by small intestinal bacteria overgrowth?. SpringerPlus, 5(1), 1551.
        Bhangle, S. D., Kramer, N., & Rosenstein, E. D. (2009). Spondylo-
        arthropathy after ampullary carcinoma resection:"post-Whipple"
        disease. JCR: Journal of Clinical Rheumatology, 15(5), 241-243.

55   Fisch, C., Schiller, P., Harr, T., & Maclachlan, D. (2001). First pre-
        sentation of intestinal bypass syndrome 18 yr after initial surgery.
        Rheumatology, 40(3), 351-353.

56   Fisch, C., Schiller, P., Harr, T., & Maclachlan, D. (2001). First presenta-
        tion of intestinal bypass syndrome 18 yr after initial surgery. Rheu-
        matology, 40(3), 351-353; Slater, G. H., Kerlin, P., Georghiou, P. R., &
        Fielding, G. A. (2004). Bowel-associated dermatosis-arthritis syndrome
        after biliopancreatic diversion. Obesity surgery, 14(1), 133-135.
        Zhao, H., Zhao, L., Shi, W., Luo, H., Duan, L., You, Y.,...& Zuo, X.
        (2016). Is it bowel-associated dermatosis-arthritis syndrome induced

by small intestinal bacteria overgrowth?. SpringerPlus, 5(1), 1551.

57   Ojetti, V., De Simone, C., Aguilar Sanchez, J., Capizzi, R., Migneco, A., Guerriero, C.,... & Gasbarrini, A. (2006). Malabsorption in psoriatic patients: cause or consequence?. Scandinavian journal of gastroenterology, 41(11), 1267-1271.
Peslyak, M., Gumayunova, N., Nesterov, A., & Potaturkina-Nesterova, N. (2012). Small intestine microflora at psoriasis. Its possible role in pathogenesis. In *3rd World Psoriasis & Psoriatic Arthritis Conference*.
Drago, F., Ciccarese, G., Indemini, E., Savarino, V., & Parodi, A. (2017). Psoriasis and small intestine bacterial overgrowth. International journal of dermatology.

58   Henriksson, A. E., Blomquist, L., Nord, C. E., Midtvedt, T., & Uribe, A. (1993). Small intestinal bacterial overgrowth in patients with rheumatoid arthritis. Annals of the rheumatic diseases, 52(7), 503.

59   Orchard, T. R., & Jewell, D. P. (1999). The importance of ileocaecal integrity in the arthritic complications of Crohn's disease. Inflammatory bowel diseases, 5(2), 92-97.

60   Pimentel, M., Wallace, D., Hallegua, D., Chow, E., Kong, Y., Park, S., & Lin, H. C. (2004). A link between irritable bowel syndrome and fibromyalgia may be related to findings on lactulose breath testing. Annals of the rheumatic diseases, 63(4), 450-452.

61   Peslyak, M., Gumayunova, N., Nesterov, A., & Potaturkina-Nesterova, N. (2012). Small intestine microflora at psoriasis. Its possible role in pathogenesis. In *3rd World Psoriasis & Psoriatic Arthritis Conference*.

62   Ramírez-Boscá, A., Navarro-López, V., Martínez-Andrés, A., Such, J., Francés, R., de la Parte, J. H., & Asín-Llorca, M. (2015). Identification of bacterial DNA in the peripheral blood of patients with active psoriasis. JAMA dermatology, 151(6), 670-671.

63   Ramírez-Boscá, A., Navarro-López, V., Martínez-Andrés, A., Such, J., Francés, R., de la Parte, J. H., & Asín-Llorca, M. (2015). Identification of bacterial DNA in the peripheral blood of patients with active psoriasis. JAMA dermatology, 151(6), 670-671.

64   Drago, F., Ciccarese, G., Indemini, E., Savarino, V., & Parodi, A. (2018). Psoriasis and small intestine bacterial overgrowth. International journal of dermatology, 57(1), 112-113.

65   Mäki-Ikola, O., Hällgren, R., Kanerud, L., Feltelius, N., Knutsson, L., & Granfors, K. (1997). Enhanced jejunal production of antibodies to Klebsiella and other Enterobacteria in patients with ankylosing spondylitis and rheumatoid arthritis. Annals of the rheumatic diseases, 56(7), 421-425.

66   Fotis, L., Shaikh, N., Baszis, K. W., Samson, C. M., Lev-Tzion, R.,
        French, A. R., & Tarr, P. I. (2017). Serologic evidence of gut-driven
        systemic inflammation in juvenile idiopathic arthritis. *The Journal
        of rheumatology*, *44*(11), 1624-1631.
        Fialho, A., Fialho, A., Thota, P., McCullough, A. J., & Shen, B.
        (2016). Small Intestinal Bacterial Overgrowth Is Associated with
        Non-Alcoholic Fatty Liver Disease. *Journal of Gastrointestinal &
        Liver Diseases*, *25*(2).
        Bauer, Tilman M., et al. "Small intestinal bacterial overgrowth in
        human cirrhosis is associated with systemic endotoxemia." The
        American journal of gastroenterology 97.9 (2002): 2364-2370

67   Dukowicz, A. C., Lacy, B. E., & Levine, G. M. (2007). Small intesti-
        nal bacterial overgrowth: a comprehensive review. Gastroenterology
        & hepatology, 3(2), 112;
        Pimentel, M., Chow, E. J., & Lin, H. C. (2000). Eradication of small
        intestinal bacterial overgrowth reduces symptoms of irritable bowel
        syndrome. The American journal of gastroenterology, 95(12), 3503-
        3506.

68   Drago, F., Ciccarese, G., Indemini, E., Savarino, V., & Parodi, A.
        (2018). Psoriasis and small intestine bacterial overgrowth. Interna-
        tional journal of dermatology, 57(1), 112-113.

69   Lauritano, E. C., Gabrielli, M., Scarpellini, E., Lupascu, A., Novi, M.,
        Sottili, S., ... & Gasbarrini, G. (2008). Small intestinal bacterial over-
        growth recurrence after antibiotic therapy. *The American journal of
        gastroenterology*, *103*(8), 2031

70   Gudjonsson, J. E., Thorarinsson, A. M., Sigurgeirsson, B., Kristins-
        son, K. G., & Valdimarsson, H. (2003). Streptococcal throat infec-
        tions and exacerbation of chronic plaque psoriasis: a prospective
        study. British journal of dermatology, 149(3), 530-534.
        Thorleifsdottir, R. H., Sigurdardottir, S. L., Sigurgeirsson, B., Olafs-
        son, J. H., Sigurdsson, M. I., Petersen, H., ... & Valdimarsson, H.
        (2012). Improvement of psoriasis after tonsillectomy is associated
        with a decrease in the frequency of circulating T cells that recognize
        streptococcal determinants and homologous skin determinants. The
        Journal of Immunology, 188(10), 5160-5165.
        Johnston, A., Gudjonsson, J. E., Sigmundsdottir, H., Love, T. J., &
        Valdimarsson, H. (2004). Peripheral blood T cell responses to kera-
        tin peptides that share sequences with streptococcal M proteins are
        largely restricted to skin-homing CD8+ T cells. Clinical & Experi-
        mental Immunology, 138(1), 83-93.

71   El-Rachkidy, R. G., Hales, J. M., Freestone, P. P., Young, H. S.,
        Griffiths, C. E., & Camp, R. D. (2007). Increased blood levels of IgG
        reactive with secreted Streptococcus pyogenes proteins in chronic
        plaque psoriasis. Journal of Investigative Dermatology, 127(6), 1337-

1342.

Rantakokko, K., Rimpiläinen, M., Uksila, J., Jansen, C., Luukkainen, R., & Toivanen, P. (1997). Antibodies to streptococcal cell wall in psoriatic arthritis and cutaneous psoriasis. Clinical and experimental rheumatology, 15(4), 399-404.

72 McFadden, J., Valdimarsson, H., & Fry, L. (1991). Cross-reactivity between streptococcal M surface antigen and human skin. British Journal of Dermatology, 125(5), 443-447.

Swerlick, R. A., Cunningham, M. W., & Hall, N. K. (1986). Monoclonal antibodies cross-reactive with group A streptococci and normal and psoriatic human skin. Journal of investigative dermatology, 87(3), 367-371.

73 Weisenseel, P., Laumbacher, B., Besgen, P., Ludolph-Hauser, D., Herzinger, T., Roecken, M., ... & Prinz, J. C. (2002). Streptococcal infection distinguishes different types of psoriasis. Journal of medical genetics, 39(10), 767-768

74 Thorleifsdottir, R. H., Sigurdardottir, S. L., Sigurgeirsson, B., Olafsson, J. H., Sigurdsson, M. I., Petersen, H., ... & Valdimarsson, H. (2012). Improvement of psoriasis after tonsillectomy is associated with a decrease in the frequency of circulating T cells that recognize streptococcal determinants and homologous skin determinants. The Journal of Immunology, 188(10), 5160-5165.

75 Thorleifsdottir, R. H., Sigurdardottir, S. L., Sigurgeirsson, B., Olafsson, J. H., Sigurdsson, M. I., Petersen, H., ... & Valdimarsson, H. (2012). Improvement of psoriasis after tonsillectomy is associated with a decrease in the frequency of circulating T cells that recognize streptococcal determinants and homologous skin determinants. The Journal of Immunology, 188(10), 5160-5165.

76 Allen, H. B., Jadeja, S., Allawh, R. M., & Goyal, K. (2018). Psoriasis, chronic tonsillitis, and biofilms: Tonsillar pathologic findings supporting a microbial hypothesis. ENT: Ear, Nose & Throat Journal, 97(3).

77 Di Pierro, F., Colombo, M., Zanvit, A., Risso, P., & Rottoli, A. S. (2014). Use of Streptococcus salivarius K12 in the prevention of streptococcal and viral pharyngotonsillitis in children. Drug, healthcare and patient safety, 6, 15.

78 Mankia, K., Cheng, Z., Do, T., Kang, J., Hunt, L., Meade, J., ... & Devine, D. (2018). OP0352 An increased prevalence of periodontal disease, porphyromonas gingivalis and aggregatibacter actinomycetemcomitans in anti-ccp positive individuals at-risk of inflammatory arthritis.

Kriebel, K., Hieke, C., Müller-Hilke, B., Nakata, M., & Kreikemeyer, B. (2018). Oral biofilms from symbiotic to pathogenic interactions and associated disease–Connection of Periodontitis and Rheumatic arthritis by peptidylarginine deiminase. *Frontiers in microbiology*, *9*, 53.

Rosenstein, E. D., Greenwald, R. A., Kushner, L. J., & Weissmann, G. (2004). Hypothesis: the humoral immune response to oral bacteria provides a stimulus for the development of rheumatoid arthritis. *Inflammation*, *28*(6), 311-318.

79   Gleńska-Olender, J., Durlik, K., Konieczna, I., Kowalska, P., Gawęda, J., & Kaca, W. (2017). Detection of human antibodies binding with smooth and rough LPSs from Proteus mirabilis O3 strains S1959, R110, R45. Antonie van Leeuwenhoek, 110(11), 1435-1443.

Ebringer, A., & Rashid, T. (2006). Rheumatoid arthritis is an autoimmune disease triggered by Proteus urinary tract infection. Journal of Immunology Research, 13(1), 41-48.

80   Ebringer, A., & Rashid, T. (2014). Rheumatoid arthritis is caused by a Proteus urinary tract infection. Apmis, 122(5), 363-368.

81   Schaffer, J. N., & Pearson, M. M. (2015). Proteus mirabilis and urinary tract infections. Microbiology spectrum, 3(5).

82   Viladomiu, M., Kivolowitz, C., Abdulhamid, A., Dogan, B., Victorio, D., Castellanos, J. G., ... & Chai, C. (2017). IgA-coated E. coli enriched in Crohn's disease spondyloarthritis promote TH17-dependent inflammation. Science Translational Medicine, 9(376), eaaf9655;

Ramírez-Boscá, A., Navarro-López, V., Martínez-Andrés, A., Such, J., Francés, R., de la Parte, J. H., & Asín-Llorca, M. (2015). Identification of bacterial DNA in the peripheral blood of patients with active psoriasis. JAMA dermatology, 151(6), 670-671

Scher, J. U., Sczesnak, A., Longman, R. S., Segata, N., Ubeda, C., Bielski, C., ... Littman, D. R. (2013). Expansion of intestinal Prevotella copri correlates with enhanced susceptibility to arthritis. eLife, 2, e01202.

Maeda, Y., Kurakawa, T., Umemoto, E., Motooka, D., Ito, Y., Gotoh, K., ... & Sakaguchi, N. (2016). Dysbiosis contributes to arthritis development via activation of autoreactive T cells in the intestine. Arthritis & Rheumatology, 68(11), 2646-2661.

Chen, J., Wright, K., Davis, J. M., Jeraldo, P., Marietta, E. V., Murray, J., ... & Taneja, V. (2016). An expansion of rare lineage intestinal microbes characterizes rheumatoid arthritis. Genome medicine, 8(1), 43.

83   Meadows, S. (2013, February 1). The Boy with the Thorn in his Joints. *The New York Times*, Magazine.

84   Kohn, D (2015, January 12). Joint Pain, from the Gut. *The Atlantic*

85   Horton, D. B., Scott, F. I., Haynes, K., Putt, M. E., Rose, C. D., Lewis, J. D., & Strom, B. L. (2015). Antibiotic exposure and juvenile idio-

pathic arthritis: a case–control study. Pediatrics, peds-2015

86   Marra, F., Marra, C. A., Richardson, K., Lynd, L. D., Kozyrskyj, A., Patrick, D. M., ... & FitzGerald, J. M. (2009). Antibiotic use in children is associated with increased risk of asthma. Pediatrics, 123(3), 1003-1010.

87   Ungaro, R., Bernstein, C. N., Gearry, R., Hviid, A., Kolho, K. L., Kronman, M. P., ... & Atreja, A. (2014). Antibiotics associated with increased risk of new-onset Crohn's disease but not ulcerative colitis: a meta-analysis. The American journal of gastroenterology, 109(11), 1728-1738.

88   Zaura, E., Brandt, B. W., de Mattos, M. J. T., Buijs, M. J., Caspers, M. P., Rashid, M. U., ... & Coates, A. R. (2015). Same exposure but two radically different responses to antibiotics: Resilience of the salivary microbiome versus long-term microbial shifts in feces. MBio, 6(6), e01693-15.

89   Song, H. J., Shim, K. N., Jung, S. A., Choi, H. J., Lee, M. A., Ryu, K. H., ... & Yoo, K. (2008). Antibiotic-associated diarrhea: candidate organisms other than Clostridium difficile. The Korean journal of internal medicine, 23(1), 9.
Högenauer, C., Hammer, H. F., Krejs, G. J., & Reisinger, C. (1998). Mechanisms and management of antibiotic-associated diarrhea. Clinical infectious diseases, 27(4), 702-710.

90   Hanson, L., VandeVusse, L., Jermé, M., Abad, C. L., & Safdar, N. (2016). Probiotics for Treatment and Prevention of Urogenital Infections in Women: A Systematic Review. Journal of Midwifery & Women's Health, 61(3), 339-355.

91   Zhang, L., Huang, Y., Zhou, Y., Buckley, T., & Wang, H. H. (2013). Antibiotic administration routes significantly influence the levels of antibiotic resistance in gut microbiota. *Antimicrobial agents and chemotherapy*, 57(8), 3659-3666.

92   FSIS RESIDUE VIOLATION INFORMATION SYSTEM, December 6, 2016. Available online at www.fsis.usda.gov

93   FSIS RESIDUE VIOLATION INFORMATION SYSTEM, December 6, 2016. Available online at www.fsis.usda.gov

Chapter 2. Rebalancing the Microbiome with Probiotics

94   Canani, R. B., Sangwan, N., Stefka, A. T., Nocerino, R., Paparo, L., Aitoro, R., ... & Nagler, C. R. (2016). Lactobacillus rhamnosus GG-supplemented formula expands butyrate-producing bacterial strains in food allergic infants. The ISME journal, 10(3), 742-750.

95   Falony, G., Vlachou, A., Verbrugghe, K., & De Vuyst, L. (2006).

Cross-feeding between Bifidobacterium longum BB536 and acetate-converting, butyrate-producing colon bacteria during growth on oligofructose. Applied and environmental microbiology, 72(12), 7835-7841.

96   Rios-Covian, D., Gueimonde, M., Duncan, S. H., Flint, H. J., & Clara, G. (2015). Enhanced butyrate formation by cross-feeding between Faecalibacterium prausnitzii and Bifidobacterium adolescentis. FEMS microbiology letters, 362(21), fnv176.
      Rivière, A., Gagnon, M., Weckx, S., Roy, D., & De Vuyst, L. (2015). Mutual cross-feeding interactions between Bifidobacterium longum subsp. longum NCC2705 and Eubacterium rectale ATCC 33656 explain the bifidogenic and butyrogenic effects of arabinoxylan oligosaccharides. Applied and environmental microbiology, 81(22), 7767-7781.
      Rivière, A., Gagnon, M., Weckx, S., Roy, D., & De Vuyst, L. (2015). Mutual cross-feeding interactions between Bifidobacterium longum subsp. longum NCC2705 and Eubacterium rectale ATCC 33656 explain the bifidogenic and butyrogenic effects of arabinoxylan oligosaccharides. Applied and environmental microbiology, 81(22), 7767-7781.

97   Falony, G., Vlachou, A., Verbrugghe, K., & De Vuyst, L. (2006). Cross-feeding between Bifidobacterium longum BB536 and acetate-converting, butyrate-producing colon bacteria during growth on oligofructose. Applied and environmental microbiology, 72(12), 7835-7841.
      Sugahara, H., Odamaki, T., Fukuda, S., Kato, T., Xiao, J. Z., Abe, F., ... & Ohno, H. (2015). Probiotic Bifidobacterium longum alters gut luminal metabolism through modification of the gut microbial community. Scientific reports, 5, 13548.
      Rios-Covian, D., Gueimonde, M., Duncan, S. H., Flint, H. J., & Clara, G. (2015). Enhanced butyrate formation by cross-feeding between Faecalibacterium prausnitzii and Bifidobacterium adolescentis. FEMS microbiology letters, 362(21), fnv176.
      Quagliariello, A., Aloisio, I., Bozzi Cionci, N., Luiselli, D., D'Auria, G., Martinez-Priego, L., ... & Di Gioia, D. (2016). Effect of Bifidobacterium breve on the Intestinal Microbiota of Coeliac Children on a Gluten Free Diet: A Pilot Study. Nutrients, 8(10), 660.

98   Leahy, S. C., Higgins, D. G., Fitzgerald, G. F., & Sinderen, D. V. (2005). Getting better with bifidobacteria. Journal of Applied Microbiology, 98(6), 1303-1315.

99   Ishibashi, N., Yaeshima, T., & Hayasawa, H. (1997). Bifidobacteria: their significance in human intestinal health. Mal J Nutr, 3, 149-159.

100   Rios-Covian, D., Gueimonde, M., Duncan, S. H., Flint, H. J., & Clara, G. (2015). Enhanced butyrate formation by cross-feeding

between Faecalibacterium prausnitzii and Bifidobacterium adolescentis. FEMS microbiology letters, 362(21), fnv176.

Rivière, A., Gagnon, M., Weckx, S., Roy, D., & De Vuyst, L. (2015). Mutual cross-feeding interactions between Bifidobacterium longum subsp. longum NCC2705 and Eubacterium rectale ATCC 33656 explain the bifidogenic and butyrogenic effects of arabinoxylan oligosaccharides. Applied and environmental microbiology, 81(22), 7767-7781.

101 Trosvik, P., & Muinck, E. J. (2015). Ecology of bacteria in the human gastrointestinal tract—identification of keystone and foundation taxa. Microbiome, 3(1), 44.

102 Mogna, L., Del Piano, M., Deidda, F., Nicola, S., Soattini, L., Debiaggi, R., ... & Mogna, G. (2012). Assessment of the in vitro inhibitory activity of specific probiotic bacteria against different Escherichia coli strains. Journal of clinical gastroenterology, 46, S29-S32.

Lemoli, E., Trabattoni, D., Parisotto, S., Borgonovo, L., Toscano, M., Rizzardini, G., ... & Piconi, S. (2012). Probiotics reduce gut microbial translocation and improve adult atopic dermatitis. Journal of clinical gastroenterology, 46, S33-S40.

Gibson, G. R., & Wang, X. (1994). Regulatory effects of bifidobacteria on the growth of other colonic bacteria. Journal of Applied Bacteriology, 77(4), 412-420.

Aloisio, I., Santini, C., Biavati, B., Dinelli, G., Cencič, A., Chingwaru, W., ... & Di Gioia, D. (2012). Characterization of Bifidobacterium spp. strains for the treatment of enteric disorders in newborns. Applied microbiology and biotechnology, 96(6), 1561-1576.

103 Bin-Nun, A., Bromiker, R., Wilschanski, M., Kaplan, M., Rudensky, B., Caplan, M., & Hammerman, C. (2005). Oral probiotics prevent necrotizing enterocolitis in very low birth weight neonates. The Journal of pediatrics, 147(2), 192-196.

Lievin, V., Peiffer, I., Hudault, S., Rochat, F., Brassart, D., Neeser, J. R., & Servin, A. L. (2000). Bifidobacterium strains from resident infant human gastrointestinal microflora exert antimicrobial activity. Gut, 47(5), 646-652.

Viswanathan, S., Lau, C., Akbari, H., Hoyen, C., & Walsh, M. C. (2016). Survey and evidence based review of probiotics used in very low birth weight preterm infants within the United States. Journal of Perinatology.

104 Athalye-Jape, G., Rao, S., & Patole, S. (2016). Lactobacillus reuteri DSM 17938 as a probiotic for preterm neonates: a strain-specific systematic review. Journal of parenteral and enteral nutrition, 40(6), 783-794.

Savino, F., Cordisco, L., Tarasco, V., Palumeri, E., Calabrese, R., Oggero, R., ... & Matteuzzi, D. (2010). Lactobacillus reuteri DSM 17938 in infantile colic: a randomized, double-blind, placebo-controlled trial. *Pediatrics*, *126*(3), e526-e533.

105   Gutierrez-Castrellon, P., Lopez-Velazquez, G., Diaz-Garcia, L., Jimenez-Gutierrez, C., Mancilla-Ramirez, J., Estevez-Jimenez, J., & Parra, M. (2014). Diarrhea in preschool children and Lactobacillus reuteri: a randomized controlled trial. *Pediatrics*, *133*(4), e904-e909

106   Ojetti, V., Petruzziello, C., Migneco, A., Gnarra, M., Gasbarrini, A., & Franceschi, F. (2017). Effect of Lactobacillus reuteri (DSM 17938) on methane production in patients affected by functional constipation: a retrospective study. *Eur Rev Med Pharmacol Sci*, *21*(7), 1702-1708.

107   Morrow, L. E., Kollef, M. H., & Casale, T. B. (2010). Probiotic prophylaxis of ventilator-associated pneumonia: a blinded, randomized, controlled trial. *American journal of respiratory and critical care medicine*, *182*(8), 1058-1064.
McFarland, L. V. (2015). Probiotics for the primary and secondary prevention of C. difficile infections: a meta-analysis and systematic review. *Antibiotics*, *4*(2), 160-178.

108   Canani, R. B., Cirillo, P., Terrin, G., Cesarano, L., Spagnuolo, M. I., De Vincenzo, A.,...& Guarino, A. (2007). Probiotics for treatment of acute diarrhoea in children: randomised clinical trial of five different preparations. *Bmj*, *335*(7615), 340.

109   McFarland, L. V. (2015). Probiotics for the primary and secondary prevention of C. difficile infections: a meta-analysis and systematic review. *Antibiotics*, *4*(2), 160-178.
Scaldaferri, F., Gerardi, V., Mangiola, F., Lopetuso, L. R., Pizzoferrato, M., Petito, V.,...& Gasbarrini, A. (2016). Role and mechanisms of action of Escherichia coli Nissle 1917 in the maintenance of remission in ulcerative colitis patients: an update. World journal of gastroenterology, 22(24), 5505

110   Auclair, J., Frappier, M., & Millette, M. (2015). Lactobacillus acidophilus CL1285, Lactobacillus casei LBC80R, and Lactobacillus rhamnosus CLR2 (Bio-K+): characterization, manufacture, mechanisms of action, and quality control of a specific probiotic combination for primary prevention of Clostridium difficile infection. Clinical Infectious Diseases, 60(suppl_2), S135-S143.

111   Beausoleil, M., Fortier, N.A., Guinette, S., L'Ecuyer, A., Savoie, M., Weiss, K., Lachaine, J., and Franco, M. (2004) Effect of a *Lactobacillus acidophilus* and *casei*-fermented milk in the primary prevention of antibiotic-associated diarrhea (lactic trial) : a randomized, double-blind, placebo-controlled trial. In *69th Annual Scientific Meeting and Post-graduate Course, November 2004*. Orlando, FL: American College of Gastroenterology.

112 Gao, X. W., Mubasher, M., Fang, C. Y., Reifer, C., & Miller, L. E. (2010). Dose–response efficacy of a proprietary probiotic formula of Lactobacillus acidophilus CL1285 and Lactobacillus casei LBC80R for antibiotic-associated diarrhea and Clostridium difficile-associated diarrhea prophylaxis in adult patients. The American journal of gastroenterology, 105(7), 1636.

113 Song, H. J., Shim, K. N., Jung, S. A., Choi, H. J., Lee, M. A., Ryu, K. H.,...& Yoo, K. (2008). Antibiotic-associated diarrhea: candidate organisms other than Clostridium difficile. The Korean journal of internal medicine, 23(1), 9.
Högenauer, C., Hammer, H. F., Krejs, G. J., & Reisinger, C. (1998). Mechanisms and management of antibiotic-associated diarrhea. Clinical infectious diseases, 27(4), 702-710

114 Millette, M., Luquet, F. M., & Lacroix, M. (2007). In vitro growth control of selected pathogens by Lactobacillus acidophilus-and Lactobacillus casei-fermented milk. Letters in applied microbiology, 44(3), 314-319.

115 Reddy, N. R., & Pierson, M. D. (1994). Reduction in antinutritional and toxic components in plant foods by fermentationa. Food Research International, 27(3), 281-290.

116 Nazareth, S., Lebwohl, B., Voyksner, J. S., & Green, P. H. (2015). 108 Widespread Contamination of Probiotics With Gluten, Detected by Liquid Chromatography-Mass Spectrometry. Gastroenterology, 148(4), S-28.

117 Millette, M., Nguyen, A., Amine, K. M., & Lacroix, M. (2013). Gastrointestinal survival of bacteria in commercial probiotic products. International Journal of Probiotics & Prebiotics, 8(4), 149.

118 Scaldaferri, F., Gerardi, V., Mangiola, F., Lopetuso, L. R., Pizzoferrato, M., Petito, V.,...& Gasbarrini, A. (2016). Role and mechanisms of action of Escherichia coli Nissle 1917 in the maintenance of remission in ulcerative colitis patients: an update. World journal of gastroenterology, 22(24), 5505.
Sonnenborn, U., & Schulze, J. (2009). The non-pathogenic Escherichia coli strain Nissle 1917–features of a versatile probiotic. Microbial Ecology in Health and Disease, 21(3-4), 122-158.

119 Kruis, W., Frič, P., Pokrotnieks, J., Lukáš, M., Fixa, B., Kaščák, M.,...& Wolff, C. (2004). Maintaining remission of ulcerative colitis with the probiotic Escherichia coli Nissle 1917 is as effective as with standard mesalazine. Gut, 53(11), 1617-1623.
Rembacken, B. J., Snelling, A. M., Hawkey, P. M., Chalmers, D. M., & Axon, A. T. R. (1999). Non-pathogenic Escherichia coli versus mesalazine for the treatment of ulcerative colitis: a randomised trial. The Lancet, 354(9179), 635-639.

120   Malchow HA. Crohn's disease and Escherichia coli. A new approach in therapy to maintain remission of colonic Crohn's disease? J Clin Gastroenterol (1997) 25(4):653–8.10.

121   Reissbrodt R, Hammes WP, dal Bello F, Prager R, Fruth A, Hantke K, Rakin A, Starcic-Erjavec M, Williams PH. Inhibition of growth of Shiga toxin-producing Escherichia coli by nonpathogenic Escherichia coli. FEMS Microbiol Lett. 2009;290:62–69.
Lasaro MA, Salinger N, Zhang J, Wang Y, Zhong Z, Goulian M, Zhu J. F1C fimbriae play an important role in biofilm formation and intestinal colonization by the Escherichia coli commensal strain Nissle 1917. Appl Environ Microbiol. 2009;75:246–251
Boudeau J, Glasser AL, Neut C, et al. Invasive ability of Escherichia coli strains isolated from ileal mucosa in Crohn's disease. Gastroenterology2000; 118(S2): A1847.
Darfeuille-Michaud A, Neut C, Barnich N, et al.Presence of adherent Escherichia coli strains in ileal mucosa of patients with Crohn's disease. Gastroenterology 1998; 115(6): 1405–13.
Lederman E, Neut C, Desreumaux P, et al. Bacterial overgrowth in the neoterminal ileum after ileocolonic resection for Crohn's disease. Gastroenterology 1997; 112: A1023
Boudeau J, Glasser AL, Masseret E, Joly B, Darfeuille-Michaud A. Invasive ability of an Escherichia coli strain isolated from the ileal mucosa of a patient with Crohn's disease. Infect Immun 1999; 67(9): 4499–509.
Swidsinski, A., Swidsinski, S., Godzun, A., Orthner, M., & Lochs, H. (2000). Therapy with E. coli Nissle reduces concentrations of mucosa associated colonic flora in patients with ulcerative colitis. Gastroenterology, 118(4), A1138.

122   Boudeau, J., Glasser, A. L., Julien, S., Colombel, J. F., & Darfeuille-Michaud, A. (2003). Inhibitory effect of probiotic Escherichia coli strain Nissle 1917 on adhesion to and invasion of intestinal epithelial cells by adherent–invasive E. coli strains isolated from patients with Crohn's disease. Alimentary pharmacology & therapeutics, 18(1), 45-56.
Huebner, C., Ding, Y., Petermann, I., Knapp, C., & Ferguson, L. R. (2011). The probiotic Escherichia coli Nissle 1917 reduces pathogen invasion and modulates cytokine expression in Caco-2 cells infected with Crohn's disease-associated E. coli LF82. Applied and environmental microbiology, 77(7), 2541-2544.

123   Hancock, V., Dahl, M., & Klemm, P. (2010). Probiotic Escherichia coli strain Nissle 1917 outcompetes intestinal pathogens during biofilm formation. Journal of medical microbiology, 59(4), 392-399.

124   Altenhoefer, A., Oswald, S., Sonnenborn, U., Enders, C., Schulze, J., Hacker, J., & Oelschlaeger, T. A. (2004). The probiotic Escherichia

coli strain Nissle 1917 interferes with invasion of human intestinal epithelial cells by different enteroinvasive bacterial pathogens. FEMS Immunology & Medical Microbiology, 40(3), 223-229.

Storm, D. W., Koff, S. A., Horvath, D. J., Li, B., & Justice, S. S. (2011). In vitro analysis of the bactericidal activity of Escherichia coli Nissle 1917 against pediatric uropathogens. The Journal of urology, 186(4), 1678-1683.

125   Lodinová-Žádníková, R., & Sonnenborn, U. (1997). Effect of preventive administration of a nonpathogenic Escherichia coli strain on the colonization of the intestine with microbial pathogens in newborn infants. Neonatology, 71(4), 224-232.

126   Kamada, N., Maeda, K., Inoue, N., Hisamatsu, T., Okamoto, S., Hong, K. S.,... & Hibi, T. (2008). Nonpathogenic Escherichia coli strain Nissle 1917 inhibits signal transduction in intestinal epithelial cells. Infection and immunity, 76(1), 214-220.

Splichalova, A., Trebichavsky, I., Rada, V., Vlkova, E., Sonnenborn, U., & Splichal, I. (2011). Interference of Bifidobacterium choerinum or Escherichia coli Nissle 1917 with Salmonella Typhimurium in gnotobiotic piglets correlates with cytokine patterns in blood and intestine. Clinical & Experimental Immunology, 163(2), 242-249

Swidsinski, A., Swidsinski, S., Godzun, A., Orthner, M., & Lochs, H. (2000). Therapy with E. coli Nissle reduces concentrations of mucosa associated colonic flora in patients with ulcerative colitis. *Gastroenterology, 118*(4), A1138.

127   FDA Memorandum to Medical Futures, Inc., Re: 75-Day Premarket Notification of New Dietary Ingredients, E.coli Nissle 1917. Dated November 16, 2011.

128   McFarland, L. V. (2010). Systematic review and meta-analysis of Saccharomyces boulardii in adult patients. World journal of gastroenterology: WJG, 16(18), 2202.

129   McFarland, L. V. (2010). Systematic review and meta-analysis of Saccharomyces boulardii in adult patients. World journal of gastroenterology: WJG, 16(18), 2202.

130   Lewis SJ, Potts LF, Barry RE. The lack of therapeutic effect of Saccharomyces boulardii in the prevention of antibiotic-related diarrhoea in elderly patients. J Infect. 1998;36:171–174.

Cremonini F, Di Caro S, Covino M, Armuzzi A, Gabrielli M, Santarelli L, Nista EC, Cammarota G, Gasbarrini G, Gasbarrini A. Effect of different probiotic preparations on anti-helicobacter pylori therapy-related side effects: a parallel group, triple blind, placebo-controlled study. Am J Gastroenterol. 2002;97:2744–2749.

Can M, Beşirbellioglu BA, Avci IY, Beker CM, Pahsa A. Prophylactic Saccharomyces boulardii in the prevention of antibiotic-associated diarrhea: a prospective study. Med Sci Monit. 2006;12:PI19–PI22.

Bravo MV, Bunout D, Leiva L, de la Maza MP, Barrera G, de la Maza J, Hirsch S. [Effect of probiotic Saccharomyces boulardii on prevention of antibiotic-associated diarrhea in adult outpatients with amoxicillin treatment] Rev Med Chil. 2008;136:981–988.

Adam J, Barret C, Barret-Bellet A, Benedetti E, Calendini A, Darchen P, Galibert JM, Guerci P, Guiot G, Haechler M, et al. Controlled double-blind clinical trials of Ultra-Levure: multi centre study by 25 physicians in 388 cases. Gazette Medicale de France. 1977;84:2072–2078

Cindoruk M, Erkan G, Karakan T, Dursun A, Unal S. Efficacy and safety of Saccharomyces boulardii in the 14-day triple anti-Helicobacter pylori therapy: a prospective randomized placebo-controlled double-blind study. Helicobacter. 2007;12:309–316.

Duman DG, Bor S, Ozütemiz O, Sahin T, Oğuz D, Iştan F, Vural T, Sandkci M, Işksal F, Simşek I, et al. Efficacy and safety of Saccharomyces boulardii in prevention of antibiotic-associated diarrhoea due to Helicobacterpylori eradication. Eur J Gastroenterol Hepatol. 2005;17:1357–1361

McFarland LV, Surawicz CM, Greenberg RN, Elmer GW, Moyer KA, Melcher SA, Bowen KE, Cox JL. Prevention of beta-lactam-associated diarrhea by Saccharomyces boulardii compared with placebo. Am J Gastroenterol. 1995;90:439–448.

McFarland, L. V. (2010). Systematic review and meta-analysis of Saccharomyces boulardii in adult patients. *World journal of gastroenterology: WJG, 16*(18), 2202.

Monteiro E, Fernandes JP, Vieira MR, Correia JP, Caetano JM, Ribeiro T, Antunes AB, Noronha R, Batista F, Reis L, et al. [Double blind clinical trial on the use of ultra-levure in the prophylaxis of antibiotic induced gastro-intestinal and mucocutaneous disorders] Acta Med Port. 1981;3:143–145.

Surawicz CM, Elmer GW, Speelman P, McFarland LV, Chinn J, van Belle G. Prevention of antibiotic-associated diarrhea by Saccharomyces boulardii: a prospective study. Gastroenterology. 1989;96:981–988.

131   Kabbani, T. A., Pallav, K., Dowd, S. E., Villafuerte-Galvez, J., Vanga, R. R., Castillo, N. E., ... & Kelly, C. P. (2017). Prospective randomized controlled study on the effects of Saccharomyces boulardii CNCM I-745 and amoxicillin-clavulanate or the combination on the gut microbiota of healthy volunteers. *Gut microbes, 8*(1), 17-32.

132   Hochter W, Chase D, Hagenhoff G. Saccharomyces boulardii in acute adult diarrhea: efficacy and tolerability of treatment. Munch Med Wschr. 1990;132:188–192.

Besirbellioglu BA, Ulcay A, Can M, Erdem H, Tanyuksel M, Avci IY, Araz E, Pahsa A. Saccharomyces boulardii and infection due to

Giardia lamblia. Scand J Infect Dis. 2006;38:479–481

Mansour-Ghanaei F, Dehbashi N, Yazdanparast K, Shafaghi A. Efficacy of saccharomyces boulardii with antibiotics in acute amoebiasis. World J Gastroenterol. 2003;9:1832–1833

Buts JP, Corthier G, Delmee M. Saccharomyces boulardii for Clostridium difficile-associated enteropathies in infants. J Pediatr Gastroenterol Nutr. 1993;16:419–425.

Surawicz CM, McFarland LV, Elmer G, Chinn J. Treatment of recurrent Clostridium difficile colitis with vancomycin and Saccharomyces boulardii. Am J Gastroenterol. 1989;84:1285–1287.

Hassett J, Meyers S, McFarland L, Mulligan ME. Recurrent Clostridium difficile infection in a patient with selective IgG1 deficiency treated with intravenous immune globulin and Saccharomyces boulardii. Clin Infect Dis. 1995;20 Suppl 2:S266–S268

Popoola J, Swann A, Warwick G. Clostridium difficile in patients with renal failure - management of an outbreak using biotherapy. Nephrol Dial Transplant. 2000;15:571–574

133   Hochter W, Chase D, Hagenhoff G. Saccharomyces boulardii in acute adult diarrhea: efficacy and tolerability of treatment. Munch Med Wschr. 1990;132:188–192.

Dinleyici, E. C., Kara, A., Dalgic, N., Kurugol, Z., Arica, V., Metin, O., ... & Bulut, S. (2015). Saccharomyces boulardii CNCM I-745 reduces the duration of diarrhoea, length of emergency care and hospital stay in children with acute diarrhoea. *Beneficial microbes*, 6(4), 415-421.

134   Ducluzeau, R., & Bensaada, M. (1982). Comparative effect of a single or continuous administration of" Saccharomyces boulardii" on the establishment of various strains of" candida" in the digestive tract of gnotobiotic mice. In *Annales de microbiologie* (Vol. 133, No. 3, pp. 491-501).

Zbinden R, Bonczi E, Altwegg M. Inhibition of Saccharomyces boulardii (nom. inval.) on cell invasion of Salmonella typhimurium and Yersinia enterocolitica. Micro Ecol Health Dis. 1999;11:158–162.

Altwegg M, Schnack J, Zbinden R. Influence of Saccharomyces boulardii on Aeromonas hemolysin. Med Microbiol Lett. 1995;4:417–425.

135   Buts JP, Dekeyser N, Stilmant C, Delem E, Smets F, Sokal E. Saccharomyces boulardii produces in rat small intestine a novel protein phosphatase that inhibits Escherichia coli endotoxin by dephosphorylation. Pediatr Res. 2006;60:24–29

Castagliuolo I, Riegler MF, Valenick L, LaMont JT, Pothoulakis C. Saccharomyces boulardii protease inhibits the effects of Clostridium difficile toxins A and B in human colonic mucosa. Infect Immun. 1999;67:302–307.

Vidon N, Huchet B, Rambaud JC. Effect of S. boulardii on water

and sodium secretions induced by cholera toxin. Gastroenterol Clin
Biol. 1986;10:1–4.
Czerucka D, Rampal P. Effect of Saccharomyces boulardii on
cAMP- and Ca2+ -dependent Cl- secretion in T84 cells. Dig Dis
Sci. 1999;44:2359–2368

136   Ducluzeau, R., & Bensaada, M. (1982). Comparative effect of a
single or continuous administration of" Saccharomyces boulardii"
on the establishment of various strains of" candida" in the digestive
tract of gnotobiotic mice. In *Annales de microbiologie* (Vol. 133,
No. 3, pp. 491-501).

137   Krasowska, A., Murzyn, A., Dyjankiewicz, A., Łukaszewicz, M., &
Dziadkowiec, D. (2009). The antagonistic effect of Saccharomyces
boulardii on Candida albicans filamentation, adhesion and biofilm
formation. *FEMS yeast research*, *9*(8), 1312-1321.
Murzyn, A., Krasowska, A., Stefanowicz, P., Dziadkowiec, D., &
Łukaszewicz, M. (2010). Capric acid secreted by S. boulardii inhibits
C. albicans filamentous growth, adhesion and biofilm formation. *PloS one*, *5*(8), e12050.
Jawhara S, Poulain D. *Saccharomyces boulardii* decreases inflammation and intestinal colonization by Candida albicans in a mouse
model of chemically-induced colitis. Med Mycol. 2007;45(8):691–700

138   Kumamoto, C. A. (2011). Inflammation and gastrointestinal Candida colonization. *Current opinion in microbiology*, *14*(4), 386-391.

139   Sokol, H., Leducq, V., Aschard, H., Pham, H. P., Jegou, S., Landman,
C.,…& Cosnes, J. (2016). Fungal microbiota dysbiosis in IBD. *Gut*,
gutjnl-2015.
Liguori, G., Lamas, B., Richard, M. L., Brandi, G., Da Costa, G.,
Hoffmann, T. W.,…& Campieri, M. (2015). Fungal dysbiosis in
mucosa-associated microbiota of Crohn's disease patients. *Journal
of Crohn's and Colitis*, *10*(3), 296-305.

140   Kumamoto, C. A. (2011). Inflammation and gastrointestinal Candida colonization. *Current opinion in microbiology*, *14*(4), 386-391.

141   Garcia Vilela E, De Lourdes De Abreu Ferrari M, Oswaldo Da
Gama Torres H, Guerra Pinto A, Carolina Carneiro Aguirre A,
Paiva Martins F, Marcos Andrade Goulart E, Sales Da Cunha A.
Influence of Saccharomyces boulardii on the intestinal permeability
of patients with Crohn's disease in remission. Scand J Gastroen-
terol. 2008;43:842–848.

142   Guslandi, M., Mezzi, G., Sorghi, M., & Testoni, P. A. (2000). Saccharomyces boulardii in maintenance treatment of Crohn's disease. *Digestive diseases and sciences*, *45*(7), 1462-1464.

143   Plein K, Hotz J. Therapeutic effects of Saccharomyces boulardii on
mild residual symptoms in a stable phase of Crohn's disease with

special respect to chronic diarrhea—a pilot study. Z Gastroenterol. 1993;31:129–134.

144 Lherm, T., Monet, C., Nougière, B., Soulier, M., Larbi, D., Le Gall, C.,... & Malbrunot, C. (2002). Seven cases of fungemia with Saccharomyces boulardii in critically ill patients. *Intensive care medicine, 28*(6), 797-801.

145 Kwak, D. S., Jun, D. W., Seo, J. G., Chung, W. S., Park, S. E., Lee, K. N.,... & Choi, H. S. (2014). Short-term probiotic therapy alleviates small intestinal bacterial overgrowth, but does not improve intestinal permeability in chronic liver disease. *European journal of gastroenterology & hepatology, 26*(12), 1353-1359.

146 Soifer, L. O., Peralta, D., Dima, G., & Besasso, H. (2010). Comparative clinical efficacy of a probiotic vs. an antibiotic in the treatment of patients with intestinal bacterial overgrowth and chronic abdominal functional distension: a pilot study. *Acta gastroenterologica Latinoamericana, 40*(4), 323-327

147 Gabrielli M, Lauritano EC, Scarpellini E, Lupascu A, Ojetti V, Gasbarrini G, Silveri NG, Gasbarrini A. Bacillus clausii as a treatment of small intestinal bacterial overgrowth. Am J Gastroenterol. 2009;104:1327–1328.
Khalighi, A. R., Khalighi, M. R., Behdani, R., Jamali, J., Khosravi, A., Kouhestani, S.,... & Khalighi, N. (2014). Evaluating the efficacy of probiotic on treatment in patients with small intestinal bacterial overgrowth (SIBO)-A pilot study. *The Indian journal of medical research, 140*(5), 604.
Barrett, J. S., Canale, K. E., Gearry, R. B., Irving, P. M., & Gibson, P. R. (2008). Probiotic effects on intestinal fermentation patterns in patients with irritable bowel syndrome. *World journal of gastroenterology: WJG, 14*(32), 5020.

148 Uribarri, J., Oh, M. S., & Carroll, H. J. (1998). D-lactic acidosis: a review of clinical presentation, biochemical features, and pathophysiologic mechanisms. *MEDICINE-BALTIMORE-, 77*, 73-82

149 Sheedy, J. R., Wettenhall, R. E., Scanlon, D., Gooley, P. R., Lewis, D. P., Mcgregor, N.,... & De Meirleir, K. L. (2009). Increased d-lactic acid intestinal bacteria in patients with chronic fatigue syndrome. *in vivo, 23*(4), 621-628.

150 Bures, J., Cyrany, J., Kohoutova, D., Förstl, M., Rejchrt, S., Kvetina, J.,... & Kopacova, M. (2010). Small intestinal bacterial overgrowth syndrome. *World journal of gastroenterology: WJG, 16*(24), 2978.
Yamaguchi, N., Sugita, R., Miki, A., Takemura, N., Kawabata, J., Watanabe, J., & Sonoyama, K. (2006). Gastrointestinal Candida colonisation promotes sensitisation against food antigens by affecting the mucosal barrier in mice. *Gut, 55*(7), 954-960.

151   Canani, R. B., Costanzo, M. D., Leone, L., Pedata, M., Meli, R., & Calignano, A. (2011). Potential beneficial effects of butyrate in intestinal and extraintestinal diseases. World J Gastroenterol, 17(12), 1519-1528.

Plöger, S., Stumpff, F., Penner, G. B., Schulzke, J. D., Gäbel, G., Martens, H.,...& Aschenbach, J. R. (2012). Microbial butyrate and its role for barrier function in the gastrointestinal tract. Annals of the New York Academy of Sciences, 1258(1), 52-59.

Willemsen, L. E. M., Koetsier, M. A., Van Deventer, S. J. H., & Van Tol, E. A. F. (2003). Short chain fatty acids stimulate epithelial mucin 2 expression through differential effects on prostaglandin E1 and E2 production by intestinal myofibroblasts. Gut, 52(10), 1442-1447.

Burger-van Paassen, N., Vincent, A., Puiman, P. J., Van Der Sluis, M., Bouma, J., Boehm, G.,...& Renes, I. B. (2009). The regulation of intestinal mucin MUC2 expression by short-chain fatty acids: implications for epithelial protection. Biochemical Journal, 420(2), 211-219.

Kripke, S. A., Fox, A. D., Berman, J. M., Settle, R. G., & Rombeau, J. L. (1989). Stimulation of intestinal mucosal growth with intracolonic infusion of short-chain fatty acids. Journal of Parenteral and Enteral Nutrition, 13(2), 109-116.

Johansson, M. E., Gustafsson, J. K., Holmén-Larsson, J., Jabbar, K. S., Xia, L., Xu, H.,...& Hansson, G. C. (2013). Bacteria penetrate the normally impenetrable inner colon mucus layer in both murine colitis models and patients with ulcerative colitis. Gut, gutjnl-2012

152   Canani, R. B., Costanzo, M. D., Leone, L., Pedata, M., Meli, R., & Calignano, A. (2011). Potential beneficial effects of butyrate in intestinal and extraintestinal diseases. World J Gastroenterol, 17(12), 1519-1528.

Plöger, S., Stumpff, F., Penner, G. B., Schulzke, J. D., Gäbel, G., Martens, H.,...& Aschenbach, J. R. (2012). Microbial butyrate and its role for barrier function in the gastrointestinal tract. Annals of the New York Academy of Sciences, 1258(1), 52-59.

Willemsen, L. E. M., Koetsier, M. A., Van Deventer, S. J. H., & Van Tol, E. A. F. (2003). Short chain fatty acids stimulate epithelial mucin 2 expression through differential effects on prostaglandin E1 and E2 production by intestinal myofibroblasts. Gut, 52(10), 1442-1447.

Burger-van Paassen, N., Vincent, A., Puiman, P. J., Van Der Sluis, M., Bouma, J., Boehm, G.,...& Renes, I. B. (2009). The regulation of intestinal mucin MUC2 expression by short-chain fatty acids: implications for epithelial protection. Biochemical Journal, 420(2), 211-219.

Kripke, S. A., Fox, A. D., Berman, J. M., Settle, R. G., & Rombeau, J. L. (1989). Stimulation of intestinal mucosal growth with intracolonic infusion of short-chain fatty acids. Journal of Parenteral and Enteral Nutrition, 13(2), 109-116.

Hsieh, C. Y., Osaka, T., Moriyama, E., Date, Y., Kikuchi, J., & Tsuneda, S. (2015). Strengthening of the intestinal epithelial tight junction by Bifidobacterium bifidum. Physiological reports, 3(3), e12327.

Ewaschuk, J. B., Diaz, H., Meddings, L., Diederichs, B., Dmytrash, A., Backer, J., ... & Madsen, K. L. (2008). Secreted bioactive factors from Bifidobacterium infantis enhance epithelial cell barrier function. American Journal of Physiology-Gastrointestinal and Liver Physiology, 295(5), G1025-G1034.

Suzuki, T., Yoshida, S., & Hara, H. (2008). Physiological concentrations of short-chain fatty acids immediately suppress colonic epithelial permeability. British journal of nutrition, 100(02), 297-305;

153 Ewaschuk, J. B., Diaz, H., Meddings, L., Diederichs, B., Dmytrash, A., Backer, J., ... & Madsen, K. L. (2008). Secreted bioactive factors from Bifidobacterium infantis enhance epithelial cell barrier function. American Journal of Physiology-Gastrointestinal and Liver Physiology, 295(5), G1025-G1034.

Ohland, C. L., & MacNaughton, W. K. (2010). Probiotic bacteria and intestinal epithelial barrier function. American Journal of Physiology-Gastrointestinal and Liver Physiology, 298(6), G807-G819.

Hsieh, C. Y., Osaka, T., Moriyama, E., Date, Y., Kikuchi, J., & Tsuneda, S. (2015). Strengthening of the intestinal epithelial tight junction by Bifidobacterium bifidum. Physiological reports, 3(3), e12327.

Zyrek, A. A., Cichon, C., Helms, S., Enders, C., Sonnenborn, U., & Schmidt, M. A. (2007). Molecular mechanisms underlying the probiotic effects of Escherichia coli Nissle 1917 involve ZO-2 and PKCζ redistribution resulting in tight junction and epithelial barrier repair. *Cellular microbiology*, 9(3), 804-816.

Ukena, S. N., Singh, A., Dringenberg, U., Engelhardt, R., Seidler, U., Hansen, W., ... & Suerbaum, S. (2007). Probiotic Escherichia coli Nissle 1917 inhibits leaky gut by enhancing mucosal integrity. *PloS one*, 2(12), e1308

154 Ohland, C. L., & MacNaughton, W. K. (2010). Probiotic bacteria and intestinal epithelial barrier function. American Journal of Physiology-Gastrointestinal and Liver Physiology, 298(6), G807-G819.

Bron, P. A., Kleerebezem, M., Brummer, R. J., Cani, P. D., Mercenier, A., MacDonald, T. T., ... & Wells, J. M. (2017). Can probiotics modulate human disease by impacting intestinal barrier function?. *British Journal of Nutrition*, 117(1), 93-107.

Ewaschuk, J. B., Diaz, H., Meddings, L., Diederichs, B., Dmytrash, A., Backer, J., ... & Madsen, K. L. (2008). Secreted bioactive factors from Bifidobacterium infantis enhance epithelial cell barrier function. American Journal of Physiology-Gastrointestinal and Liver Physiology, 295(5), G1025-G1034.

Mack, D. R., Ahrné, S., Hyde, L., Wei, S., & Hollingsworth, M. A.

(2003). Extracellular MUC3 mucin secretion follows adherence of Lactobacillus strains to intestinal epithelial cells in vitro. *Gut, 52*(6), 827-833

Zyrek, A. A., Cichon, C., Helms, S., Enders, C., Sonnenborn, U., & Schmidt, M. A. (2007). Molecular mechanisms underlying the probiotic effects of Escherichia coli Nissle 1917 involve ZO-2 and PKCζ redistribution resulting in tight junction and epithelial barrier repair. *Cellular microbiology, 9*(3), 804-816.

Ukena, S. N., Singh, A., Dringenberg, U., Engelhardt, R., Seidler, U., Hansen, W., ... & Suerbaum, S. (2007). Probiotic Escherichia coli Nissle 1917 inhibits leaky gut by enhancing mucosal integrity. *PloS one, 2*(12), e1308.

Karczewski, J., Troost, F. J., Konings, I., Dekker, J., Kleerebezem, M., Brummer, R. J. M., & Wells, J. M. (2010). Regulation of human epithelial tight junction proteins by Lactobacillus plantarum in vivo and protective effects on the epithelial barrier. *American Journal of Physiology-Gastrointestinal and Liver Physiology, 298*(6), G851-G859.

Yan, F., Cao, H., Cover, T. L., Washington, M. K., Shi, Y., Liu, L., ... & Polk, D. B. (2011). Colon-specific delivery of a probiotic-derived soluble protein ameliorates intestinal inflammation in mice through an EGFR-dependent mechanism. *The Journal of clinical investigation, 121*(6), 2242-2253.

155   Sagar, S., Vos, A. P., Morgan, M. E., Garssen, J., Georgiou, N. A., Boon, L., ... & Folkerts, G. (2014). The combination of Bifidobacterium breve with non-digestible oligosaccharides suppresses airway inflammation in a murine model for chronic asthma. Biochimica et Biophysica Acta (BBA)-Molecular Basis of Disease, 1842(4), 573-583.

Drago, L., De Vecchi, E., Gabrieli, A., De Grandi, R., & Toscano, M. (2015). Immunomodulatory effects of Lactobacillus salivarius LS01 and Bifidobacterium breve BR03, alone and in combination, on peripheral blood mononuclear cells of allergic asthmatics. Allergy, asthma & immunology research, 7(4), 409-413.

Jeon, S. G., Kayama, H., Ueda, Y., Takahashi, T., Asahara, T., Tsuji, H., ... & Okumura, R. (2012). Probiotic Bifidobacterium breve induces IL-10-producing Tr1 cells in the colon. PLoS Pathog, 8(5), e1002714.

Khokhlova, E. V., Smeianov, V. V., Efimov, B. A., Kafarskaia, L. I., Pavlova, S. I., & Shkoporov, A. N. (2012). Anti-inflammatory properties of intestinal Bifidobacterium strains isolated from healthy infants. Microbiology and immunology, 56(1), 27-39.

Zheng, B., van Bergenhenegouwen, J., Overbeek, S., van de Kant, H. J., Garssen, J., Folkerts, G., ... & Kraneveld, A. D. (2014). Bifidobacterium breve attenuates murine dextran sodium sulfate-induced colitis and increases regulatory T cell responses. PloS one, 9(5), e95441

Konieczna, P., Groeger, D., Ziegler, M., Frei, R., Ferstl, R., Shanahan, F., ... & O'mahony, L. (2011). Bifidobacterium infantis 35624 administration induces Foxp3 T regulatory cells in human peripheral blood: potential role for myeloid and plasmacytoid dendritic cells. Gut, gutjnl-2011

Groeger, D., O'Mahony, L., Murphy, E. F., Bourke, J. F., Dinan, T. G., Kiely, B., ... & Quigley, E. M. (2013). Bifidobacterium infantis 35624 modulates host inflammatory processes beyond the gut. Gut microbes, 4(4), 325-339.

Kwon, H. K., Lee, C. G., So, J. S., Chae, C. S., Hwang, J. S., Sahoo, A., ... & Im, S. H. (2010). Generation of regulatory dendritic cells and CD4+ Foxp3+ T cells by probiotics administration suppresses immune disorders. Proceedings of the National Academy of Sciences, 107(5), 2159-2164.

Thomas, S., Metzke, D., Schmitz, J., Dörffel, Y., & Baumgart, D. C. (2011). Anti-inflammatory effects of Saccharomyces boulardii mediated by myeloid dendritic cells from patients with Crohn's disease and ulcerative colitis. *American Journal of Physiology-Gastrointestinal and Liver Physiology, 301*(6), G1083-G1092.

Spaiser, S. J., Culpepper, T., Nieves Jr, C., Ukhanova, M., Mai, V., Percival, S. S., ... & Langkamp-Henken, B. (2015). Lactobacillus gasseri KS-13, Bifidobacterium bifidum G9-1, and Bifidobacterium longum MM-2 ingestion induces a less inflammatory cytokine profile and a potentially beneficial shift in gut microbiota in older adults: a randomized, double-blind, placebo-controlled, crossover study. Journal of the American College of Nutrition, 34(6), 459-469

Mizuta, M., Yamamoto, S., Inokawa, H., ... & Xiao, J. Z. (2016). Perioperative supplementation with bifidobacteria improves postoperative nutritional recovery, inflammatory response, and fecal microbiota in patients undergoing colorectal surgery: a prospective, randomized clinical trial. Bioscience of microbiota, food and health, 35(2), 77-87.

156   Sagar, S., Vos, A. P., Morgan, M. E., Garssen, J., Georgiou, N. A., Boon, L., ... & Folkerts, G. (2014). The combination of Bifidobacterium breve with non-digestible oligosaccharides suppresses airway inflammation in a murine model for chronic asthma. Biochimica et Biophysica Acta (BBA)-Molecular Basis of Disease, 1842(4), 573-583.

Drago, L., De Vecchi, E., Gabrieli, A., De Grandi, R., & Toscano, M. (2015). Immunomodulatory effects of Lactobacillus salivarius LS01 and Bifidobacterium breve BR03, alone and in combination, on peripheral blood mononuclear cells of allergic asthmatics. Allergy, asthma & immunology research, 7(4), 409-413.

Jeon, S. G., Kayama, H., Ueda, Y., Takahashi, T., Asahara, T., Tsuji, H., ... & Okumura, R. (2012). Probiotic Bifidobacterium breve induces IL-10-producing Tr1 cells in the colon. PLoS Pathog, 8(5), e1002714.

Khokhlova, E. V., Smeianov, V. V., Efimov, B. A., Kafarskaia, L. I., Pavlova, S. I., & Shkoporov, A. N. (2012). Anti-inflammatory properties of intestinal Bifidobacterium strains isolated from healthy infants. Microbiology and immunology, 56(1), 27-39.

Zheng, B., van Bergenhenegouwen, J., Overbeek, S., van de Kant, H. J., Garssen, J., Folkerts, G.,... & Kraneveld, A. D. (2014). Bifidobacterium breve attenuates murine dextran sodium sulfate-induced colitis and increases regulatory T cell responses. PloS one, 9(5), e95441

Konieczna, P., Groeger, D., Ziegler, M., Frei, R., Ferstl, R., Shanahan, F.,... & O'mahony, L. (2011). Bifidobacterium infantis 35624 administration induces Foxp3 T regulatory cells in human peripheral blood: potential role for myeloid and plasmacytoid dendritic cells. Gut, gutjnl-2011

Groeger, D., O'Mahony, L., Murphy, E. F., Bourke, J. F., Dinan, T. G., Kiely, B.,... & Quigley, E. M. (2013). Bifidobacterium infantis 35624 modulates host inflammatory processes beyond the gut. Gut microbes, 4(4), 325-339.

Kwon, H. K., Lee, C. G., So, J. S., Chae, C. S., Hwang, J. S., Sahoo, A.,... & Im, S. H. (2010). Generation of regulatory dendritic cells and CD4+ Foxp3+ T cells by probiotics administration suppresses immune disorders. Proceedings of the National Academy of Sciences, 107(5), 2159-2164.

157 Van der Aa, L. B., Van Aalderen, W. M. C., Heymans, H. S. A., Henk Sillevis Smitt, J., Nauta, A. J., Knippels, L. M. J.,... & Sprikkelman, A. B. (2011). Synbiotics prevent asthma-like symptoms in infants with atopic dermatitis. Allergy, 66(2), 170-177.

Abramson, S. L. (2011). Synbiotics Prevent Asthma-Like Symptoms in Infants With Atopic Dermatitis. Pediatrics, 128(Supplement 3), S138-S138.

Van De Pol, M. A., Lutter, R., Smids, B. S., Weersink, E. J., & Van Der Zee, J. S. (2011). Synbiotics reduce allergen-induced T-helper 2 response and improve peak expiratory flow in allergic asthmatics. Allergy, 66(1), 39-47.

Lemoli, E., Trabattoni, D., Parisotto, S., Borgonovo, L., Toscano, M., Rizzardini, G.,... & Piconi, S. (2012). Probiotics reduce gut microbial translocation and improve adult atopic dermatitis. Journal of clinical gastroenterology, 46, S33-S40.

Kruis, W., Frič, P., Pokrotnieks, J., Lukáš, M., Fixa, B., Kaščák, M.,... & Wolff, C. (2004). Maintaining remission of ulcerative colitis with the probiotic Escherichia coli Nissle 1917 is as effective as with standard mesalazine. Gut, 53(11), 1617-1623.

Rembacken, B. J., Snelling, A. M., Hawkey, P. M., Chalmers, D. M., & Axon, A. T. R. (1999). Non-pathogenic Escherichia coli versus mesalazine for the treatment of ulcerative colitis: a randomised trial. The Lancet, 354(9179), 635-639

Miraglia, D. G. M., Maiello, N., Decimo, F., Fusco, N., D'Agostino, B., Sullo, N.,...& Marseglia, G. L. (2012). Airways allergic inflammation and L. reuterii treatment in asthmatic children. Journal of biological regulators and homeostatic agents, 26(1 Suppl), S35-40.

Tamaki, H., Nakase, H., Inoue, S., Kawanami, C., Itani, T., Ohana, M.,...& Noda, T. (2016). Efficacy of probiotic treatment with Bifidobacterium longum 536 for induction of remission in active ulcerative colitis: A randomized, double-blinded, placebo-controlled multicenter trial. Digestive Endoscopy, 28(1), 67-74.

del Campo, R., Garriga, M., Pérez-Aragón, A., Guallarte, P., Lamas, A., Máiz, L.,...& Baquero, F. (2014). Improvement of digestive health and reduction in proteobacterial populations in the gut microbiota of cystic fibrosis patients using a Lactobacillus reuteri probiotic preparation: a double blind prospective study. Journal of Cystic Fibrosis, 13(6), 716-722.

158   Lucaciu, L., Ilies, M., Iuga, C., & Seicean, A. (2018). P136 Serum IL-17 and IL-23 levels can distinguish between severe and non-severe inflammatory bowel disease. *Journal of Crohn's and Colitis, 12*(supplement_1), S163-S163.

Kuwabara, T., Ishikawa, F., Kondo, M., & Kakiuchi, T. (2017). The role of IL-17 and related cytokines in inflammatory autoimmune diseases. *Mediators of inflammation, 2017.*

Krueger, J. G., & Brunner, P. M. (2018). Interleukin-17 alters the biology of many cell types involved in the genesis of psoriasis, systemic inflammation and associated comorbidities. *Experimental dermatology, 27*(2), 115-123.

Sakkas, L. I., & Bogdanos, D. P. (2017). Are psoriasis and psoriatic arthritis the same disease? The IL-23/IL-17 axis data. *Autoimmunity reviews, 16*(1), 10-15.

Poddubnyy, D., & Sieper, J. (2017). What is the best treatment target in axial spondyloarthritis: tumour necrosis factor α, interleukin 17, or both?. *Rheumatology.*

159   Tan, T. G., Sefik, E., Geva-Zatorsky, N., Kua, L., Naskar, D., Teng, F.,...& Kasper, D. L. (2016). Identifying species of symbiont bacteria from the human gut that, alone, can induce intestinal Th17 cells in mice. Proceedings of the National Academy of Sciences, 201617460.

Cosorich, I., Dalla-Costa, G., Sorini, C., Ferrarese, R., Messina, M. J., Dolpady, J.,...& Comi, G. (2017). High frequency of intestinal TH17 cells correlates with microbiota alterations and disease activity in multiple sclerosis. *Science Advances, 3*(7), e1700492.

Curtis, M. M., & Way, S. S. (2009). Interleukin-17 in host defence against bacterial, mycobacterial and fungal pathogens. *Immunology, 126*(2), 177-185.

160   Indrio, F., Riezzo, G., Tafuri, S., Ficarella, M., Carlucci, B., Bisceglia,
       M.,...& Francavilla, R. (2017). Probiotic supplementation in pre-
       term: Feeding intolerance and hospital cost. Nutrients, 9(9), 965.
       Savino, F., Garro, M., Montanari, P., Galliano, I., & Bergallo, M.
       (2018). Crying Time and RORγ/FOXP3 Expression in Lactobacillus
       reuteri DSM17938-Treated Infants with Colic: A Randomized Trial.
       The Journal of pediatrics, 192, 171-177.
       Miraglia, D. G. M., Maiello, N., Decimo, F., Fusco, N., D'Agostino,
       B., Sullo, N.,...& Marseglia, G. L. (2012). Airways allergic inflam-
       mation and L. reuterii treatment in asthmatic children. Journal of
       biological regulators and homeostatic agents, 26(1 Suppl), S35-40.
       Tanabe, S., Kinuta, Y., & Saito, Y. (2008). Bifidobacterium infantis
       suppresses proinflammatory interleukin-17 production in murine
       splenocytes and dextran sodium sulfate-induced intestinal inflamma-
       tion. International journal of molecular medicine, 22(2), 181-185.
       Ghadimi, D., Helwig, U., Schrezenmeir, J., Heller, K. J., & Vrese, M.
       (2012). Epigenetic imprinting by commensal probiotics inhibits the
       IL-23/IL-17 axis in an in vitro model of the intestinal mucosal im-
       mune system. Journal of leukocyte biology, 92(4), 895-911.

161   Consoli, M. L. D., da Silva, R. S., Nicoli, J. R., Bruña-Romero, O.,
       da Silva, R. G., de Vasconcelos Generoso, S., & Correia, M. I. T.
       (2016). Randomized clinical trial: impact of oral administration of
       Saccharomyces boulardii on gene expression of intestinal cytokines
       in patients undergoing colon resection. Journal of Parenteral and
       Enteral Nutrition, 40(8), 1114-1121.
       López, P., Gueimonde, M., Margolles, A., & Suárez, A. (2010).
       Distinct Bifidobacterium strains drive different immune responses
       in vitro. International journal of food microbiology, 138(1-2),
       157-165.
       Jeon, S. G., Kayama, H., Ueda, Y., Takahashi, T., Asahara, T., Tsuji,
       H.,...& Okumura, R. (2012). Probiotic Bifidobacterium breve in-
       duces IL-10-producing Tr1 cells in the colon. PLoS pathogens, 8(5),
       e1002714.

162   López, P., González-Rodríguez, I., Gueimonde, M., Margolles, A.,
       & Suárez, A. (2011). Immune response to Bifidobacterium bifidum
       strains support Treg/Th17 plasticity. PloS one, 6(9), e24776.
       López, P., Gueimonde, M., Margolles, A., & Suárez, A. (2010).
       Distinct Bifidobacterium strains drive different immune responses
       in vitro. International journal of food microbiology, 138(1-2),
       157-165.

163   Curtis, M. M., & Way, S. S. (2009). Interleukin-17 in host defence
       against bacterial, mycobacterial and fungal pathogens. Immunol-
       ogy, 126(2), 177-185.
       Tan, T. G., Sefik, E., Geva-Zatorsky, N., Kua, L., Naskar, D., Teng,

F.,...& Kasper, D. L. (2016). Identifying species of symbiont bacteria from the human gut that, alone, can induce intestinal Th17 cells in mice. Proceedings of the National Academy of Sciences, 201617460

Cosorich, I., Dalla-Costa, G., Sorini, C., Ferrarese, R., Messina, M. J., Dolpady, J.,...& Comi, G. (2017). High frequency of intestinal TH17 cells correlates with microbiota alterations and disease activity in multiple sclerosis. *Science Advances, 3*(7), e1700492.

164 López, P., González-Rodríguez, I., Gueimonde, M., Margolles, A., & Suárez, A. (2011). Immune response to Bifidobacterium bifidum strains support Treg/Th17 plasticity. *PloS one, 6*(9), e24776.

López, P., Gueimonde, M., Margolles, A., & Suárez, A. (2010). Distinct Bifidobacterium strains drive different immune responses in vitro. *International journal of food microbiology, 138*(1-2), 157-165.

165 Kwon, H. K., Lee, C. G., So, J. S., Chae, C. S., Hwang, J. S., Sahoo, A.,...& Im, S. H. (2010). Generation of regulatory dendritic cells and CD4+ Foxp3+ T cells by probiotics administration suppresses immune disorders. Proceedings of the National Academy of Sciences, 107(5), 2159-2164.

166 Llana, M. N., Sarnacki, S. H., Castañeda, M. D. R. A., Bernal, M. I., Giacomodonato, M. N., & Cerquetti, M. C. (2013). Consumption of Lactobacillus casei fermented milk prevents Salmonella reactive arthritis by modulating IL-23/IL-17 expression. *PLoS One, 8*(12), e82588.

167 Sun, D., Luo, F., Xing, J. C., Zhang, F., Xu, J. Z., & Zhang, Z. H. (2018). 1, 25 (OH) 2 D3 inhibited Th17 cells differentiation via regulating the NF-κB activity and expression of IL-17. *Cell proliferation*, e12461-e12461.

Marinho, A., Carvalho, C., Boleixa, D., Bettencourt, A., Leal, B., Guimarães, J.,...& Costa, P. P. (2017). Vitamin D supplementation effects on FoxP3 expression in T cells and FoxP3+/IL-17A ratio and clinical course in systemic lupus erythematosus patients: a study in a Portuguese cohort. *Immunologic research, 65*(1), 197-206.

Tejón, G., Manríquez, V., De Calisto, J., Flores-Santibáñez, F., Hidalgo, Y., Crisóstomo, N.,...& Rosemblatt, M. (2015). Vitamin A impairs the reprogramming of Tregs into IL-17-producing cells during intestinal inflammation. *BioMed research international, 2015.*

Tang, J., Zhou, R. U., Luger, D., Zhu, W., Silver, P. B., Grajewski, R. S.,...& Caspi, R. R. (2009). Calcitriol suppresses antiretinal autoimmunity through inhibitory effects on the Th17 effector response. *The Journal of Immunology, 182*(8), 4624-4632.

Chen, X., Su, W., Wan, T., Yu, J., Zhu, W., Tang, F.,...& Zheng, S. G. (2017). Sodium butyrate regulates Th17/Treg cell balance to ameliorate uveitis via the Nrf2/HO-1 pathway. *Biochemical pharmacol-*

ogy, 142, 111-119.

Zhu, C., Song, K., Shen, Z., Quan, Y., Tan, B., Luo, W., ... & Wang, X. (2018). Roseburia intestinalis inhibits interleukin-17 excretion and promotes regulatory T cells differentiation in colitis. *Molecular medicine reports, 17*(6), 7567-7574.

Kim, J. Y., Lim, K., Kim, K. H., Kim, J. H., Choi, J. S., & Shim, S. C. (2018). N-3 polyunsaturated fatty acids restore Th17 and Treg balance in collagen antibody-induced arthritis. *PloS one, 13*(3), e0194331.

168   Gezginc, Y., Akyol, I., Kuley, E., & Özogul, F. (2013). Biogenic amines formation in Streptococcus thermophilus isolated from home-made natural yogurt. *Food chemistry, 138*(1), 655-662.

169   Priyadarshani, D., Mesthri, W., & Rakshit, S. K. (2011). Screening selected strains of probiotic lactic acid bacteria for their ability to produce biogenic amines (histamine and tyramine). International journal of food science & technology, 46(10), 2062-2069.

170   Cifone, M. G., Cinque, B., La Torre, C., Lombardi, F., Palumbo, P., van den Rest, M. E., ... & Donelli, G. (2017). Complexities and pitfalls in the production of multispecies probiotics: the paradigmatic case of VSL# 3 formulation and visbiome. In The Microbiota in Gastrointestinal Pathophysiology (pp. 171-178).

171   Barcik, W., Pugin, B., Westermann, P., Perez, N. R., Ferstl, R., Wawrzyniak, M., ... & Akdis, C. A. (2016). Histamine-secreting microbes are increased in the gut of adult asthma patients. Journal of Allergy and Clinical Immunology, 138(5), 1491-1494.

Özoğul, F. (2004). Production of biogenic amines by Morganella morganii, Klebsiella pneumoniae and Hafnia alvei using a rapid HPLC method. European Food Research and Technology, 219(5), 465-469.

Pugin, B., Barcik, W., Westermann, P., Heider, A., Wawrzyniak, M., Hellings, P., ... & O'Mahony, L. (2017). A wide diversity of bacteria from the human gut produces and degrades biogenic amines. Microbial ecology in health and disease, 28(1), 1353881.

172   Matsumoto, N., Riley, S., Fraser, D., Al-Assaf, S., Ishimura, E., Wolever, T., ... & Phillips, A. O. (2006). Butyrate modulates TGF-β1 generation and function: Potential renal benefit for Acacia (sen) SUPERGUM™(gum arabic)?. *Kidney international, 69*(2), 257-265.

Daguet, D., Pinheiro, I., Verhelst, A., Possemiers, S., & Marzorati, M. (2015). Acacia gum improves the gut barrier functionality in vitro. *AGRO FOOD INDUSTRY HI-TECH, 26*(4), 29-33.

Calame, W., Weseler, A. R., Viebke, C., Flynn, C., & Siemensma, A. D. (2008). Gum arabic establishes prebiotic functionality in healthy human volunteers in a dose-dependent manner. British journal of nutrition, 100(06), 1269-1275.

Marzorati, M., Qin, B., Hildebrand, F., Klosterbuer, A., Roughead, Z., Roessle, C.,... & Possemiers, S. (2015). Addition of acacia gum to a FOS/inulin blend improves its fermentation profile in the Simulator of the Human Intestinal Microbial Ecosystem (SHIME®). Journal of Functional Foods, 16, 211-222.

Cherbut, C., Michel, C., Raison, V., Kravtchenko, T., & Severine, M. (2003). Acacia gum is a bifidogenic dietary fibre with high digestive tolerance in healthy humans. *Microbial Ecology in Health and Disease, 15*(1), 43-50.

Wyatt, G. M., Bayliss, C. E., & Holcroft, J. D. (1986). A change in human faecal flora in response to inclusion of gum arabic in the diet. *British Journal of Nutrition, 55*(2), 261-266.

173   Calame, W., Weseler, A. R., Viebke, C., Flynn, C., & Siemensma, A. D. (2008). Gum arabic establishes prebiotic functionality in healthy human volunteers in a dose-dependent manner. British journal of nutrition, 100(06), 1269-1275.

Marzorati, M., Qin, B., Hildebrand, F., Klosterbuer, A., Roughead, Z., Roessle, C.,... & Possemiers, S. (2015). Addition of acacia gum to a FOS/inulin blend improves its fermentation profile in the Simulator of the Human Intestinal Microbial Ecosystem (SHIME®). Journal of Functional Foods, 16, 211-222.

Cherbut, C., Michel, C., Raison, V., Kravtchenko, T., & Severine, M. (2003). Acacia gum is a bifidogenic dietary fibre with high digestive tolerance in healthy humans. *Microbial Ecology in Health and Disease, 15*(1), 43-50.

Wyatt, G. M., Bayliss, C. E., & Holcroft, J. D. (1986). A change in human faecal flora in response to inclusion of gum arabic in the diet. *British Journal of Nutrition, 55*(2), 261-266.

174   Van Laere, K. M., Hartemink, R., Bosveld, M., Schols, H. A., & Voragen, A. G. (2000). Fermentation of plant cell wall derived polysaccharides and their corresponding oligosaccharides by intestinal bacteria. *Journal of Agricultural and Food Chemistry, 48*(5), 1644-1652.

175   Cherbut, C., Michel, C., Raison, V., Kravtchenko, T., & Severine, M. (2003). Acacia gum is a bifidogenic dietary fibre with high digestive tolerance in healthy humans. *Microbial Ecology in Health and Disease, 15*(1), 43-50.

Calame, W., Weseler, A. R., Viebke, C., Flynn, C., & Siemensma, A. D. (2008). Gum arabic establishes prebiotic functionality in healthy human volunteers in a dose-dependent manner. British journal of nutrition, 100(06), 1269-1275.

176   Min, Y. W., Park, S. U., Jang, Y. S., Kim, Y. H., Rhee, P. L., Ko, S. H.,... & Chang, D. K. (2012). Effect of composite yogurt enriched with acacia fiber and Bifidobacterium lactis. *World Journal of Gastroenterology: WJG, 18*(33), 4563.

Bliss, D. Z., Jung, H. J., Savik, K., Lowry, A., LeMoine, M., Jensen, L., ... & Schaffer, K. (2001). Supplementation with dietary fiber improves fecal incontinence. *Nursing research*, *50*(4), 203-213.

177   Macfarlane, G. T., Steed, H., & Macfarlane, S. (2008). Bacterial metabolism and health-related effects of galacto-oligosaccharides and other prebiotics. *Journal of applied microbiology*, *104*(2), 305-344.

178   Davis, L. M., Martínez, I., Walter, J., Goin, C., & Hutkins, R. W. (2011). Barcoded pyrosequencing reveals that consumption of galactooligosaccharides results in a highly specific bifidogenic response in humans. *PLoS One*, *6*(9), e25200.

Fanaro, S., Marten, B., Bagna, R., Vigi, V., Fabris, C., Peña-Quintana, L., ... & Schrezenmeir, J. (2009). Galacto-oligosaccharides are bifidogenic and safe at weaning: a double-blind randomized multicenter study. *Journal of pediatric gastroenterology and nutrition*, *48*(1), 82-88.

Azcarate-Peril, M. A., Ritter, A. J., Savaiano, D., Monteagudo-Mera, A., Anderson, C., Magness, S. T., & Klaenhammer, T. R. (2017). Impact of short-chain galactooligosaccharides on the gut microbiome of lactose-intolerant individuals. Proceedings of the National Academy of Sciences, 201606722.

179   Knol, J., Boehm, G., Lidestri, M., Negretti, F., Jelinek, J., Agosti, M., ... & Mosca, F. (2005). Increase of faecal bifidobacteria due to dietary oligosaccharides induces a reduction of clinically relevant pathogen germs in the faeces of formula-fed preterm infants. *Acta Paediatrica*, *94*(s449), 31-33.

180   Azcarate-Peril, M. A., Ritter, A. J., Savaiano, D., Monteagudo-Mera, A., Anderson, C., Magness, S. T., & Klaenhammer, T. R. (2017). Impact of short-chain galactooligosaccharides on the gut microbiome of lactose-intolerant individuals. Proceedings of the National Academy of Sciences, 201606722.

181   Scher, J. U., Sczesnak, A., Longman, R. S., Segata, N., Ubeda, C., Bielski, C., ... & Huttenhower, C. (2013). Expansion of intestinal Prevotella copri correlates with enhanced susceptibility to arthritis. *elife*, *2*.

182   Macfarlane, G. T., Steed, H., & Macfarlane, S. (2008). Bacterial metabolism and health-related effects of galacto-oligosaccharides and other prebiotics. *Journal of applied microbiology*, *104*(2), 305-344.

183   Ohashi, Y., Sumitani, K., Tokunaga, M., Ishihara, N., Okubo, T., & Fujisawa, T. (2015). Consumption of partially hydrolysed guar gum stimulates Bifidobacteria and butyrate-producing bacteria in the human large intestine. Beneficial microbes, 6(4), 451-455.

Okubo, T., Ishihara, N., Takahashi, H., Fujisawa, T., Mujo, K., Yamamoto, T., & Mitsuoka, T. (1994). Effects of partially hydrolyzed guar gum intake on human intestinal microflora and its metabolism. Bioscience, biotechnology, and biochemistry, 58(8), 1364-1369.

184   Noack, J., Timm, D., Hospattankar, A., & Slavin, J. (2013). Fermentation profiles of wheat dextrin, inulin and partially hydrolyzed guar gum using an in vitro digestion pretreatment and in vitro batch fermentation system model. *Nutrients*, 5(5), 1500-1510.

185   McDonald, D. E., Pethick, D. W., Pluske, J. R., & Hampson, D. J. (1999). Adverse effects of soluble non-starch polysaccharide (guar gum) on piglet growth and experimental colibacillosis immediately after weaning. Research in veterinary science, 67(3), 245-250.

Vulevic, J., Rastall, R. A., & Gibson, G. R. (2004). Developing a quantitative approach for determining the in vitro prebiotic potential of dietary oligosaccharides. *FEMS microbiology letters*, 236(1), 153-159.

186   Giannini, E. G., Mansi, C., Dulbecco, P., & Savarino, V. (2006). Role of partially hydrolyzed guar gum in the treatment of irritable bowel syndrome. *Nutrition*, 22(3), 334-342.

Parisi, G. C., Zilli, M., Miani, M. P., Carrara, M., Bottona, E., Verdianelli, G., ... & Tonon, A. (2002). High-fiber diet supplementation in patients with irritable bowel syndrome (IBS): a multicenter, randomized, open trial comparison between wheat bran diet and partially hydrolyzed guar gum (PHGG). *Digestive diseases and sciences*, 47(8), 1697-1704.

Furnari, M., Parodi, A., Gemignani, L., Giannini, E. G., Marenco, S., Savarino, E., ... & Savarino, V. (2010). Clinical trial: the combination of rifaximin with partially hydrolysed guar gum is more effective than rifaximin alone in eradicating small intestinal bacterial overgrowth. Alimentary pharmacology & therapeutics, 32(8), 1000-1006.

187   Dr. Allyson Siebecker, interview with Dr. Michael Ruscio, February 2016, https://drruscio.com/prebiotics-fodmaps-treating-sibo-episode-51/

188   Fernandez-Banares, F., Hinojosa, J., Sanchez-Lombrana, J. L., Navarro, E., Martinez-Salmeron, J. F., Garcia-Puges, A., ... & Gine, J. J. (1999). Randomized clinical trial of Plantago ovata seeds (dietary fiber) as compared with mesalamine in maintaining remission in ulcerative colitis. The American journal of gastroenterology, 94(2), 427-433.

Nordgaard, I., Hove, H., Clausen, M. R., & Mortensen, P. B. (1996). Colonic production of butyrate in patients with previous colonic cancer during long-term treatment with dietary fibre (Plantago ovata seeds). Scandinavian journal of gastroenterology, 31(10), 1011-1020.

Hayden, U. L., Mcguirk, S. M., West, S. E., & Carey, H. V. (1998). Psyllium improves fecal consistency and prevents enhanced secretory responses in jejunal tissues of piglets infected with ETEC. Digestive diseases and sciences, 43(11), 2536-2541.

Yakoob, J., Jafri, W., Mehmood, M. H., Abbas, Z., & Tariq, K. (2017). Cytokine changes in gastric and colonic epithelial cell in response to Planta ovata extract. Journal of Complementary and Integrative Medicine.

Rodríguez-Cabezas, M. E., Galvez, J., Camuesco, D., Lorente, M. D., Concha, A., Martinez-Augustin, O.,...& Zarzuelo, A. (2003). Intestinal anti-inflammatory activity of dietary fiber (Plantago ovata seeds) in HLA-B27 transgenic rats. Clinical nutrition, 22(5), 463-471.

Van Laere, K. M., Hartemink, R., Bosveld, M., Schols, H. A., & Voragen, A. G. (2000). Fermentation of plant cell wall derived polysaccharides and their corresponding oligosaccharides by intestinal bacteria. *Journal of Agricultural and Food Chemistry, 48*(5), 1644-1652.

189   Dewulf, E. M., Cani, P. D., Claus, S. P., Fuentes, S., Puylaert, P. G., Neyrinck, A. M.,...& Delzenne, N. M. (2012). Insight into the prebiotic concept: lessons from an exploratory, double blind intervention study with inulin-type fructans in obese women. Gut, gutjnl-2012.

Furrie, E., Macfarlane, S., Kennedy, A., Cummings, J. H., Walsh, S. V., O'neil, D. A., & Macfarlane, G. T. (2005). Synbiotic therapy (Bifidobacterium longum/Synergy 1) initiates resolution of inflammation in patients with active ulcerative colitis: a randomised controlled pilot trial. Gut, 54(2), 242-249.

Lindsay, J. O., Whelan, K., Stagg, A. J., Gobin, P., Al-Hassi, H. O., Rayment, N.,...& Forbes, A. (2006). Clinical, microbiological, and immunological effects of fructo-oligosaccharide in patients with Crohn's disease. Gut, 55(3), 348-355.

Fujimori S., Gudis K., Mitsui K., et al. A randomized controlled trial on the efficacy of synbiotic versus probiotic or prebiotic treatment to improve the quality of life in patients with ulcerative colitis. Nutrition. 2009;25(5):520–525. doi: 10.1016/j.nut.2008.11.017

Casellas, F., Borruel, N., Torrejon, A., Varela, E., Antolin, M., Guarner, F., & MALAGELADA, J. R. (2007). Oral oligofructose-enriched inulin supplementation in acute ulcerative colitis is well tolerated and associated with lowered faecal calprotectin. Alimentary pharmacology & therapeutics, 25(9), 1061-1067

190   Hartemink, R., Van Laere, K. M. J., & Rombouts, F. M. (1997). Growth of enterobacteria on fructo-oligosaccharides. Journal of Applied Microbiology, 83(3), 367-374.

Loh, G., Eberhard, M., Brunner, R. M., Hennig, U., Kuhla, S., Kleessen, B., & Metges, C. C. (2006). Inulin alters the intestinal microbiota and short-chain fatty acid concentrations in growing pigs regardless of their basal diet. *The Journal of nutrition*, *136*(5), 1198-1202.

Rycroft, C. E., Jones, M. R., Gibson, G. R., & Rastall, R. A. (2001). A comparative in vitro evaluation of the fermentation properties of prebiotic oligosaccharides. *Journal of applied microbiology*, *91*(5), 878-887.

Chapter 3. Additional Strategies to Combat Bacterial Overgrowth

191 Lauritano, E. C., Gabrielli, M., Scarpellini, E., Lupascu, A., Novi, M., Sottili, S., ... & Gasbarrini, G. (2008). Small intestinal bacterial overgrowth recurrence after antibiotic therapy. *The American journal of gastroenterology*, *103*(8), 2031

192 Drago, F., Ciccarese, G., Indemini, E., Savarino, V., & Parodi, A. (2018). Psoriasis and small intestine bacterial overgrowth. International journal of dermatology, 57(1), 112-113.

193 Cedars Sinai Patient Handout. http://www.siboinfo.com/uploads/5/4/8/4/5484269/low_fermentation_diet.pdf

194 Urdaneta, V., & Casadesús, J. (2017). interactions between Bacteria and Bile Salts in the Gastrointestinal and Hepatobiliary Tracts. *Frontiers in medicine*, *4*, 163.
Lorenzo-Zúñiga, V., Bartoli, R., Planas, R., Hofmann, A. F., Viñado, B., Hagey, L. R., ... & Gassull, M. A. (2003). Oral bile acids reduce bacterial overgrowth, bacterial translocation, and endotoxemia in cirrhotic rats. *Hepatology*, *37*(3), 551-557.

195 Cahill, C. J., Pain, J. A., & Bailey, M. E. (1987). Bile salts, endotoxin and renal function in obstructive jaundice. *Surgery, gynecology & obstetrics*, *165*(6), 519-522.
Cahill, C. J. (1983). Prevention of postoperative renal failure in patients with obstructive jaundice—the role of bile salts. *British journal of surgery*, *70*(10), 590-595.
Lorenzo-Zúñiga, V., Bartoli, R., Planas, R., Hofmann, A. F., Viñado, B., Hagey, L. R., ... & Gassull, M. A. (2003). Oral bile acids reduce bacterial overgrowth, bacterial translocation, and endotoxemia in cirrhotic rats. *Hepatology*, *37*(3), 551-557.
Kocsar, L. T., Bertok, L., & Varteresz, V. (1969). Effect of bile acids on the intestinal absorption of endotoxin in rats. *Journal of bacteriology*, *100*(1), 220-223.

196 Gyurcsovics, K., & Bertók, L. (2003). Pathophysiology of psoriasis: coping endotoxins with bile acid therapy. *Pathophysiology*, *10*(1), 57-61.
Ely, P. H. (2018). Is psoriasis a bowel disease? Successful treatment

with bile acids and bioflavonoids suggest it is. *Clinics in Dermatology*.

197   Madisch, A., Vinson, B. R., Abdel-Aziz, H., Kelber, O., Nieber, K., Kraft, K., & Storr, M. (2017). Modulation of gastrointestinal motility beyond metoclopramide and domperidone. *Wiener Medizinische Wochenschrift*, *167*(7-8), 160-168.

198   Ottillinger, B., Storr, M., Malfertheiner, P., & Allescher, H. D. (2013). STW 5 (Iberogast®)—a safe and effective standard in the treatment of functional gastrointestinal disorders. Wiener Medizinische Wochenschrift, 163(3-4), 65-72.

199   Ottillinger, B., Storr, M., Malfertheiner, P., & Allescher, H. D. (2013). STW 5 (Iberogast®)—a safe and effective standard in the treatment of functional gastrointestinal disorders. Wiener Medizinische Wochenschrift, 163(3-4), 65-72.

200   Chen, P. W., Jheng, T. T., Shyu, C. L., & Mao, F. C. (2013). Antimicrobial potential for the combination of bovine lactoferrin or its hydrolysate with lactoferrin-resistant probiotics against foodborne pathogens. *Journal of dairy science*, *96*(3), 1438-1446.
      Bellamy, W., Takase, M., Wakabayashi, H., Kawase, K., & Tomita, M. (1992). Antibacterial spectrum of lactoferricin B, a potent bactericidal peptide derived from the N-terminal region of bovine lactoferrin. Journal of Applied Microbiology, 73(6), 472-479.
      Yuan, Y., Wu, Q., Cheng, G., Liu, X., Liu, S., Luo, J.,...& Dong, X. (2015). Recombinant human lactoferrin enhances the efficacy of triple therapy in mice infected with Helicobacter pylori. International journal of molecular medicine, 36(2), 363-368
      Griffiths, E. A., Duffy, L. C., Schanbacher, F. L., Dryja, D., Leavens, A., Neiswander, R. L.,...& Ogra, P. (2003). In vitro growth responses of bifidobacteria and enteropathogens to bovine and human lactoferrin. Digestive diseases and sciences, 48(7), 1324-1332.

201   Griffiths, E. A., Duffy, L. C., Schanbacher, F. L., Dryja, D., Leavens, A., Neiswander, R. L.,...& Ogra, P. (2003). In vitro growth responses of bifidobacteria and enteropathogens to bovine and human lactoferrin. Digestive diseases and sciences, 48(7), 1324-1332.

202   Bertuccini, L., Costanzo, M., Iosi, F., Tinari, A., Terruzzi, F., Stronati, L.,...& Superti, F. (2014). Lactoferrin prevents invasion and inflammatory response following E. coli strain LF82 infection in experimental model of Crohn's disease. Digestive and Liver Disease, 46(6), 496-504.
      Ammons, M. C., & Copié, V. (2013). Mini-review: Lactoferrin: a bioinspired, anti-biofilm therapeutic. Biofouling, 29(4), 443-455.

203   Chen, P. W., Liu, Z. S., Kuo, T. C., Hsieh, M. C., & Li, Z. W. (2017). Prebiotic effects of bovine lactoferrin on specific probiotic bacteria.

BioMetals, 30(2), 237-248.

Oda, H., Wakabayashi, H., Yamauchi, K., & Abe, F. (2014). Lactoferrin and bifidobacteria. *Biometals*, 27(5), 915-922.

204   Oda, H., Wakabayashi, H., Yamauchi, K., & Abe, F. (2014). Lactoferrin and bifidobacteria. Biometals, 27(5), 915-922.

Akin, I. M., Atasay, B., Dogu, F., Okulu, E., Arsan, S., Karatas, H. D.,... & Turmen, T. (2014). Oral lactoferrin to prevent nosocomial sepsis and necrotizing enterocolitis of premature neonates and effect on T-regulatory cells. Am J Perinatol, 31(12), 1111-1120.

205   Abubakar, E. M. M. (2009). Efficacy of crude extracts of garlic (Allium sativum Linn.) against nosocomial Escherichia coli, Staphylococcus aureus, Streptococcus pneumoniea and Pseudomonas aeruginosa. *Journal of Medicinal Plants Research*, 3(4), 179-185.

206   Ankri, S., & Mirelman, D. (1999). Antimicrobial properties of allicin from garlic. *Microbes and infection*, 1(2), 125-129.

Gebreyohannes, G., & Gebreyohannes, M. (2013). Medicinal values of garlic: A review. *International Journal of Medicine and Medical Sciences*, 5(9), 401-408.

Ranjbar-Omid, M., Arzanlou, M., Amani, M., Shokri Al-Hashem, S. K., Amir Mozafari, N., & Peeri Doghaheh, H. (2015). Allicin from garlic inhibits the biofilm formation and urease activity of Proteus mirabilis in vitro. *FEMS microbiology letters*, 362(9).

Ruiz, R., García, M. P., Lara, A., & Rubio, L. A. (2010). Garlic derivatives (PTS and PTS-O) differently affect the ecology of swine faecal microbiota in vitro. Veterinary microbiology, 144(1-2), 110-117.

207   Yin, M. C., Chang, H. C., & Tsao, S. M. (2002). Inhibitory effects of aqueous garlic extract, garlic oil and four diallyl sulphides against four enteric pathogens. Journal of Food and Drug Analysis, 10(2).

Saravanan, P., Ramya, V., Sridhar, H., Balamurugan, V., & Umamaheswari, S. (2010). Antibacterial activity of Allium sativum L. on pathogenic bacterial strains. Global veterinaria, 4(5), 519-522.

208   Khodavandi, A., Alizadeh, F., Harmal, N. S., Sidik, S. M., Othman, F., Sekawi, Z.,... & Chong, P. P. (2011). Comparison between efficacy of allicin and fluconazole against Candida albicans in vitro and in a systemic candidiasis mouse model. *FEMS microbiology letters*, 315(2), 87-93.

Khodavandi, A., Alizadeh, F., Aala, F., Sekawi, Z., & Chong, P. P. (2010). In vitro investigation of antifungal activity of allicin alone and in combination with azoles against Candida species. *Mycopathologia*, 169(4), 287-295.

Gebreyohannes, G., & Gebreyohannes, M. (2013). Medicinal values of garlic: A review. *International Journal of Medicine and Medical Sciences*, 5(9), 401-408.

209   Ruiz, R., García, M. P., Lara, A., & Rubio, L. A. (2010). Garlic deriva-
       tives (PTS and PTS-O) differently affect the ecology of swine faecal
       microbiota in vitro. *Veterinary microbiology*, *144*(1-2), 110-117.
       Filocamo, A., Nueno-Palop, C., Bisignano, C., Mandalari, G., & Nar-
       bad, A. (2012). Effect of garlic powder on the growth of commensal
       bacteria from the gastrointestinal tract. *Phytomedicine*, *19*(8-9),
       707-711.
       Booyens, J., & Thantsha, M. S. (2013). Antibacterial effect of hydro-
       soluble extracts of garlic (Allium sativum) against Bifidobacterium
       spp. and Lactobacillus acidophilus. *African Journal of Microbiology
       Research*, *7*(8), 669-677.

210   Liu, S., He, L., Jiang, Q., Duraipandiyan, V., Al-Dhabi, N. A., Liu,
       G.,...& Yin, Y. (2018). Effect of Dietary α-ketoglutarate and Allicin
       Supplementation on the Cecal Microbial Community Composition
       and Diversity in Growing Pigs. *Journal of the Science of Food and
       Agriculture*.
       Busquet, M., Calsamiglia, S., Ferret, A., Cardozo, P. W., & Kamel, C.
       (2005). Effects of cinnamaldehyde and garlic oil on rumen microbial
       fermentation in a dual flow continuous culture. *Journal of Dairy
       Science*, *88*(7), 2508-2516.

211   Lan, J., Zhao, Y., Dong, F., Yan, Z., Zheng, W., Fan, J., & Sun, G.
       (2015). Meta-analysis of the effect and safety of berberine in the
       treatment of type 2 diabetes mellitus, hyperlipemia and hyperten-
       sion. *Journal of ethnopharmacology*, *161*, 69-81.

212   Zhang, X., Zhao, Y., Zhang, M., Pang, X., Xu, J., Kang, C.,...& Li,
       X. (2012). Structural changes of gut microbiota during berberine-
       mediated prevention of obesity and insulin resistance in high-fat
       diet-fed rats. PloS one, 7(8), e42529.
       Kong, W. J., Xing, X. Y., Xiao, X. H., Zhao, Y. L., Wei, J. H., Wang, J.
       B.,...& Yang, M. H. (2012). Effect of berberine on Escherichia coli,
       Bacillus subtilis, and their mixtures as determined by isothermal
       microcalorimetry. Applied microbiology and biotechnology, 96(2),
       503-510.
       Han, J., Lin, H., & Huang, W. (2011). Modulating gut microbiota as
       an anti-diabetic mechanism of berberine. Medical science monitor:
       international medical journal of experimental and clinical research,
       17(7), RA164.

213   Rabbani, G. H., Butler, T., Knight, J., Sanyal, S. C., & Alam, K.
       (1987). Randomized controlled trial of berberine sulfate therapy for
       diarrhea due to enterotoxigenic Escherichia coli and Vibrio chol-
       erae. Journal of infectious diseases, 155(5), 979-984.
       Zorić, N., Kosalec, I., Tomić, S., Bobnjarić, I., Jug, M., Vlainić, T., &
       Vlainić, J. (2017). Membrane of Candida albicans as a target of ber-
       berine. BMC complementary and alternative medicine, 17(1), 268.

Dhamgaye S, Devaux F, Vandeputte P, Khandelwal NK, Sanglard D, Mukhopadhyay G, Prasad R. Molecular mechanisms of action of herbal antifungal alkaloid berberine in Candida albicans. PloS ONE. 2014. doi:10.1371/journal.pone.0104554.

da Silva AR, de Andrade Neto JB, da Silva CR, Campos RDS, Costa Silva RA, Freitas DD, do Nascimento FBSA, de Andrade LND, Sampaio LS, Grangeiro TB, Magalhães HIF, Cavalcanti BC, de Moraes MO, Nobre Júnior HV. Berberine antifungal activity in fluconazole-resistant pathogenic yeasts: action mechanism evaluated by flow cytometry and biofilm growth inhibition in Candida spp. Antimicrob Agents Chemother. 2016. doi:10.1128/AAC.01846-15.

214   Wang, L. L., Guo, H. H., Huang, S., Feng, C. L., Han, Y. X., & Jiang, J. D. (2017). Comprehensive evaluation of SCFA production in the intestinal bacteria regulated by berberine using gas-chromatography combined with polymerase chain reaction. Journal of Chromatography B, 1057, 70-80.

Zhu, L., Zhang, D., Zhu, H., Zhu, J., Weng, S., Dong, L.,...& Shen, X. (2018). Berberine treatment increases Akkermansia in the gut and improves high-fat diet-induced atherosclerosis in Apoe−/− mice. *Atherosclerosis, 268*, 117-126.

Xu, J. H., Liu, X. Z., Pan, W., & Zou, D. J. (2017). Berberine protects against diet-induced obesity through regulating metabolic endotoxemia and gut hormone levels. Molecular medicine reports, 15(5), 2765-2787

Zhang, X., Zhao, Y., Zhang, M., Pang, X., Xu, J., Kang, C.,...& Li, X. (2012). Structural changes of gut microbiota during berberine-mediated prevention of obesity and insulin resistance in high-fat diet-fed rats. PloS one, 7(8), e42529.

215   Yue, M., Xia, Y., Shi, C., Guan, C., Li, Y., Liu, R.,...& Dai, Y. (2017). Berberine ameliorates collagen-induced arthritis in rats by suppressing Th17 cell responses via inducing cortistatin in the gut. *The FEBS journal, 284*(17), 2786-2801.

Wang, X., He, X., Zhang, C. F., Guo, C. R., Wang, C. Z., & Yuan, C. S. (2017). Anti-arthritic effect of berberine on adjuvant-induced rheumatoid arthritis in rats. Biomedicine & Pharmacotherapy, 89, 887-893.

Yue, J., Xu, J., Li, H., Wang, J., Zheng, N., Yao, H.,...& Qin, L. (2018). THU0078 Berberine ameliorates bone erosions in collagen-induced arthritis rat models via suppressing the expression of il-17a.

216   Qin, X., Guo, B. T., Wan, B., Fang, L., Lu, L., Wu, L.,...& Zhang, J. Z. (2010). Regulation of Th1 and Th17 cell differentiation and amelioration of experimental autoimmune encephalomyelitis by natural product compound berberine. The Journal of Immunology, 0903853.

Yang, Y., Qi, J., Wang, Q., Du, L., Zhou, Y., Yu, H.,...& Yang, P. (2013). Berberine suppresses Th17 and dendritic cell responses. Investigative ophthalmology & visual science, 54(4), 2516-2522.

Yang, Y., Wang, Q., Xie, M., Liu, P., Qi, X., Liu, X., & Li, Z. (2017). Berberine exerts an anti-inflammatory role in ocular Behcet's disease. Molecular medicine reports, 15(1), 97-102.

217   Guo, Y., Chen, Y., Tan, Z. R., Klaassen, C. D., & Zhou, H. H. (2012). Repeated administration of berberine inhibits cytochromes P450 in humans. *European journal of clinical pharmacology, 68*(2), 213-217. https://www.rxlist.com/berberine/supplements.htm

218   Lan, J., Zhao, Y., Dong, F., Yan, Z., Zheng, W., Fan, J., & Sun, G. (2015). Meta-analysis of the effect and safety of berberine in the treatment of type 2 diabetes mellitus, hyperlipemia and hypertension. *Journal of ethnopharmacology, 161*, 69-81.

219   Williams, D. W., Kuriyama, T., Silva, S., Malic, S., & Lewis, M. A. (2011). Candida biofilms and oral candidosis: treatment and prevention. *Periodontology 2000, 55*(1), 250-265.
       Harriott, M. M., Lilly, E. A., Rodriguez, T. E., Fidel Jr, P. L., & Noverr, M. C. (2010). Candida albicans forms biofilms on the vaginal mucosa. *Microbiology, 156*(12), 3635-3644.
       Ganguly, S., & Mitchell, A. P. (2011). Mucosal biofilms of Candida albicans. *Current opinion in microbiology, 14*(4), 380-385.

Chapter 4. A Microbiome-Restoring Diet

220   Hou, J. K., Abraham, B., & El-Serag, H. (2011). Dietary intake and risk of developing inflammatory bowel disease: a systematic review of the literature. *The American journal of gastroenterology, 106*(4), 563.
       Penagini, F., Dilillo, D., Borsani, B., Cococcioni, L., Galli, E., Bedogni, G.,...& Zuccotti, G. V. (2016). Nutrition in Pediatric Inflammatory Bowel Disease: From Etiology to Treatment. A Systematic Review. Nutrients, 8(6), 334.
       Minami, Y., Hirabayashi, Y., Nagata, C., Ishii, T., Harigae, H., & Sasaki, T. (2011). Intakes of vitamin B6 and dietary fiber and clinical course of systemic lupus erythematosus: a prospective study of Japanese female patients. Journal of epidemiology, 21(4), 246-254.
       Trompette, A., Gollwitzer, E. S., Yadava, K., Sichelstiel, A. K., Sprenger, N., Ngom-Bru, C.,...& Marsland, B. J. (2014). Gut microbiota metabolism of dietary fiber influences allergic airway disease and hematopoiesis. Nature medicine, 20(2), 159-166.
       Reif, S., Klein, I., Lubin, F., Farbstein, M., Hallak, A., & Gilat, T. (1997). Pre-illness dietary factors in inflammatory bowel disease. *Gut, 40*(6), 754-760.

221 De Filippo, C., Cavalieri, D., Di Paola, M., Ramazzotti, M., Poullet, J. B., Massart, S., ... & Lionetti, P. (2010). Impact of diet in shaping gut microbiota revealed by a comparative study in children from Europe and rural Africa. Proceedings of the National Academy of Sciences, 107(33), 14691-14696.

222 O'Keefe, S. J. D., Li, J. V., Lahti, L., Ou, J., Carbonero, F., Mohammed, K., ... Zoetendal, E. G. (2015). Fat, Fiber and Cancer Risk in African Americans and Rural Africans. Nature Communications, 6, 6342. http://doi.org/10.1038/ncomms7342

223 Hou, J. K., Abraham, B., & El-Serag, H. (2011). Dietary intake and risk of developing inflammatory bowel disease: a systematic review of the literature. *The American journal of gastroenterology*, 106(4), 563.
Penagini, F., Dilillo, D., Borsani, B., Cococcioni, L., Galli, E., Bedogni, G., ... & Zuccotti, G. V. (2016). Nutrition in Pediatric Inflammatory Bowel Disease: From Etiology to Treatment. A Systematic Review. Nutrients, 8(6), 334.
Minami, Y., Hirabayashi, Y., Nagata, C., Ishii, T., Harigae, H., & Sasaki, T. (2011). Intakes of vitamin B6 and dietary fiber and clinical course of systemic lupus erythematosus: a prospective study of Japanese female patients. Journal of epidemiology, 21(4), 246-254.
Trompette, A., Gollwitzer, E. S., Yadava, K., Sichelstiel, A. K., Sprenger, N., Ngom-Bru, C., ... & Marsland, B. J. (2014). Gut microbiota metabolism of dietary fiber influences allergic airway disease and hematopoiesis. Nature medicine, 20(2), 159-166.
Reif, S., Klein, I., Lubin, F., Farbstein, M., Hallak, A., & Gilat, T. (1997). Pre-illness dietary factors in inflammatory bowel disease. *Gut*, 40(6), 754-760.

224 Ajani, U. A., Ford, E. S., & Mokdad, A. H. (2004). Dietary fiber and C-reactive protein: findings from national health and nutrition examination survey data. The Journal of nutrition, 134(5), 1181-1185.
Ma, Y., Hébert, J. R., Li, W., Bertone-Johnson, E. R., Olendzki, B., Pagoto, S. L., ... & Griffith, J. A. (2008). Association between dietary fiber and markers of systemic inflammation in the Women's Health Initiative Observational Study. Nutrition, 24(10), 941-949.

225 Ma, Y., Hébert, J. R., Li, W., Bertone-Johnson, E. R., Olendzki, B., Pagoto, S. L., ... & Griffith, J. A. (2008). Association between dietary fiber and markers of systemic inflammation in the Women's Health Initiative Observational Study. Nutrition, 24(10), 941-949.

226 Holscher, H. D. (2017). Dietary fiber and prebiotics and the gastrointestinal microbiota. *Gut Microbes*, 8(2), 172-184.

227 Lupton, J. R. (2004). Microbial degradation products influence colon cancer risk: the butyrate controversy. *The Journal of nutri-*

tion, 134(2), 479-482.

228   Dominianni, C., Sinha, R., Goedert, J. J., Pei, Z., Yang, L., Hayes, R.
B., & Ahn, J. (2015). Sex, body mass index, and dietary fiber intake
influence the human gut microbiome. PloS one, 10(4), e0124599.

229   Tanaka: relationship of Enhanced Butyrate Production by Colonic
Butyrate-Producing Bacteria to Immunomodulatory Effects in Normal Mice Fed an Insoluble Fraction o fBrassica rapa L.

230   Waldecker, M., Kautenburger, T., Daumann, H., Veeriah, S., Will, F.,
Dietrich, H.,...& Schrenk, D. (2008). Histone-deacetylase inhibition
and butyrate formation: Fecal slurry incubations with apple pectin
and apple juice extracts. *Nutrition, 24*(4), 366-374.

231   Anhê, F. F., Varin, T. V., Le Barz, M., Desjardins, Y., Levy, E., Roy, D.,
& Marette, A. (2015). *Gut Microbiota Dysbiosis in Obesity-Linked
Metabolic Diseases and Prebiotic Potential of Polyphenol-Rich
Extracts.* Current Obesity Reports, 389–400;
Roopchand, D. E., Carmody, R. N., Kuhn, P., Moskal, K., Rojas-Sil-
va, P., Turnbaugh, P. J., & Raskin, I. (2015). Dietary Polyphenols Pro-
mote Growth of the Gut Bacterium Akkermansia muciniphila and
Attenuate High-Fat Diet–Induced Metabolic Syndrome. Diabetes,
64(8), 2847-2858.
Henning, S. M., Summanen, P. H., Lee, R. P., Yang, J., Finegold, S. M.,
Heber, D., & Li, Z. (2017). Pomegranate ellagitannins stimulate the
growth of Akkermansia muciniphila in vivo. Anaerobe, 43, 56-60.

232   de Vos, W. M. (2017). Microbe profile: Akkermansia muciniphila:
a conserved intestinal symbiont that acts as the gatekeeper of our
mucosa. Microbiology, 163(5), 646-648.

233   Castaldo G., Galdo G., Rotondi Aufiero F., Cereda E. Very low-calorie ketogenic diet may allow restoring response to systemic therapy
in relapsing plaque psoriasis. Obes. Res. Clin. Pract. 2015
Ebringer, A., & Wilson, C. (1996). The use of a low starch diet in the
treatment of patients suffering from ankylosing spondylitis. Clinical
rheumatology, 15(1), 62-66

234   http://www.phoenixhelix.com/2013/11/03/charles-story/

235   Fletcher, A. A. (1922). Chronic Arthritis—Some Phases in its Etiology
and Treatment. Canadian Medical Association journal, 12(9), 633.

236   Pemberton, R., & TOMPKINS, E. H. (1920). Studies on Arthritis in
the Army Based on Four Hundred Cases: II. Observations on the
Basal Metabolism. Archives of Internal Medicine, 25(3), 241-242.

237   Fletcher, A. A. (1922). Chronic Arthritis—Some Phases in its Etiology
and Treatment. Canadian Medical Association journal, 12(9), 633.

238   Ebringer, A., & Wilson, C. (1996). The use of a low starch diet in the
treatment of patients suffering from ankylosing spondylitis. Clinical

rheumatology, 15(1), 62-66

239 Rashid, T., & Ebringer, A. (2007). Ankylosing spondylitis is linked to Klebsiella—the evidence. Clinical rheumatology, 26(6), 858-864.

240 Ebringer, A., & Wilson, C. (1996). The use of a low starch diet in the treatment of patients suffering from ankylosing spondylitis. Clinical rheumatology, 15(1), 62-66

241 Ebringer, A., & Wilson, C. (1996). The use of a low starch diet in the treatment of patients suffering from ankylosing spondylitis. Clinical rheumatology, 15(1), 62-66

242 Ochuba, G. U., & von Riesen, V. L. (1980). Fermentation of polysac-charides by Klebsielleae and other facultative bacilli. *Applied and environmental microbiology, 39*(5), 988-992.

243 Puccetti, A., Dolcino, M., Tinazzi, E., Moretta, F., D'Angelo, S., Oliv-ieri, I., & Lunardi, C. (2017). Antibodies Directed against a Peptide Epitope of a Klebsiella pneumoniae-Derived Protein Are Present in Ankylosing Spondylitis. PloS one, 12(1), e0171073.

244 Puccetti, A., Dolcino, M., Tinazzi, E., Moretta, F., D'Angelo, S., Oliv-ieri, I., & Lunardi, C. (2017). Antibodies Directed against a Peptide Epitope of a Klebsiella pneumoniae-Derived Protein Are Present in Ankylosing Spondylitis. PloS one, 12(1), e0171073.

245 Castaldo, G., Galdo, G., Aufiero, F. R., & Cereda, E. (2016). Very low-calorie ketogenic diet may allow restoring response to systemic therapy in relapsing plaque psoriasis. *Obesity research & clinical practice, 10*(3), 348-352.
Suskind, D. L., Wahbeh, G., Cohen, S. A., Damman, C. J., Klein, J., Braly, K.,...& Lee, D. (2016). Patients Perceive Clinical Benefit with the Specific Carbohydrate Diet for Inflammatory Bowel Disease. Digestive diseases and sciences, 61(11), 3255-3260.
Kakodkar, S., Farooqui, A. J., Mikolaitis, S. L., & Mutlu, E. A. (2015). The specific carbohydrate diet for inflammatory bowel disease: a case series. Journal of the Academy of Nutrition and Dietetics, 115(8), 1226-1232.
Khandalavala, B. N., & Nirmalraj, M. C. (2015). Resolution of severe ulcerative colitis with the specific carbohydrate diet. Case reports in gastroenterology, 9(2), 291-295
Obih, C., Wahbeh, G., Lee, D., Braly, K., Giefer, M., Shaffer, M. L.,...& Suskind, D. L. (2016). Specific carbohydrate diet for pe-diatric inflammatory bowel disease in clinical practice within an academic IBD center. Nutrition, 32(4), 418-425;
Suskind, D. L., Wahbeh, G., Gregory, N., Vendettuoli, H., & Christie, D. (2014). Nutritional therapy in pediatric Crohn disease: the specific carbohydrate diet. Journal of pediatric gastroenterology and nutrition, 58(1), 87-91.

Cohen, S. A., Gold, B. D., Oliva, S., Lewis, J., Stallworth, A., Koch, B.,...& Mason, D. (2014). Clinical and mucosal improvement with specific carbohydrate diet in pediatric Crohn disease. Journal of pediatric gastroenterology and nutrition, 59(4), 516-521.

Burgis, J. C., Nguyen, K., Park, K. T., & Cox, K. (2016). Response to strict and liberalized specific carbohydrate diet in pediatric Crohn's disease. World journal of gastroenterology, 22(6), 2111

246   Viladomiu, M., Kivolowitz, C., Abdulhamid, A., Dogan, B., Victorio, D., Castellanos, J. G.,...& Chai, C. (2017). IgA-coated E. coli enriched in Crohn's disease spondyloarthritis promote TH17-dependent inflammation. Science Translational Medicine, 9(376), eaaf9655.

Kivolowitz, C., Abdulhamid, A., Victorio, D., Castellanos, J., Simpson, K., Scherl, E., & Longman, R. (2016). O-006 Expansion of Immunologically-Relevant E. Coli in the Intestinal Microbiota of Patients with IBD-Associated Spondyloarthritis Promotes Mucosal RORgt-Dependent Immunity. Inflammatory bowel diseases, 22, S3.

247   Nickerson, K. P., Chanin, R., & McDonald, C. (2015). Deregulation of intestinal anti-microbial defense by the dietary additive, maltodextrin. Gut microbes, 6(1), 78-83.

248   Dr. Allyson Siebecker (2014), SIBO Specific Food Guide. http://www.siboinfo.com/uploads/5/4/8/4/5484269/sibo_specific_diet_food_guide_sept_2014.pdf

249   Penagini, F., Dilillo, D., Borsani, B., Cococcioni, L., Galli, E., Bedogni, G.,...& Zuccotti, G. V. (2016). Nutrition in Pediatric Inflammatory Bowel Disease: From Etiology to Treatment. A Systematic Review. Nutrients, 8(6), 334.

Burgis, J. C., Nguyen, K., Park, K. T., & Cox, K. (2016). Response to strict and liberalized specific carbohydrate diet in pediatric Crohn's disease. World journal of gastroenterology, 22(6), 2111.

250   Suskind, D. L., Wahbeh, G., Cohen, S. A., Damman, C. J., Klein, J., Braly, K.,...& Lee, D. (2016). Patients Perceive Clinical Benefit with the Specific Carbohydrate Diet for Inflammatory Bowel Disease. Digestive diseases and sciences, 61(11), 3255-3260.

Kakodkar, S., Farooqui, A. J., Mikolaitis, S. L., & Mutlu, E. A. (2015). The specific carbohydrate diet for inflammatory bowel disease: a case series. Journal of the Academy of Nutrition and Dietetics, 115(8), 1226-1232.

Khandalavala, B. N., & Nirmalraj, M. C. (2015). Resolution of severe ulcerative colitis with the specific carbohydrate diet. Case reports in gastroenterology, 9(2), 291-295

Obih, C., Wahbeh, G., Lee, D., Braly, K., Giefer, M., Shaffer, M. L.,...& Suskind, D. L. (2016). Specific carbohydrate diet for pediatric inflammatory bowel disease in clinical practice within an academic IBD center. Nutrition, 32(4), 418-425;

Suskind, D. L., Wahbeh, G., Gregory, N., Vendettuoli, H., & Christie, D. (2014). Nutritional therapy in pediatric Crohn disease: the specific carbohydrate diet. Journal of pediatric gastroenterology and nutrition, 58(1), 87-91.

Cohen, S. A., Gold, B. D., Oliva, S., Lewis, J., Stallworth, A., Koch, B., ... & Mason, D. (2014). Clinical and mucosal improvement with specific carbohydrate diet in pediatric Crohn disease. Journal of pediatric gastroenterology and nutrition, 59(4), 516-521.

Burgis, J. C., Nguyen, K., Park, K. T., & Cox, K. (2016). Response to strict and liberalized specific carbohydrate diet in pediatric Crohn's disease. World journal of gastroenterology, 22(6), 2111.

251   Suskind, D. (2016). Nutrition in Immune Balance (NIMBAL) Therapy: Using Diet to Treat Inflammatory Bowel Disease. Seattle, Washington. Nimbal Publishing .

252   Suskind, D. L., Cohen, S. A., Brittnacher, M. J., Wahbeh, G., Lee, D., Shaffer, M. L., ... & Giefer, M. (2017). Clinical and Fecal Microbial Changes With Diet Therapy in Active Inflammatory Bowel Disease. Journal of Clinical Gastroenterology.

253   Walters, S. S., Quiros, A., Rolston, M., Grishina, I., Li, J., Fenton, A., ... & Nieves, R. (2014). Analysis of gut microbiome and diet modification in patients with Crohn's disease. SOJ Microbiol Infect Dis, 2(3), 1-13.

254   James, M. J., Gibson, R. A., & Cleland, L. G. (2000). Dietary poly-unsaturated fatty acids and inflammatory mediator production. The American journal of clinical nutrition, 71(1), 343s-348s.

Sperling, R. I. (1991). Effects of Dietary Fish Oil on Leukocyte Leu-kotriene and PAF Generation and on Neutrophil Chemotaxis1. In Health Effects of Omega 3 Polyunsaturated Fatty Acids in Seafoods (pp. 391-400). Karger Publishers.

Barrea L., Balato N., Di Somma C., Macchia P.E., Napolitano M., Savanelli M.C., Esposito K., Colao A., Savastano S. Nutrition and psoriasis: Is there any association between the severity of the disease and adherence to the Mediterranean diet? J. Transl. Med. 2015;13:18. doi: 10.1186/s12967-014-0372-1.)

Hayashi, H., Satoi, K., Sato-Mito, N., Kaburagi, T., Yoshino, H., Higaki, M., ... & Sato, K. (2012). Nutritional status in relation to adipokines and oxidative stress is associated with disease activity in patients with rheumatoid arthritis. Nutrition, 28(11), 1109-1114.

Skoldstam, L., Hagfors, L., & Johansson, G. (2003). An experimental study of a Mediterranean diet intervention for patients with rheu-matoid arthritis. Annals of the Rheumatic Diseases, 62(3), 208–214. http://doi.org/10.1136/ard.62.3.208

Guida, B., Napoleone, A., Trio, R., Nastasi, A., Balato, N., Laccetti,

R., & Cataldi, M. (2014). Energy-restricted, n-3 polyunsaturated fatty acids-rich diet improves the clinical response to immuno-modulating drugs in obese patients with plaque-type psoriasis: a randomized control clinical trial. Clinical Nutrition, 33(3), 399-405.

Hansen, G. V. O., Nielsen, L., Kluger, E., Thysen, M., Emmertsen, H., Stengaard-Pedersen, K.,... & Andersen, P. W. (1996). Nutritional status of Danish rheumatoid arthritis patients and effects of a diet adjusted in energy intake, fish-meal, and antioxidants. Scandinavian journal of rheumatology, 25(5), 325-333.

255   Barrea L., Balato N., Di Somma C., Macchia P.E., Napolitano M., Savanelli M.C., Esposito K., Colao A., Savastano S. Nutrition and psoriasis: Is there any association between the severity of the disease and adherence to the Mediterranean diet? J. Transl. Med. 2015;13:18. doi: 10.1186/s12967-014-0372-1.)

Hayashi, H., Satoi, K., Sato-Mito, N., Kaburagi, T., Yoshino, H., Higaki, M.,... & Sato, K. (2012). Nutritional status in relation to adipokines and oxidative stress is associated with disease activity in patients with rheumatoid arthritis. Nutrition, 28(11), 1109-1114.

Skoldstam, L., Hagfors, L., & Johansson, G. (2003). An experimental study of a Mediterranean diet intervention for patients with rheu-matoid arthritis. Annals of the Rheumatic Diseases, 62(3), 208–214. http://doi.org/10.1136/ard.62.3.208

Guida, B., Napoleone, A., Trio, R., Nastasi, A., Balato, N., Laccetti, R., & Cataldi, M. (2014). Energy-restricted, n-3 polyunsaturated fatty acids-rich diet improves the clinical response to immuno-modulating drugs in obese patients with plaque-type psoriasis: a randomized control clinical trial. Clinical Nutrition, 33(3), 399-405.

Hansen, G. V. O., Nielsen, L., Kluger, E., Thysen, M., Emmertsen, H., Stengaard-Pedersen, K.,... & Andersen, P. W. (1996). Nutritional status of Danish rheumatoid arthritis patients and effects of a diet adjusted in energy intake, fish-meal, and antioxidants. Scandinavian journal of rheumatology, 25(5), 325-333.

256   Serra-Majem, L., Ribas, L., García, A., Pérez-Rodrigo, C., & Arance-ta, J. (2003). Nutrient adequacy and Mediterranean Diet in Spanish school children and adolescents. European journal of clinical nutri-tion, 57, S35-S39.

Castro-Quezada, I., Román-Viñas, B., & Serra-Majem, L. (2014). The Mediterranean diet and nutritional adequacy: a review. Nutri-ents, 6(1), 231-248.

257   Agarwal, S., Reider, C., Brooks, J. R., & Fulgoni III, V. L. (2015). Comparison of prevalence of inadequate nutrient intake based on body weight status of adults in the United States: an analysis of NHANES 2001–2008. Journal of the American College of Nutrition, 34(2), 126-134.

Rosanoff, A., Weaver, C. M., & Rude, R. K. (2012). Suboptimal magnesium status in the United States: are the health consequences underestimated?. Nutrition reviews, 70(3), 153-164.

258   Rosanoff, A., Weaver, C. M., & Rude, R. K. (2012). Suboptimal magnesium status in the United States: are the health consequences underestimated?. Nutrition reviews, 70(3), 153-164.

Dibaba, D. T., Xun, P., & He, K. (2014). Dietary magnesium intake is inversely associated with serum C-reactive protein levels: meta-analysis and systematic review. European journal of clinical nutrition, 68(4), 510.

King, D. E. (2009). Inflammation and elevation of C-reactive protein: does magnesium play a key role?. Magnesium Research, 22(2), 57-59.

Almoznino-Sarafian, D., Berman, S., Mor, A., Shteinshnaider, M., Gorelik, O., Tzur, I., ... & Cohen, N. (2007). Magnesium and C-reactive protein in heart failure: an anti-inflammatory effect of magnesium administration?. European journal of nutrition, 46(4), 230-237.

Kim, D. J., Xun, P., Liu, K., Loria, C., Yokota, K., Jacobs, D. R., & He, K. (2010). Magnesium intake in relation to systemic inflammation, insulin resistance, and the incidence of diabetes. Diabetes care, 33(12), 2604-2610.

Chacko, S. A., Song, Y., Nathan, L., Tinker, L., De Boer, I. H., Tylavsky, F., ... & Liu, S. (2010). Relations of dietary magnesium intake to biomarkers of inflammation and endothelial dysfunction in an ethnically diverse cohort of postmenopausal women. Diabetes care, 33(2), 304-310.

Song, Y., Li, T. Y., van Dam, R. M., Manson, J. E., & Hu, F. B. (2007). Magnesium intake and plasma concentrations of markers of systemic inflammation and endothelial dysfunction in women. The American journal of clinical nutrition, 85(4), 1068-1074.

Nielsen, F. H., Johnson, L. K., & Zeng, H. (2010). Magnesium supplementation improves indicators of low magnesium status and inflammatory stress in adults older than 51 years with poor quality sleep. Magnesium Research, 23(4), 158-168.

Chacko, S. A., Sul, J., Song, Y., Li, X., LeBlanc, J., You, Y., ... & Liu, S. (2011). Magnesium supplementation, metabolic and inflammatory markers, and global genomic and proteomic profiling: a randomized, double-blind, controlled, crossover trial in overweight individuals. The American journal of clinical nutrition, 93(2), 463-473.

259   Murr, C., Pilz, S., Grammer, T. B., Kleber, M. E., Böhm, B. O., März, W., & Fuchs, D. (2012). Low serum zinc levels in patients undergoing coronary angiography correlate with immune activation and inflammation. Journal of Trace Elements in Medicine and Biology, 26(1), 26-30;

De Paula, R. C., Aneni, E. C., Costa, A. P. R., Figueiredo, V. N.,

Moura, F. A., Freitas, W. M.,... & Blaha, M. (2014). Low zinc levels is associated with increased inflammatory activity but not with atherosclerosis, arteriosclerosis or endothelial dysfunction among the very elderly. BBA clinical, 2, 1-6.

260   Preedy, V. R., & Watson, R. R. (Eds.). (2014). The Mediterranean Diet: An Evidence-Based Approach. Academic press.

261   Hagfors, L., Leanderson, P., Sköldstam, L., Andersson, J., & Johansson, G. (2003). Antioxidant intake, plasma antioxidants and oxidative stress in a randomized, controlled, parallel, Mediterranean dietary intervention study on patients with rheumatoid arthritis. Nutrition journal, 2(1), 5.
Kolomvotsou, A. I., Rallidis, L. S., Mountzouris, K. C., Lekakis, J., Koutelidakis, A., Efstathiou, S.,... & Zampelas, A. (2013). Adherence to Mediterranean diet and close dietetic supervision increase total dietary antioxidant intake and plasma antioxidant capacity in subjects with abdominal obesity. European journal of nutrition, 52(1), 37-48.
Razquin, C., Martinez, J. A., Martinez-Gonzalez, M. A., Mitjavila, M. T., Estruch, R., & Marti, A. (2009). A 3 years follow-up of a Mediterranean diet rich in virgin olive oil is associated with high plasma antioxidant capacity and reduced body weight gain. European journal of clinical nutrition, 63(12), 1387-1393.

262   Quiñonez-Flores, C. M., González-Chávez, S. A., Del Río Nájera, D., & Pacheco-Tena, C. (2016). Oxidative Stress Relevance in the Pathogenesis of the Rheumatoid Arthritis: A Systematic Review. BioMed Research International, 2016.
Mateen, S., Moin, S., Khan, A. Q., Zafar, A., & Fatima, N. (2016). Increased Reactive Oxygen Species Formation and Oxidative Stress in Rheumatoid Arthritis. PloS one, 11(4), e0152925.

263   Bae, S. C., Kim, S. J., & Sung, M. K. (2003). Inadequate antioxidant nutrient intake and altered plasma antioxidant status of rheumatoid arthritis patients. Journal of the American College of Nutrition, 22(4), 311-315.

264   Quiñonez-Flores, C. M., González-Chávez, S. A., Del Río Nájera, D., & Pacheco-Tena, C. (2016). Oxidative Stress Relevance in the Pathogenesis of the Rheumatoid Arthritis: A Systematic Review. BioMed Research International, 2016.
Datta, S., Kundu, S., Ghosh, P., De, S., Ghosh, A., & Chatterjee, M. (2014). Correlation of oxidant status with oxidative tissue damage in patients with rheumatoid arthritis. Clinical rheumatology, 33(11), 1557-1564.
Wolters M. (2005) Diet and psoriasis: experimental data and clinical evidence. Br J Dermatol. 153:706–714
Vijayakumar, D., Suresh, K., & Manoharan, S. (2006). Lipid per-

oxidation and antioxidant status in blood of rheumatoid arthritis patients. Indian Journal of Clinical Biochemistry, 21(1), 105-105.

Wolters M. (2005) Diet and psoriasis: experimental data and clinical evidence. Br J Dermatol. 153:706–714

Kundu, S., Ghosh, P., Datta, S., Ghosh, A., Chattopadhyay, S., & Chatterjee, M. (2012). Oxidative stress as a potential biomarker for determining disease activity in patients with rheumatoid arthritis. Free radical research, 46(12), 1482-1489.

Mateen, S., Moin, S., Khan, A. Q., Zafar, A., & Fatima, N. (2016). Increased Reactive Oxygen Species Formation and Oxidative Stress in Rheumatoid Arthritis. PloS one, 11(4), e0152925

Lin, X., & Huang, T. (2016). Oxidative stress in psoriasis and potential therapeutic use of antioxidants. Free radical research, 50(6), 585-595.

Wang, L., Gao, L., Jin, D., Wang, P., Yang, B., Deng, W.,... & Shen, H. (2015). The Relationship of Bone Mineral Density to Oxidant/Antioxidant Status and Inflammatory and Bone Turnover Markers in a Multicenter Cross-Sectional Study of Young Men with Ankylosing Spondylitis. Calcified tissue international, 97(1), 12-22.

Datta, S., Kundu, S., Ghosh, P., De, S., Ghosh, A., & Chatterjee, M. (2014). Correlation of oxidant status with oxidative tissue damage in patients with rheumatoid arthritis. Clinical rheumatology, 33(11), 1557-1564.

265   Root, M. M., McGinn, M. C., Nieman, D. C., Henson, D. A., Heinz, S. A., Shanely, R. A.,... & Jin, F. (2012). Combined fruit and vegetable intake is correlated with improved inflammatory and oxidant status from a cross-sectional study in a community setting. Nutrients, 4(1), 29-41;

Linos, A., Kaklamani, V. G., Kaklamani, E., Koumantaki, Y., Giziaki, E., Papazoglou, S., & Mantzoros, C. S. (1999). Dietary factors in relation to rheumatoid arthritis: a role for olive oil and cooked vegetables?. The American journal of clinical nutrition, 70(6), 1077-1082.

Valtueña, S., Pellegrini, N., Franzini, L., Bianchi, M. A., Ardigo, D., Del Rio, D.,... & Brighenti, F. (2008). Food selection based on total antioxidant capacity can modify antioxidant intake, systemic inflammation, and liver function without altering markers of oxidative stress. The American journal of clinical nutrition, 87(5), 1290-1297.

Mier-Cabrera, J., Aburto-Soto, T., Burrola-Méndez, S., Jiménez-Zamudio, L., Tolentino, M. C., Casanueva, E., & Hernández-Guerrero, C. (2009). Women with endometriosis improved their peripheral antioxidant markers after the application of a high antioxidant diet. Reproductive Biology and Endocrinology, 7(1), 54.

266   Dragsted, L. O., Pedersen, A., Hermetter, A., Basu, S., Hansen, M., Haren, G. R.,... & Jakobsen, J. (2004). The 6-a-day study: effects of fruit and vegetables on markers of oxidative stress and antioxidative

defense in healthy nonsmokers. The American journal of clinical nutrition, 79(6), 1060-1072.

Dauchet, L., Péneau, S., Bertrais, S., Vergnaud, A. C., Estaquio, C., Kesse-Guyot, E., ... & Hercberg, S. (2008). Relationships between different types of fruit and vegetable consumption and serum concentrations of antioxidant vitamins. British journal of nutrition, 100(03), 633-641.

Zino, S., Skeaff, M., Williams, S., & Mann, J. (1997). Randomised controlled trial of effect of fruit and vegetable consumption on plasma concentrations of lipids and antioxidants. Bmj, 314(7097), 1787.

267   Jiang, Y., Wu, S. H., Shu, X. O., Xiang, Y. B., Ji, B. T., Milne, G. L., ... & Yang, G. (2014). Cruciferous vegetable intake is inversely correlated with circulating levels of proinflammatory markers in women. Journal of the Academy of Nutrition and Dietetics, 114(5), 700-708.

268   Jiang, Y., Wu, S. H., Shu, X. O., Xiang, Y. B., Ji, B. T., Milne, G. L., ... & Yang, G. (2014). Cruciferous vegetable intake is inversely correlated with circulating levels of proinflammatory markers in women. Journal of the Academy of Nutrition and Dietetics, 114(5), 700-708.

269   Lu, B., Rho, Y. H., Cui, J., Iannaccone, C. K., Frits, M. L., Karlson, E. W., & Shadick, N. A. (2014). Associations of smoking and alcohol consumption with disease activity and functional status in rheumatoid arthritis. The Journal of rheumatology, 41(1), 24-30.

Lu, B., Solomon, D. H., Costenbader, K. H., Keenan, B. T., Chibnik, L. B., & Karlson, E. W. (2010). Alcohol consumption and markers of inflammation in women with preclinical rheumatoid arthritis. Arthritis & Rheumatism, 62(12), 3554-3559.

Di Giuseppe, D., Alfredsson, L., Bottai, M., Askling, J., & Wolk, A. (2012). Long term alcohol intake and risk of rheumatoid arthritis in women: a population based cohort study. Bmj, 345, e4230.

270   Purohit, V., Bode, J. C., Bode, C., Brenner, D. A., Choudhry, M. A., Hamilton, F., ... & Swanson, C. (2008). Alcohol, intestinal bacterial growth, intestinal permeability to endotoxin, and medical consequences: summary of a symposium. Alcohol, 42(5), 349-361.

271   Arsenault, B. J., Earnest, C. P., Després, J. P., Blair, S. N., & Church, T. S. (2009). Obesity, coffee consumption and CRP levels in postmenopausal overweight/obese women: importance of hormone replacement therapy use. European journal of clinical nutrition, 63(12), 1419-1424.

Kotani, K., Tsuzaki, K., Sano, Y., Maekawa, M., Fujiwara, S., Hamada, T., & Sakane, N. (2008). The relationship between usual coffee consumption and serum C-reactive protein level in a Japanese female population. Clinical chemistry and laboratory medicine, 46(10), 1434-1437.

Lopez-Garcia, E., van Dam, R. M., Qi, L., & Hu, F. B. (2006). Coffee consumption and markers of inflammation and endothelial dysfunction in healthy and diabetic women. The American journal of clinical nutrition, 84(4), 888-893.

Maki, T., Pham, N. M., Yoshida, D., Yin, G., Ohnaka, K., Takayanagi, R., & Kono, S. (2010). The relationship of coffee and green tea consumption with high-sensitivity C-reactive protein in Japanese men and women. Clinical chemistry and laboratory medicine, 48(6), 849-854.

Zampelas, A., Panagiotakos, D. B., Pitsavos, C., Chrysohoou, C., & Stefanadis, C. (2004). Associations between coffee consumption and inflammatory markers in healthy persons: the ATTICA study. The American journal of clinical nutrition, 80(4), 862-867

272   Mikuls, T. R., Cerhan, J. R., Criswell, L. A., Merlino, L., Mudano, A. S., Burma, M., ... & Saag, K. G. (2002). Coffee, tea, and caffeine consumption and risk of rheumatoid arthritis: results from the Iowa Women's Health Study. Arthritis & Rheumatism, 46(1), 83-91.

Löfvenborg, J. E., Andersson, T., Carlsson, P. O., Dorkhan, M., Groop, L., Martinell, M., ... & Carlsson, S. (2014). Coffee consumption and the risk of latent autoimmune diabetes in adults-results from a Swedish case-control study. Diabetic Medicine, 31(7), 799-805.

273   Mikuls, T. R., Cerhan, J. R., Criswell, L. A., Merlino, L., Mudano, A. S., Burma, M., ... & Saag, K. G. (2002). Coffee, tea, and caffeine consumption and risk of rheumatoid arthritis: results from the Iowa Women's Health Study. Arthritis & Rheumatism, 46(1), 83-91.

Rebello, S. A., Chen, C. H., Naidoo, N., Xu, W., Lee, J., Chia, K. S., ... & van Dam, R. M. (2011). Coffee and tea consumption in relation to inflammation and basal glucose metabolism in a multiethnic Asian population: a cross-sectional study. Nutrition journal, 10(1), 1

Kempf, K., Herder, C., Erlund, I., Kolb, H., Martin, S., Carstensen, M., ... & Jaakko, T. (2010). Effects of coffee consumption on subclinical inflammation and other risk factors for type 2 diabetes: a clinical trial. The American journal of clinical nutrition, 91(4), 950-957.

Wu, D., Wang, J., Pae, M., & Meydani, S. N. (2012). Green tea EGCG, T cells, and T cell-mediated autoimmune diseases. Molecular aspects of medicine, 33(1), 107-118.

Yang, E. J., Lee, J., Lee, S. Y., Kim, E. K., Moon, Y. M., Jung, Y. O., ... & Cho, M. L. (2014). EGCG attenuates autoimmune arthritis by inhibition of STAT3 and HIF-1α with Th17/Treg control. PLoS One, 9(2), e86062.

Lee, S. Y., Jung, Y. O., Ryu, J. G., Oh, H. J., Son, H. J., Lee, S. H., ... & Kim, H. Y. (2016). Epigallocatechin-3-gallate ameliorates autoimmune arthritis by reciprocal regulation of T helper-17 regulatory

T cells and inhibition of osteoclastogenesis by inhibiting STAT3 signaling. Journal of leukocyte biology, jlb-3A0514.

Alghadir, A. H., Gabr, S. A., & Al-Eisa, E. S. (2016). Green tea and exercise interventions as nondrug remedies in geriatric patients with rheumatoid arthritis. Journal of physical therapy science, 28(10), 2820-2829.

274   Dumas, J. A., Bunn, J. Y., Nickerson, J., Crain, K. I., Ebenstein, D. B., Tarleton, E. K., ... & Kien, C. L. (2016). Dietary saturated fat and monounsaturated fat have reversible effects on brain function and the secretion of pro-inflammatory cytokines in young women. Metabolism, 65(10), 1582-1588.

Gupta, S., Knight, A. G., Gupta, S., Keller, J. N., & Bruce-Keller, A. J. (2012). Saturated long-chain fatty acids activate inflammatory signaling in astrocytes. Journal of neurochemistry, 120(6), 1060-1071.

Håversen, Liliana, et al. "Induction of proinflammatory cytokines by long-chain saturated fatty acids in human macrophages." Atherosclerosis 202.2 (2009): 382-393.

Kien, C. L., Bunn, J. Y., Fukagawa, N. K., Anathy, V., Matthews, D. E., Crain, K. I., ... & Poynter, M. E. (2015). Lipidomic evidence that lowering the typical dietary palmitate to oleate ratio in humans decreases the leukocyte production of proinflammatory cytokines and muscle expression of redox-sensitive genes. The Journal of nutritional biochemistry, 26(12), 1599-1606.

Soto-Vaca, A., Losso, J. N., McDonough, K., & Finley, J. W. (2013). Differential effect of 14 free fatty acids in the expression of inflammation markers on human arterial coronary cells. Journal of agricultural and food chemistry, 61(42), 10074-10079.

Rocha, D. M., Caldas, A. P., Oliveira, L. L., Bressan, J., & Hermsdorff, H. H. (2016). Saturated fatty acids trigger TLR4-mediated inflammatory response. Atherosclerosis, 244, 211-215.

Snodgrass, R. G., Huang, S., Choi, I. W., Rutledge, J. C., & Hwang, D. H. (2013). Inflammasome-mediated secretion of IL-1β in human monocytes through TLR2 activation; modulation by dietary fatty acids. The Journal of Immunology, 191(8), 4337-4347.

Robblee, M. M., Kim, C. C., Abate, J. P., Valdearcos, M., Sandlund, K. L., Shenoy, M. K., ... & Koliwad, S. K. (2016). Saturated fatty acids engage an IRE1α-dependent pathway to activate the NLRP3 inflammasome in myeloid cells. Cell reports, 14(11), 2611-2623.

Reynolds, C. M., McGillicuddy, F. C., Harford, K. A., Finucane, O. M., Mills, K. H., & Roche, H. M. (2012). Dietary saturated fatty acids prime the NLRP3 inflammasome via TLR4 in dendritic cells—implications for diet-induced insulin resistance. Molecular nutrition & food research, 56(8), 1212-1222.

Yang, X., Haghiac, M., Glazebrook, P., Minium, J., Catalano, P. M., & Hauguel-de Mouzon, S. (2015). Saturated fatty acids enhance TLR4 immune pathways in human trophoblasts. Human Reproduction, dev173.

Gupta, S., Knight, A. G., Gupta, S., Keller, J. N., & Bruce-Keller, A. J. (2012). Saturated long-chain fatty acids activate inflammatory signaling in astrocytes. Journal of neurochemistry, 120(6), 1060-1071.

275 Lyte, J. M., Gabler, N. K., & Hollis, J. H. (2016). Postprandial serum endotoxin in healthy humans is modulated by dietary fat in a randomized, controlled, cross-over study. Lipids in Health and Disease, 15(1), 186.

Mani, V., Hollis, J. H., & Gabler, N. K. (2013). Dietary oil composition differentially modulates intestinal endotoxin transport and postprandial endotoxemia. Nutrition & metabolism, 10(1), 6.

Chapter 5. The Low-Starch Diet in Practice

276 Tommasini, A., Not, T., Kiren, V., Baldas, V., Santon, D., Trevisiol, C.,…& Lenhardt, A. (2004). Mass screening for coeliac disease using antihuman transglutaminase antibody assay. *Archives of disease in childhood*, *89*(6), 512-515.

277 Bhatia, B. K., Millsop, J. W., Debbaneh, M., Koo, J., Linos, E., & Liao, W. (2014). Diet and psoriasis, part II: celiac disease and role of a gluten-free diet. Journal of the American Academy of Dermatology, 71(2), 350-358.

Wu, J. J., Nguyen, T. U., Poon, K. Y. T., & Herrinton, L. J. (2012). The association of psoriasis with autoimmune diseases. Journal of the American Academy of Dermatology, 67(5), 924-930.

278 Al-Mayouf, S. M., Al-Mehaidib, A. I., & Alkaff, M. A. (2003). The significance of elevated serologic markers of celiac disease in children with juvenile rheumatoid arthritis. Saudi Journal of Gastroenterology, 9(2), 75.

279 Woo WK, McMillan SA, Watson RG, McCluggage WG, Sloan JM, McMillan JC. Coeliac disease-associated antibodies correlate with psoriasis activity. Br J Dermatol. 2004;151:891–4; 26.

Lindqvist U, Rudsander A, Boström A, Nilsson B, Michaëlsson G. IgA antibodies to gliadin and coeliac disease in psoriatic arthritis. Rheumatology (Oxford) 2002;41:31–7. [PubMed])

280 Michaëlsson G, Gerdén B, Hagforsen E, Nilsson B, Pihl-Lundin I, Kraaz W, et al. Psoriasis patients with antibodies to gliadin can be improved by a gluten-free diet. Br J Dermatol. 2000;142:44–51)

281 Addolorato, G., Parente, A., de Lorenzi, G., D'angelo Di Paola, M. E., Abenavoli, L., Leggio, L.,…& Gasbarrini, G. (2003). Rapid regression of psoriasis in a coeliac patient after gluten-free diet. Digestion, 68(1), 9-12.

Frikha F, Snoussi M, Bahloul Z. Osteomalacia associated with cutaneous psoriasis as the presenting feature of coeliac disease: a case report. Pan Afr Med J. 2012;11:58.)

282   Hafström, I., Ringertz, B., Spångberg, A., Von Zweigbergk, L., Brannemark, S., Nylander, I.,... & Klareskog, L. (2001). A vegan diet free of gluten improves the signs and symptoms of rheumatoid arthritis: the effects on arthritis correlate with a reduction in antibodies to food antigens. Rheumatology, 40(10), 1175-1179.

283   Hollon, J., Puppa, E. L., Greenwald, B., Goldberg, E., Guerrerio, A., & Fasano, A. (2015). Effect of gliadin on permeability of intestinal biopsy explants from celiac disease patients and patients with non-celiac gluten sensitivity. Nutrients, 7(3), 1565-1576.
Drago, S., El Asmar, R., Di Pierro, M., Grazia Clemente, M., Sapone, A. T. A., Thakar, M.,... & Zampini, L. (2006). Gliadin, zonulin and gut permeability: Effects on celiac and non-celiac intestinal mucosa and intestinal cell lines. Scandinavian journal of gastroenterology, 41(4), 408-419.
Lammers, K. M., Lu, R., Brownley, J., Lu, B., Gerard, C., Thomas, K.,... & Netzel–Arnett, S. (2008). Gliadin induces an increase in intestinal permeability and zonulin release by binding to the chemokine receptor CXCR3. Gastroenterology, 135(1), 194-204.

284   Drago, S., El Asmar, R., Di Pierro, M., Grazia Clemente, M., Sapone, A. T. A., Thakar, M.,... & Zampini, L. (2006). Gliadin, zonulin and gut permeability: Effects on celiac and non-celiac intestinal mucosa and intestinal cell lines. Scandinavian journal of gastroenterology, 41(4), 408-419.
De Punder, K., & Pruimboom, L. (2013). The dietary intake of wheat and other cereal grains and their role in inflammation. Nutrients, 5(3), 771-787.
Lammers, K. M., Lu, R., Brownley, J., Lu, B., Gerard, C., Thomas, K.,... & Netzel–Arnett, S. (2008). Gliadin induces an increase in intestinal permeability and zonulin release by binding to the chemokine receptor CXCR3. Gastroenterology, 135(1), 194-204.

285   Fasano, A. (2011). Zonulin and its regulation of intestinal barrier function: the biological door to inflammation, autoimmunity, and cancer. Physiological reviews, 91(1), 151-175.

286   Uhde, M., Ajamian, M., Caio, G., De Giorgio, R., Indart, A., Green, P. H.,... & Alaedini, A. (2016). Intestinal cell damage and systemic immune activation in individuals reporting sensitivity to wheat in the absence of coeliac disease. Gut, 65(12), 1930-1937.

287   Hollon, J. R., Cureton, P. A., Martin, M. L., Puppa, E. L. L., & Fasano, A. (2013). Trace gluten contamination may play a role in mucosal and clinical recovery in a subgroup of diet-adherent non-responsive celiac disease patients. BMC gastroenterology, 13(1), 1.

288 Hollon, J. R., Cureton, P. A., Martin, M. L., Puppa, E. L. L., & Fasano, A. (2013). Trace gluten contamination may play a role in mucosal and clinical recovery in a subgroup of diet-adherent non-responsive celiac disease patients. BMC gastroenterology, 13(1), 1.

289 Thompson, T., Lee, A. R., & Grace, T. (2010). Gluten contamination of grains, seeds, and flours in the United States: a pilot study. Journal of the American Dietetic Association, 110(6), 937-940.

290 Lee, H. J., Anderson, Z., & Ryu, D. (2014). Gluten contamination in foods labeled as "gluten free" in the United States. Journal of Food Protection®, 77(10), 1830-1833.

291 Zevallos, V. F., Ellis, H. J., Šuligoj, T., Herencia, L. I., & Ciclitira, P. J. (2012). Variable activation of immune response by quinoa (Chenopodium quinoa Willd.) prolamins in celiac disease. The American journal of clinical nutrition, 96(2), 337-344.
    Ortiz-Sánchez, J. P., Cabrera-Chávez, F., & de la Barca, A. M. C. (2013). Maize prolamins could induce a gluten-like cellular immune response in some celiac disease patients. Nutrients, 5(10), 4174-4183.
    Giménez, M. J., Real, A., García-Molina, M. D., Sousa, C., & Barro, F. (2017). Characterization of celiac disease related oat proteins: bases for the development of high quality oat varieties suitable for celiac patients. *Scientific reports*, 7, 42588.

292 Hollon, J. R., Cureton, P. A., Martin, M. L., Puppa, E. L. L., & Fasano, A. (2013). Trace gluten contamination may play a role in mucosal and clinical recovery in a subgroup of diet-adherent non-responsive celiac disease patients. BMC gastroenterology, 13(1), 1.

293 De Punder, K., & Pruimboom, L. (2013). The dietary intake of wheat and other cereal grains and their role in inflammation. Nutrients, 5(3), 771-787.
    Shibasaki, M., Sumazaki, R., Isoyama, S., & Takita, H. (1992). Interaction of lectins with human IgE: IgE-binding property and histamine-releasing activity of twelve plant lectins. International archives of allergy and immunology, 98(1), 18-25.
    Nachbar, M. S., & Oppenheim, J. D. (1980). Lectins in the United States diet: a survey of lectins in commonly consumed foods and a review of the literature. The American journal of clinical nutrition, 33(11), 2338-2345;
    Matucci, A., Veneri, G., Dalla Pellegrina, C., Zoccatelli, G., Vincenzi, S., Chignola, R.,...& Rizzi, C. (2004). Temperature-dependent decay of wheat germ agglutinin activity and its implications for food processing and analysis. Food Control, 15(5), 391-395.
    Rizzi, C., Galeoto, L., Zoccatelli, G., Vincenzi, S., Chignola, R., & Peruffo, A. D. (2003). Active soybean lectin in foods: quantitative determination by ELISA using immobilised asialofetuin. Food

research international, 36(8), 815-821.

Pramod, S. N., Venkatesh, Y. P., & Mahesh, P. A. (2007). Potato lectin activates basophils and mast cells of atopic subjects by its interaction with core chitobiose of cell-bound non-specific immunoglobulin E. Clinical & Experimental Immunology, 148(3), 391-401

294   Pan, L., Qin, G., Zhao, Y., Wang, J., Liu, F., & Che, D. (2013). Effects of soybean agglutinin on mechanical barrier function and tight junction protein expression in intestinal epithelial cells from piglets. International journal of molecular sciences, 14(11), 21689-21704.

Nachbar, M. S., & Oppenheim, J. D. (1980). Lectins in the United States diet: a survey of lectins in commonly consumed foods and a review of the literature. The American journal of clinical nutrition, 33(11), 2338-2345;

Pusztai, A., & Bardocz, S. (1996). Biological effects of plant lectins on the gastrointestinal tract: metabolic consequences and applications. Trends in glycoscience and glycotechnology, 8, 149-166.

Dalla Pellegrina, C., Perbellini, O., Scupoli, M. T., Tomelleri, C., Zanetti, C., Zoccatelli, G.,...& Chignola, R. (2009). Effects of wheat germ agglutinin on human gastrointestinal epithelium: insights from an experimental model of immune/epithelial cell interaction. Toxicology and applied pharmacology, 237(2), 146-153

Pan, L., Qin, G., Zhao, Y., Wang, J., Liu, F., & Che, D. (2013). Effects of soybean agglutinin on mechanical barrier function and tight junction protein expression in intestinal epithelial cells from piglets. International journal of molecular sciences, 14(11), 21689-21704.

295   Patel, B., Schutte, R., Sporns, P., Doyle, J., Jewel, L., & Fedorak, R. N. (2002). Potato glycoalkaloids adversely affect intestinal permeability and aggravate inflammatory bowel disease. Inflammatory bowel diseases, 8(5), 340-346.

296   Kamo, S., Suzuki, S., & Sato, T. (2014). The content of soyasaponin and soyasapogenol in soy foods and their estimated intake in the Japanese. Food science & nutrition, 2(3), 289-297.

Francis, G., Kerem, Z., Makkar, H. P., & Becker, K. (2002). The biological action of saponins in animal systems: a review. British journal of Nutrition, 88(06), 587-605.

Nickel, J., Spanier, L. P., Botelho, F. T., Gularte, M. A., & Helbig, E. (2016). Effect of different types of processing on the total phenolic compound content, antioxidant capacity, and saponin content of Chenopodium quinoa Willd grains. Food chemistry, 209, 139-143.

297   Gee, J. M., Price, K. R., Ridout, C. L., Wortley, G. M., Hurrell, R. F., & Johnson, I. T. (1993). Saponins of quinoa (Chenopodium quinoa): effects of processing on their abundance in quinoa products and their biological effects on intestinal mucosal tissue. Journal of the Science of Food and Agriculture, 63(2), 201-209.

Knudsen, D., Jutfelt, F., Sundh, H., Sundell, K., Koppe, W., & Frøkiær, H. (2008). Dietary soya saponins increase gut permeability and play a key role in the onset of soyabean-induced enteritis in Atlantic salmon (Salmo salar L.). British Journal of Nutrition, 100(01), 120-129.

298   Reddy, N. R., & Pierson, M. D. (1994). Reduction in antinutritional and toxic components in plant foods by fermentationa. *Food Research International, 27*(3), 281-290.

299   Messina, V. (2014). Nutritional and health benefits of dried beans. The American journal of clinical nutrition, 100(Supplement 1), 437S-442S.

300   Carlini, C. R., & Udedibie, A. B. (1997). Comparative effects of processing methods on hemagglutinating and antitryptic activities of Canavalia ensiformis and Canavalia braziliensis seeds. Journal of Agricultural and Food Chemistry, 45(11), 4372-4377.

301   Thomson, L. U., Rea, R. L., & Jenkins, D. J. (1983). Effect of heat processing on hemagglutinin activity in red kidney beans. Journal of Food Science, 48(1), 235-236.
       Carlini, C. R., & Udedibie, A. B. (1997). Comparative effects of processing methods on hemagglutinating and antitryptic activities of Canavalia ensiformis and Canavalia braziliensis seeds. Journal of Agricultural and Food Chemistry, 45(11), 4372-4377.

302   Atkinson, F. S., Foster-Powell, K., & Brand-Miller, J. C. (2008). International tables of glycemic index and glycemic load values: 2008. *Diabetes care, 31*(12), 2281-2283.

303   Katschinski, B., Logan, R. F., Edmond, M., & Langman, M. J. (1988). Smoking and sugar intake are separate but interactive risk factors in Crohn's disease. Gut, 29(9), 1202-1206.

304   Hu, Y., Costenbader, K. H., Gao, X., Al-Daabil, M., Sparks, J. A., Solomon, D. H.,...& Lu, B. (2014). Sugar-sweetened soda consumption and risk of developing rheumatoid arthritis in women. The American journal of clinical nutrition, 100(3), 959-967.

305   Gibson, P. R., Newnham, E., Barrett, J. S., Shepherd, S. J., & Muir, J. G. (2007). Review article: fructose malabsorption and the bigger picture. Alimentary pharmacology & therapeutics, 25(4), 349-363.

306   Payne, A. N., Chassard, C., & Lacroix, C. (2012). Gut microbial adaptation to dietary consumption of fructose, artificial sweeteners and sugar alcohols: implications for host–microbe interactions contributing to obesity. *Obesity reviews, 13*(9), 799-809.

307   Bian, X., Chi, L., Gao, B., Tu, P., Ru, H., & Lu, K. (2017). The artificial sweetener acesulfame potassium affects the gut microbiome and body weight gain in CD-1 mice. *PloS one, 12*(6), e0178426.

Rodriguez-Palacios, A., Harding, A., Menghini, P., Himmelman, C., Retuerto, M., Nickerson, K. P., ... & Pizarro, T. T. (2018). The artificial sweetener Splenda promotes gut proteobacteria, dysbiosis, and myeloperoxidase reactivity in Crohn's disease–like ileitis. *Inflammatory bowel diseases*, 24(5), 1005-1020.

308   Hvatum, M., Kanerud, L., Hällgren, R., & Brandtzaeg, P. (2006). The gut–joint axis: cross reactive food antibodies in rheumatoid arthritis. Gut, 55(9), 1240-1247.

Cabrera-Chávez, F., & de la Barca, A. M. C. (2009). Bovine milk intolerance in celiac disease is related to IgA reactivity to α-and β-caseins. *Nutrition*, 25(6), 715-716.

309   Nickerson, K. P., & McDonald, C. (2012). Crohn's disease-associated adherent-invasive Escherichia coli adhesion is enhanced by exposure to the ubiquitous dietary polysaccharide maltodextrin. *PLoS One*, 7(12), e52132.

Munyaka, P. M., Sepehri, S., Ghia, J. E., & Khafipour, E. (2016). Carrageenan gum and adherent invasive Escherichia coli in a piglet model of inflammatory bowel disease: impact on intestinal mucosa-associated microbiota. *Frontiers in microbiology*, 7, 462.

Shang, Q., Sun, W., Shan, X., Jiang, H., Cai, C., Hao, J., ... & Yu, G. (2017). Carrageenan-induced colitis is associated with decreased population of anti-inflammatory bacterium, akkermansia muciniphila, in the gut microbiota of c57bl/6j mice. *Toxicology letters*, 279, 87-95.

Necas, J., & Bartosikova, L. (2013). Carrageenan: a review. *Veterinarni Medicina*, 58(4).

310   De Filippo, Carlotta et al. "Impact of Diet in Shaping Gut Microbiota Revealed by a Comparative Study in Children from Europe and Rural Africa." Proceedings of the National Academy of Sciences of the United States of America 107.33 (2010): 14691–14696.

311   Roberts, C. L., Keita, Å. V., Duncan, S. H., O'kennedy, N., Söderholm, J. D., Rhodes, J. M., & Campbell, B. J. (2010). Translocation of Crohn's disease Escherichia coli across M-cells: contrasting effects of soluble plant fibres and emulsifiers. Gut, 59(10), 1331-1339.

312   Castaldo, G., Galdo, G., Aufiero, F. R., & Cereda, E. (2016). Very low-calorie ketogenic diet may allow restoring response to systemic therapy in relapsing plaque psoriasis. Obesity research & clinical practice, 10(3), 348-352.

313   O'Hearn, L. A. (2017). Ketogenic Diets, Caloric Restriction, and Hormones. *Journal of Evolution* and *Health*, 2(3), 13.

314   Jensen, P., Egeberg, A., Thyssen, J. P., Gislason, G., & Skov, L. (2017). Psoriatic Arthritis, but not Psoriasis, is Associated with Primary Adrenal Insufficiency. *Acta dermato-venereologica*, 97(4), 519-521.

Kebapcilar, L., Bilgir, O., Alacacioglu, A., Yildiz, Y., Taylan, A., Gunaydin, R., ... & Sari, I. (2010). Impaired hypothalamo-pituitary-adrenal axis in patients with ankylosing spondylitis. *Journal of endocrinological investigation, 33*(1), 42-47.

315 Kossoff, E. H., Cervenka, M. C., Henry, B. J., Haney, C. A., & Turner, Z. (2013). A decade of the modified Atkins diet (2003–2013): results, insights, and future directions. *Epilepsy & Behavior, 29*(3), 437-442.

316 Kossoff, E. H., Cervenka, M. C., Henry, B. J., Haney, C. A., & Turner, Z. (2013). A decade of the modified Atkins diet (2003–2013): results, insights, and future directions. *Epilepsy & Behavior, 29*(3), 437-442.

317 Pendyala, S., Walker, J. M., & Holt, P. R. (2012). A high-fat diet is associated with endotoxemia that originates from the gut. *Gastroenterology, 142*(5), 1100-1101.

Lyte, J. M., Gabler, N. K., & Hollis, J. H. (2016). Postprandial serum endotoxin in healthy humans is modulated by dietary fat in a randomized, controlled, cross-over study. *Lipids in health and disease, 15*(1), 186.

Cani, P. D., Amar, J., Iglesias, M. A., Poggi, M., Knauf, C., Bastelica, D., ... & Waget, A. (2007). Metabolic endotoxemia initiates obesity and insulin resistance. *Diabetes, 56*(7), 1761-1772.

Cani, P. D., Bibiloni, R., Knauf, C., Waget, A., Neyrinck, A. M., Delzenne, N. M., & Burcelin, R. (2008). Changes in gut microbiota control metabolic endotoxemia-induced inflammation in high-fat diet–induced obesity and diabetes in mice. *Diabetes, 57*(6), 1470-1481.

Lam, Y. Y., Ha, C. W., Hoffmann, J., Oscarsson, J., Dinudom, A., Mather, T. J., ... & Storlien, L. H. (2015). Effects of dietary fat profile on gut permeability and microbiota and their relationships with metabolic changes in mice. *Obesity, 23*(7), 1429-1439.

Erridge, C., Attina, T., Spickett, C. M., & Webb, D. J. (2007). A high-fat meal induces low-grade endotoxemia: evidence of a novel mechanism of postprandial inflammation–. *The American journal of clinical nutrition, 86*(5), 1286-1292.

Moreira, A. P. B., Texeira, T. F. S., Ferreira, A. B., Peluzio, M. D. C. G., & Alfenas, R. D. C. G. (2012). Influence of a high-fat diet on gut microbiota, intestinal permeability and metabolic endotoxaemia. *British Journal of Nutrition, 108*(5), 801-809.

Serino, M., Luche, E., Gres, S., Baylac, A., Bergé, M., Cenac, C., ... & Mariette, J. (2012). Metabolic adaptation to a high-fat diet is associated with a change in the gut microbiota. *Gut, 61*(4), 543-553.

Lyte, J. M., Gabler, N. K., & Hollis, J. H. (2016). Postprandial serum endotoxin in healthy humans is modulated by dietary fat in a randomized, controlled, cross-over study. *Lipids in health and disease, 15*(1), 186.

Chapter 6. Anti-inflammatory Fats and Oils

318 Estruch, R., Ros, E., Salas-Salvadó, J., Covas, M. I., Corella, D., Arós, F., . . . & Lamuela-Raventos, R. M. (2013). Primary prevention of cardiovascular disease with a Mediterranean diet. New England Journal of Medicine, 368(14), 1279-1290.

Sofi, F., Abbate, R., Gensini, G. F., & Casini, A. (2010). Accruing evidence on benefits of adherence to the Mediterranean diet on health: an updated systematic review and meta-analysis. The American journal of clinical nutrition, 92(5), 1189-1196.

Schwingshackl, L., & Hoffmann, G. (2014). Adherence to Mediterranean diet and risk of cancer: A systematic review and meta-analysis of observational studies. International journal of cancer, 135(8), 1884-1897.

Tresserra-Rimbau, A., Rimm, E. B., Medina-Remón, A., Martínez-González, M. A., López-Sabater, M. C., Covas, M. I., . . . & Arós, F. (2014). Polyphenol intake and mortality risk: a re-analysis of the PREDIMED trial. BMC medicine, 12(1), 77.

Martínez-González, M. Á., De la Fuente-Arrillaga, C., Nuñez-Cordoba, J. M., Basterra-Gortari, F. J., Beunza, J. J., Vazquez, Z., . . . & Bes-Rastrollo, M. (2008). Adherence to Mediterranean diet and risk of developing diabetes: prospective cohort study. Bmj, 336(7657), 1348-1351.

319 Chrysohoou, C., Panagiotakos, D. B., Pitsavos, C., Das, U. N., & Stefanadis, C. (2004). Adherence to the Mediterranean diet attenuates inflammation and coagulation process in healthy adults: The ATTICA Study. Journal of the American College of Cardiology, 44(1), 152-158.

Richard, C., Couture, P., Desroches, S., & Lamarche, B. (2013). Effect of the Mediterranean diet with and without weight loss on markers of inflammation in men with metabolic syndrome. Obesity, 21(1), 51-57.

Sköldstam, L., Hagfors, L., & Johansson, G. (2003). An experimental study of a Mediterranean diet intervention for patients with rheumatoid arthritis. Annals of the rheumatic diseases, 62(3), 208-214.

320 Skoldstam, L., Hagfors, L., & Johansson, G. (2003). An experimental study of a Mediterranean diet intervention for patients with rheumatoid arthritis. Annals of the Rheumatic Diseases, 62(3), 208–214; Abendroth, A., Michalsen, A., Luedtke, R., Rueffer, A., Musial, F., Dobos, G. J., & Langhorst, J. (2010). Changes of intestinal microflora in patients with rheumatoid arthritis during fasting or a Mediterranean diet. Forschende Komplementärmedizin/Research in Complementary Medicine, 17(6), 307-313; McKellar, G., Morrison, E., McEntegart, A., Hampson, R., Tierney, A., Mackle, G., . . . & Capell, H. A. (2007). A pilot study of a Mediterranean-type diet intervention in female patients with rheumatoid

arthritis living in areas of social deprivation in Glasgow. Annals of the rheumatic diseases, 66(9), 1239-1243.

Preedy, V. R., & Watson, R. R. (Eds.). (2014). The Mediterranean Diet: An Evidence-Based Approach. Academic press.

Barrea, L., Balato, N., Di Somma, C., Macchia, P. E., Napolitano, M., Savanelli, M. C., ... & Savastano, S. (2015). Nutrition and psoriasis: is there any association between the severity of the disease and adherence to the Mediterranean diet?. Journal of translational medicine, 13(1), 18.

321   Barrea L., Balato N., Di Somma C., Macchia P.E., Napolitano M., Savanelli M.C., Esposito K., Colao A., Savastano S. Nutrition and psoriasis: Is there any association between the severity of the disease and adherence to the Mediterranean diet? J. Transl. Med. 2015;13:18. doi: 10.1186/s12967-014-0372-1.)

Hayashi, H., Satoi, K., Sato-Mito, N., Kaburagi, T., Yoshino, H., Higaki, M., ... & Sato, K. (2012). Nutritional status in relation to adipokines and oxidative stress is associated with disease activity in patients with rheumatoid arthritis. Nutrition, 28(11), 1109-1114.

Skoldstam, L., Hagfors, L., & Johansson, G. (2003). An experimental study of a Mediterranean diet intervention for patients with rheumatoid arthritis. Annals of the Rheumatic Diseases, 62(3), 208–214. http://doi.org/10.1136/ard.62.3.208

Guida, B., Napoleone, A., Trio, R., Nastasi, A., Balato, N., Laccetti, R., & Cataldi, M. (2014). Energy-restricted, n-3 polyunsaturated fatty acids-rich diet improves the clinical response to immuno-modulating drugs in obese patients with plaque-type psoriasis: a randomized control clinical trial. Clinical Nutrition, 33(3), 399-405.

Hansen, G. V. O., Nielsen, L., Kluger, E., Thysen, M., Emmertsen, H., Stengaard-Pedersen, K., ... & Andersen, P. W. (1996). Nutritional status of Danish rheumatoid arthritis patients and effects of a diet adjusted in energy intake, fish-meal, and antioxidants. Scandinavian journal of rheumatology, 25(5), 325-333.

322   Skoldstam, L., Hagfors, L., & Johansson, G. (2003). An experimental study of a Mediterranean diet intervention for patients with rheumatoid arthritis. Annals of the Rheumatic Diseases, 62(3), 208–214.

323   Hagfors, L., Nilsson, I., Sköldstam, L., & Johansson, G. (2005). Fat intake and composition of fatty acids in serum phospholipids in a randomized, controlled, Mediterranean dietary intervention study on patients with rheumatoid arthritis. Nutrition & metabolism, 2(1), 26.

324   Guida, B., Napoleone, A., Trio, R., Nastasi, A., Balato, N., Laccetti, R., & Cataldi, M. (2014). Energy-restricted, n-3 polyunsaturated fatty acids-rich diet improves the clinical response to immuno-modulating drugs in obese patients with plaque-type psoriasis: a randomized control clinical trial. Clinical Nutrition, 33(3), 399-405.

325 Barrea, L., Balato, N., Di Somma, C., Macchia, P. E., Napolitano, M., Savanelli, M. C.,... & Savastano, S. (2015). Nutrition and psoriasis: is there any association between the severity of the disease and adherence to the Mediterranean diet?. Journal of translational medicine, 13(1), 18.

326 Miles, E. A., & Calder, P. C. (2012). Influence of marine n-3 polyunsaturated fatty acids on immune function and a systematic review of their effects on clinical outcomes in rheumatoid arthritis. British Journal of Nutrition, 107(S2), S171-S184.
   van den Elsen, L. W., Nusse, Y., Balvers, M., Redegeld, F. A., Knol, E. F., Garssen, J., & Willemsen, L. E. (2013). n-3 Long-chain PUFA reduce allergy-related mediator release by human mast cells in vitro via inhibition of reactive oxygen species. British Journal of Nutrition, 109(10), 1821-1831;
   Murata, M., Kaneniwa, M., Saito, H., Shinohara, K., Maeda-Yamamoto, M.,... & Ooizumi, T. (1998). Effect of tetracosahexaenoic acid on the content and release of histamine, and eicosanoid production in MC/9 mouse mast cell. Lipids, 33(11), 1107-1114
   Liu, Y., Chen, F., Odle, J., Lin, X., Jacobi, S. K., Zhu, H.,... & Hou, Y. (2012). Fish oil enhances intestinal integrity and inhibits TLR4 and NOD2 signaling pathways in weaned pigs after LPS challenge. The Journal of nutrition, 142(11), 2017-2024.

327 Berbert, A. A., Kondo, C. R. M., Almendra, C. L., Matsuo, T., & Dichi, I. (2005). Supplementation of fish oil and olive oil in patients with rheumatoid arthritis. Nutrition, 21(2), 131-136.
   Beauchamp, G. K., Keast, R. S., Morel, D., Lin, J., Pika, J., Han, Q.,... & Breslin, P. A. (2005). Phytochemistry: ibuprofen-like activity in extra-virgin olive oil. Nature, 437(7055), 45-46.

328 Bogani, P., Galli, C., Villa, M., & Visioli, F. (2007). Postprandial anti-inflammatory and antioxidant effects of extra virgin olive oil. Atherosclerosis, 190(1), 181-186.

329 Kremer, J. M., Lawrence, D. A., Jubiz, W., Digiacomo, R., Rynes, R., Bartholomew, L. E., & Sherman, M. (1990). Dietary fish oil and olive oil supplementation in patients with Rheumatoid Arthritis clinical and immunologic effects. Arthritis & Rheumatology, 33(6), 810-820.

330 Kremer, J. M., Lawrence, D. A., Jubiz, W., Digiacomo, R., Rynes, R., Bartholomew, L. E., & Sherman, M. (1990). Dietary fish oil and olive oil supplementation in patients with Rheumatoid Arthritis clinical and immunologic effects. Arthritis & Rheumatology, 33(6), 810-820.

331 Berbert, A. A., Kondo, C. R. M., Almendra, C. L., Matsuo, T., & Dichi, I. (2005). Supplementation of fish oil and olive oil in patients with rheumatoid arthritis. Nutrition, 21(2), 131-136.

332 Adam, O., Beringer, C., Kless, T., Lemmen, C., Adam, A., Wiseman,

M., ... & Forth, W. (2003). Anti-inflammatory effects of a low arachidonic acid diet and fish oil in patients with rheumatoid arthritis. Rheumatology international, 23(1), 27-36.

333 Gerster, H. (1998). Can adults adequately convert a-linolenic acid (18: 3n-3) to eicosapentaenoic acid (20: 5n-3) and docosahexaenoic acid (22: 6n-3)?. International Journal for Vitamin and Nutrition Research, 68(3), 159-173.

Lane, K., Derbyshire, E., Li, W., & Brennan, C. (2014). Bioavailability and potential uses of vegetarian sources of omega-3 fatty acids: a review of the literature. Critical reviews in food science and nutrition, 54(5), 572-579.

334 Karimi, R., Fitzgerald, T. P., & Fisher, N. S. (2012). A quantitative synthesis of mercury in commercial seafood and implications for exposure in the United States. Environmental health perspectives, 120(11), 1512. Supplemental Material. Available at http://www.stonybrook.edu/commcms/gelfond/docs/Seafood%20Mercury%20Database.pdf

USDA data, available at https://health.gov/dietaryguidelines/dga2005/report/html/table_g2_adda2.htm

335 Blanchet, C., Lucas, M., Julien, P., Morin, R., Gingras, S., & Dewailly, É. (2005). Fatty acid composition of wild and farmed Atlantic salmon (Salmo salar) and rainbow trout (Oncorhynchus mykiss). Lipids, 40(5), 529-531.

336 Ponnampalam, E. N., Mann, N. J., & Sinclair, A. J. (2006). Effect of feeding systems on omega-3 fatty acids, conjugated linoleic acid and trans fatty acids in Australian beef cuts: potential impact on human health. Asia Pacific Journal of Clinical Nutrition, 15(1), 21.

Daley, C. A., Abbott, A., Doyle, P. S., Nader, G. A., & Larson, S. (2010). A review of fatty acid profiles and antioxidant content in grass-fed and grain-fed beef. Nutrition journal, 9(1), 10.

337 Senftleber, N. K., Nielsen, S. M., Andersen, J. R., Bliddal, H., Tarp, S., Lauritzen, L., ... & Christensen, R. (2017). Marine Oil Supplements for Arthritis Pain: A Systematic Review and Meta-Analysis of Randomized Trials. Nutrients, 9(1), 42.

338 Millsop, J. W., Bhatia, B. K., Debbaneh, M., Koo, J., & Liao, W. (2014). Diet and psoriasis, part III: role of nutritional supplements. Journal of the American Academy of Dermatology, 71(3), 561-569.

339 Miles, E. A., & Calder, P. C. (2012). Influence of marine n-3 polyunsaturated fatty acids on immune function and a systematic review of their effects on clinical outcomes in rheumatoid arthritis. British Journal of Nutrition, 107(S2), S171-S184.

340 Sundström, B., Stålnacke, K., Hagfors, L., & Johansson, G. (2006). Supplementation of omega-3 fatty acids in patients with ankylosing

spondylitis. Scandinavian journal of rheumatology, 35(5), 359-362.

341   Belluzzi, A., Brignola, C., Campieri, M., Pera, A., Boschi, S., &
       Miglioli, M. (1996). Effect of an enteric-coated fish-oil preparation
       on relapses in Crohn's disease. New England Journal of Medicine,
       334(24), 1557-1560.

342   Gheita, T., Kamel, S., Helmy, N., El-Laithy, N., & Monir, A. (2012).
       Omega-3 fatty acids in juvenile idiopathic arthritis: effect on
       cytokines (IL-1 and TNF-α), disease activity and response criteria.
       Clinical rheumatology, 31(2), 363-366.

343   Paoli, A., Moro, T., Bosco, G., Bianco, A., Grimaldi, K. A., Campore-
       si, E., & Mangar, D. (2015). Effects of n-3 polyunsaturated fatty acids
       (ω-3) supplementation on some cardiovascular risk factors with a
       ketogenic Mediterranean diet. Marine drugs, 13(2), 996-1009.

344   Endres, S., Ghorbani, R., Kelley, V. E., Georgilis, K., Lonnemann, G.,
       van der Meer, J. W.,...& Schaefer, E. J. (1989). The effect of dietary
       supplementation with n—3 polyunsaturated fatty acids on the syn-
       thesis of interleukin-1 and tumor necrosis factor by mononuclear
       cells. New England Journal of Medicine, 320(5), 265-271.

345   Albert, B. B., Cameron-Smith, D., Hofman, P. L., & Cutfield, W.
       S. (2013). Oxidation of marine omega-3 supplements and human
       health. BioMed research international, 2013.

346   Albert, B. B., Cameron-Smith, D., Hofman, P. L., & Cutfield, W.
       S. (2013). Oxidation of marine omega-3 supplements and human
       health. BioMed research international, 2013;
       Albert, B. B., Derraik, J. G., Cameron-Smith, D., Hofman, P. L.,
       Tumanov, S., Villas-Boas, S. G.,...& Cutfield, W. S. (2015). Fish oil
       supplements in New Zealand are highly oxidised and do not meet
       label content of n-3 PUFA. Scientific reports, 5, 7928.

347   Albert, B. B., Cameron-Smith, D., Hofman, P. L., & Cutfield, W.
       S. (2013). Oxidation of marine omega-3 supplements and human
       health. BioMed research international, 2013;
       Albert, B. B., Derraik, J. G., Cameron-Smith, D., Hofman, P. L.,
       Tumanov, S., Villas-Boas, S. G.,...& Cutfield, W. S. (2015). Fish oil
       supplements in New Zealand are highly oxidised and do not meet
       label content of n-3 PUFA. Scientific reports, 5, 7928.

348   Senftleber, N. K., Nielsen, S. M., Andersen, J. R., Bliddal, H., Tarp,
       S., Lauritzen, L.,...& Christensen, R. (2017). Marine Oil Supple-
       ments for Arthritis Pain: A Systematic Review and Meta-Analysis of
       Randomized Trials. Nutrients, 9(1), 42.
       Millsop, J. W., Bhatia, B. K., Debbaneh, M., Koo, J., & Liao, W.
       (2014). Diet and psoriasis, part III: role of nutritional supplements.
       Journal of the American Academy of Dermatology, 71(3), 561-569

349 Halvorsen, B. L., & Blomhoff, R. (2011). Determination of lipid oxidation products in vegetable oils and marine omega-3 supplements. Food & nutrition research, 55.

350 Kragballe, K., & Fogh, K. (1988). A low-fat diet supplemented with dietary fish oil (Max-EPA) results in improvement of psoriasis and in formation of leukotriene B5. Acta dermato-venereologica, 69(1), 23-28.

351 Proudman, S. M., James, M. J., Spargo, L. D., Metcalf, R. G., Sullivan, T. R., Rischmueller, M., ... & Cleland, L. G. (2013). Fish oil in recent onset rheumatoid arthritis: a randomised, double-blind controlled trial within algorithm-based drug use. Annals of the rheumatic diseases, annrheumdis-2013.

352 Cleland, L. G., James, M. J., & Proudman, S. M. (2005). Fish oil: what the prescriber needs to know. Arthritis research & therapy, 8(1), 202.

353 Gheita, T., Kamel, S., Helmy, N., El-Laithy, N., & Monir, A. (2012). Omega-3 fatty acids in juvenile idiopathic arthritis: effect on cytokines (IL-1 and TNF-α), disease activity and response criteria. Clinical rheumatology, 31(2), 363-366.

354 Halvorsen, B. L., & Blomhoff, R. (2011). Determination of lipid oxidation products in vegetable oils and marine omega-3 supplements. Food & nutrition research, 55.

355 Jackowski, S. A., Alvi, A. Z., Mirajkar, A., Imani, Z., Gamalevych, Y., Shaikh, N. A., & Jackowski, G. (2015). Oxidation levels of North American over-the-counter n-3 (omega-3) supplements and the influence of supplement formulation and delivery form on evaluating oxidative safety. Journal of nutritional science, 4, e30.

356 Jackowski, S. A., Alvi, A. Z., Mirajkar, A., Imani, Z., Gamalevych, Y., Shaikh, N. A., & Jackowski, G. (2015). Oxidation levels of North American over-the-counter n-3 (omega-3) supplements and the influence of supplement formulation and delivery form on evaluating oxidative safety. Journal of nutritional science, 4, e30.

357 Dyerberg, J., Madsen, P., Møller, J. M., Aardestrup, I., & Schmidt, E. B. (2010). Bioavailability of marine n-3 fatty acid formulations. Prostaglandins, Leukotrienes and Essential Fatty Acids, 83(3), 137-141.

358 Eritsland, J. (2000). Safety considerations of polyunsaturated fatty acids. The American journal of clinical nutrition, 71(1), 197S-201S.

359 http://olivecenter.ucdavis.edu/research/files/oliveoilfinal071410updated.pdf

360 Silva, L., Pinto, J., Carrola, J., & Paiva-Martins, F. (2010). Oxidative stability of olive oil after food processing and comparison with other vegetable oils. Food Chemistry, 121(4), 1177-1187;
Casal, S., Malheiro, R., Sendas, A., Oliveira, B. P., & Pereira, J. A.

(2010). Olive oil stability under deep-frying conditions. Food and chemical toxicology, 48(10), 2972-2979.

361 Berasategi, I., Barriuso, B., Ansorena, D., & Astiasarán, I. (2012). Stability of avocado oil during heating: Comparative study to olive oil. Food Chemistry, 132(1), 439-446.
Werman, M. J., & Neeman, I. (1986). Oxidative stability of avocado oil. Journal of the American Oil Chemists' Society, 63(3), 355-360.

362 Frankel EN, Smith LM, Hamblin CL, Creveling RK, Clifford AJ. Occurrence of cyclic fatty acid monomers in frying oils used for fast foods. J Am Oil Chem Soc. 1984;61:87-90.
Koski, A., Psomiadou, E., Tsimidou, M., Hopia, A., Kefalas, P., Wähälä, K., & Heinonen, M. (2002). Oxidative stability and minor constituents of virgin olive oil and cold-pressed rapeseed oil. European Food Research and Technology, 214(4), 294-298.
Halvorsen, B. L., & Blomhoff, R. (2011). Determination of lipid oxidation products in vegetable oils and marine omega-3 supplements. Food & nutrition research, 55.

363 Halvorsen, B. L., & Blomhoff, R. (2011). Determination of lipid oxidation products in vegetable oils and marine omega-3 supplements. Food & nutrition research, 55.

364 Chen, C., & Khismatullin, D. B. (2015). Oxidized low-density lipoprotein contributes to atherogenesis via co-activation of macrophages and mast cells. PloS one, 10(3), e0123088;
Meng, Z., Yan, C., Deng, Q., Dong, X., Duan, Z. M., Gao, D. F., & Niu, X. L. (2013). Oxidized low-density lipoprotein induces inflammatory responses in cultured human mast cells via Toll-like receptor 4. Cellular Physiology and Biochemistry, 31(6), 842-853;
Shaik-Dasthagirisaheb, Y. B., Varvara, G., Murmura, G., Saggini, A., Caraffa, A., Antinolfi, P., ... & Toniato, E. (2012). Role of vitamins D, E and C in immunity and inflammation. Journal of biological regulators and homeostatic agents, 27(2), 291-295.
Kanner, J. (2007). Dietary advanced lipid oxidation endproducts are risk factors to human health. Molecular nutrition & food research, 51(9), 1094-1101.
Staprans I, Rapp JH, Pan XM, Kim KY, Feingold KR. Oxidized lipids in the diet are a source of oxidized lipid in chylomicrons of human serum. Arterioscler Thromb. 1994;14:1900-1905.

365 Halvorsen, B. L., & Blomhoff, R. (2011). Determination of lipid oxidation products in vegetable oils and marine omega-3 supplements. Food & nutrition research, 55.

366 Frankel EN, Smith LM, Hamblin CL, Creveling RK, Clifford AJ. Occurrence of cyclic fatty acid monomers in frying oils used for fast foods. J Am Oil Chem Soc. 1984;61:87-90.

Koski, A., Psomiadou, E., Tsimidou, M., Hopia, A., Kefalas, P., Wähälä, K., & Heinonen, M. (2002). Oxidative stability and minor constituents of virgin olive oil and cold-pressed rapeseed oil. European Food Research and Technology, 214(4), 294-298.

Halvorsen, B. L., & Blomhoff, R. (2011). Determination of lipid oxidation products in vegetable oils and marine omega-3 supplements. Food & nutrition research, 55.

367   Mozaffarian, D., Aro, A., & Willett, W. C. (2009). Health effects of trans-fatty acids: experimental and observational evidence. European journal of clinical nutrition, 63, S5-S21.

Kanner, J. (2007). Dietary advanced lipid oxidation endproducts are risk factors to human health. Molecular nutrition & food research, 51(9), 1094-1101.

368   Kochhar, S. P., & Henry, C. J. K. (2009). Oxidative stability and shelf-life evaluation of selected culinary oils. International journal of food sciences and nutrition, 60(sup7), 289-296.

369   Ramsden, C. E., Zamora, D., Majchrzak-Hong, S., Faurot, K. R., Broste, S. K., Frantz, R. P., ... & Hibbeln, J. R. (2016). Re-evaluation of the traditional diet-heart hypothesis: analysis of recovered data from Minnesota Coronary Experiment (1968-73). bmj, 353, i1246; Siri-Tarino, P. W., Sun, Q., Hu, F. B., & Krauss, R. M. (2010). Meta-analysis of prospective cohort studies evaluating the association of saturated fat with cardiovascular disease. The American journal of clinical nutrition, ajcn-27725.

370   Dumas, J. A., Bunn, J. Y., Nickerson, J., Crain, K. I., Ebenstein, D. B., Tarleton, E. K., ... & Kien, C. L. (2016). Dietary saturated fat and monounsaturated fat have reversible effects on brain function and the secretion of pro-inflammatory cytokines in young women. Metabolism, 65(10), 1582-1588.

371   Kien, C. L., Bunn, J. Y., Fukagawa, N. K., Anathy, V., Matthews, D. E., Crain, K. I., ... & Poynter, M. E. (2015). Lipidomic evidence that lowering the typical dietary palmitate to oleate ratio in humans decreases the leukocyte production of proinflammatory cytokines and muscle expression of redox-sensitive genes. The Journal of nutritional biochemistry, 26(12), 1599-1606.

372   Rocha, D. M., Caldas, A. P., Oliveira, L. L., Bressan, J., & Hermsdorff, H. H. (2016). Saturated fatty acids trigger TLR4-mediated inflammatory response. Atherosclerosis, 244, 211-215.

Snodgrass, R. G., Huang, S., Choi, I. W., Rutledge, J. C., & Hwang, D. H. (2013). Inflammasome-mediated secretion of IL-1β in human monocytes through TLR2 activation; modulation by dietary fatty acids. The Journal of Immunology, 191(8), 4337-4347.

Robblee, M. M., Kim, C. C., Abate, J. P., Valdearcos, M., Sandlund,

K. L., Shenoy, M. K., ... & Koliwad, S. K. (2016). Saturated fatty acids engage an IRE1α-dependent pathway to activate the NLRP3 inflammasome in myeloid cells. Cell reports, 14(11), 2611-2623.

373   Reynolds, C. M., McGillicuddy, F. C., Harford, K. A., Finucane, O. M., Mills, K. H., & Roche, H. M. (2012). Dietary saturated fatty acids prime the NLRP3 inflammasome via TLR4 in dendritic cells—implications for diet-induced insulin resistance. Molecular nutrition & food research, 56(8), 1212-1222.

374   Kien, C. L., Bunn, J. Y., Fukagawa, N. K., Anathy, V., Matthews, D. E., Crain, K. I., ... & Poynter, M. E. (2015). Lipidomic evidence that lowering the typical dietary palmitate to oleate ratio in humans decreases the leukocyte production of proinflammatory cytokines and muscle expression of redox-sensitive genes. The Journal of nutritional biochemistry, 26(12), 1599-1606.

375   Soto-Vaca, A., Losso, J. N., McDonough, K., & Finley, J. W. (2013). Differential effect of 14 free fatty acids in the expression of inflammation markers on human arterial coronary cells. Journal of agricultural and food chemistry, 61(42), 10074-10079.

376   Yang, X., Haghiac, M., Glazebrook, P., Minium, J., Catalano, P. M., & Hauguel-de Mouzon, S. (2015). Saturated fatty acids enhance TLR4 immune pathways in human trophoblasts. Human Reproduction, dev173.

377   Gupta, S., Knight, A. G., Gupta, S., Keller, J. N., & Bruce-Keller, A. J. (2012). Saturated long-chain fatty acids activate inflammatory signaling in astrocytes. Journal of neurochemistry, 120(6), 1060-1071.

378   Gupta, S., Knight, A. G., Gupta, S., Keller, J. N., & Bruce-Keller, A. J. (2012). Saturated long-chain fatty acids activate inflammatory signaling in astrocytes. Journal of neurochemistry, 120(6), 1060-1071. Håversen, Liliana, et al. "Induction of proinflammatory cytokines by long-chain saturated fatty acids in human macrophages." Atherosclerosis 202.2 (2009): 382-393.
Soto-Vaca, A., Losso, J. N., McDonough, K., & Finley, J. W. (2013). Differential effect of 14 free fatty acids in the expression of inflammation markers on human arterial coronary cells. Journal of agricultural and food chemistry, 61(42), 10074-10079.

379   Soto-Vaca, A., Losso, J. N., McDonough, K., & Finley, J. W. (2013). Differential effect of 14 free fatty acids in the expression of inflammation markers on human arterial coronary cells. Journal of agricultural and food chemistry, 61(42), 10074-10079;
Huang, S., Rutkowsky, J. M., Snodgrass, R. G., Ono-Moore, K. D., Schneider, D. A., Newman, J. W., ... & Hwang, D. H. (2012). Saturated fatty acids activate TLR-mediated proinflammatory signaling pathways. Journal of lipid research, 53(9), 2002-2013.

380 Lyte, J. M., Gabler, N. K., & Hollis, J. H. (2016). Postprandial serum endotoxin in healthy humans is modulated by dietary fat in a randomized, controlled, cross-over study. Lipids in Health and Disease, 15(1), 186.

381 Lyte, J. M., Gabler, N. K., & Hollis, J. H. (2016). Postprandial serum endotoxin in healthy humans is modulated by dietary fat in a randomized, controlled, cross-over study. Lipids in Health and Disease, 15(1), 186.

382 Mani, V., Hollis, J. H., & Gabler, N. K. (2013). Dietary oil composition differentially modulates intestinal endotoxin transport and postprandial endotoxemia. Nutrition & metabolism, 10(1), 6.

383 Mani, V., Hollis, J. H., & Gabler, N. K. (2013). Dietary oil composition differentially modulates intestinal endotoxin transport and postprandial endotoxemia. Nutrition & metabolism, 10(1), 6.

384 Johnson, G. H., & Fritsche, K. (2012). Effect of dietary linoleic acid on markers of inflammation in healthy persons: a systematic review of randomized controlled trials. Journal of the Academy of Nutrition and Dietetics, 112(7), 1029-1041;
Pischon, T., Hankinson, S. E., Hotamisligil, G. S., Rifai, N., Willett, W. C., & Rimm, E. B. (2003). Habitual dietary intake of n-3 and n-6 fatty acids in relation to inflammatory markers among US men and women. Circulation, 108(2), 155-160

385 Liou, Y. A., & Innis, S. M. (2009). Dietary linoleic acid has no effect on arachidonic acid, but increases n-6 eicosadienoic acid, and lowers dihomo-γ-linolenic and eicosapentaenoic acid in plasma of adult men. Prostaglandins, Leukotrienes and Essential Fatty Acids, 80(4), 201-206.
Liou, Y. A., King, D. J., Zibrik, D., & Innis, S. M. (2007). Decreasing linoleic acid with constant α-linolenic acid in dietary fats increases (n-3) eicosapentaenoic acid in plasma phospholipids in healthy men. The Journal of nutrition, 137(4), 945-952.

386 Millsop, J. W., Bhatia, B. K., Debbaneh, M., Koo, J., & Liao, W. (2014). Diet and psoriasis, part III: role of nutritional supplements. Journal of the American Academy of Dermatology, 71(3), 561-569.

387 Sköldstam, L., Larsson, L., & Lindström, F. D. (1979). Effects of fasting and lactovegetarian diet on rheumatoid arthritis. Scandinavian journal of rheumatology, 8(4), 249-255.
Hafstrom I, Ringertz B, Spangberg A, von Zweigbergk L, Brannemark S, Nylander I, et al. A vegan diet free of gluten improves the signs and symptoms of rheumatoid arthritis: the effects on arthritis correlate with a reduction in antibodies to food antigens. Rheumatology 2001; 40:1175-9.

388 Hafstorm.

389   Adam, O., Beringer, C., Kless, T., Lemmen, C., Adam, A., Wiseman, M., ... & Forth, W. (2003). Anti-inflammatory effects of a low arachidonic acid diet and fish oil in patients with rheumatoid arthritis. Rheumatology international, 23(1), 27-36.

390   Adam, O., Beringer, C., Kless, T., Lemmen, C., Adam, A., Wiseman, M., ... & Forth, W. (2003). Anti-inflammatory effects of a low arachidonic acid diet and fish oil in patients with rheumatoid arthritis. Rheumatology international, 23(1), 27-36.

Chapter 7. Troubleshooting and Customizing the Keystone Diet

391   Williams, R. (1981). Rheumatoid arthritis and food: a case study. British medical journal (Clinical research ed.), 283(6290), 563.

392   Beri, D., Malaviya, A. N., Shandilya, R., & Singh, R. R. (1988). Effect of dietary restrictions on disease activity in rheumatoid arthritis. Annals of the Rheumatic Diseases, 47(1), 69–72.
      Williams, R. (1981). Rheumatoid arthritis and food: a case study. British medical journal (Clinical research ed.), 283(6290), 563.
      Pacor, M. L., Lunardi, C., Di Lorenzo, G., Biasi, D., & Corrocher, R. (2001). Food allergy and seronegative arthritis: report of two cases. Clinical rheumatology, 20(4), 279-281.
      Parke, A. L., & Hughes, G. R. V. (1981). Rheumatoid arthritis and food: a case study. Br Med J (Clin Res Ed), 282(6281), 2027-2029.
      Hvatum, M., Kanerud, L., Hällgren, R., & Brandtzaeg, P. (2006). The gut-joint axis: cross reactive food antibodies in rheumatoid arthritis. Gut, 55(9), 1240-1247.

393   Ratner, D., Vigder, K., & Eshel, E. (1985). Juvenile rheumatoid arthritis and milk allergy. Journal of the Royal Society of Medicine, 78(5), 410-413.
      Schrander, J. J., Marcelis, C., De Vries, M. P., & van Santen-Hoeufft, H. M. (1997). Does food intolerance play a role in juvenile chronic arthritis?. Rheumatology, 36(8), 905-908.

394   Appelboom, T., & Durez, P. (1994). Effect of milk product deprivation on spondyloarthropathy. Annals of the Rheumatic Diseases, 53(7), 481–482.

395   Van de Laar, M. A., Aalbers, M., Bruins, F. G., van Dinther-Janssen, A. C., Van Der Korst, J. K., & Meijer, C. J. (1992). Food intolerance in rheumatoid arthritis. II. Clinical and histological aspects. Annals of the rheumatic diseases, 51(3), 303-306

396   Hvatum, M., Kanerud, L., Hällgren, R., & Brandtzaeg, P. (2006). The gut-joint axis: cross reactive food antibodies in rheumatoid arthritis. Gut, 55(9), 1240-1247.

397 Panush, R. S., Stroud, R. M., & Webster, E. M. (1986). Food-induced (allergic) arthritis. Inflammatory arthritis exacerbated by milk. Arthritis & Rheumatism, 29(2), 220-226.

398 Titchenal, C. A., & Dobbs, J. (2007). A system to assess the quality of food sources of calcium. Journal of Food Composition and Analysis, 20(8), 717-724;
Wien, E. M., & Schwartz, R. (1983). Comparison of in vitro and in vivo measurements of dietary Ca exchangeability and bioavailability. The Journal of nutrition, 113(2), 388-393.

399 Rodríguez del Río, P., Sánchez-García, S., Escudero, C., Pastor-Vargas, C., Sánchez Hernández, J. J., Pérez-Rangel, I., & Ibáñez, M. D. (2012). Allergy to goat's and sheep's milk in a population of cow's milk–allergic children treated with oral immunotherapy. Pediatric Allergy and Immunology, 23(2), 128-132.

400 Hodge, L., Swain, A., & Faulkner-Hogg, K. (2009). Food allergy and intolerance. Australian family physician, 38(9), 705.

401 Malakar, S., Gibson, P. R., Barrett, J. S., & Muir, J. G. (2017). Naturally occurring dietary salicylates: A closer look at common Australian foods. Journal of Food Composition and Analysis, 57, 31-39.

402 Swain, A. R., Soutter, V. L., & Loblay, R. H. (2011). RPAH elimination diet handbook: with food & shopping guide. Allergy Unit, Royal Prince Alfred Hospital.

403 Swain, A. R., Dutton, S. P., & Truswell, A. S. (1985). Salicylates in foods. J Am Diet Assoc, 85(8), 950-60.
Hodge, L., Swain, A., & Faulkner-Hogg, K. (2009). Food allergy and intolerance. Australian family physician, 38(9), 705.

404 Skypala, I. J., Williams, M., Reeves, L., Meyer, R., & Venter, C. (2015). Sensitivity to food additives, vaso-active amines and salicylates: a review of the evidence. Clinical and translational allergy, 5(1), 34.

405 Swain, A. R., Soutter, V. L., & Loblay, R. H. (2011). RPAH elimination diet handbook: with food & shopping guide. Allergy Unit, Royal Prince Alfred Hospital.

406 http://www.fedup.com.au/images/stories/SCarthritis.pdf

407 Panush, R. S., Carter, R. L., Katz, P., Kowsari, B., Longley, S., & Finnie, S. (1983). Diet therapy for rheumatoid arthritis. Arthritis & Rheumatology, 26(4), 462-471.

408 Jemima, E. A., Prema, A., & Thangam, E. B. (2014). Functional characterization of histamine H4 receptor on human mast cells. Molecular immunology, 62(1), 19-28.
Steinke, J. W., Negri, J., Liu, L., Payne, S. C., & Borish, L. (2014). Aspirin activation of eosinophils and mast cells: implications in the

pathogenesis of aspirin-exacerbated respiratory disease. The Journal of Immunology, 193(1), 41-47.

Mita, H., Endoh, S., Kudoh, M., Kawagishi, Y., Kobayashi, M., Taniguchi, M., & Akiyama, K. (2001). Possible involvement of mast-cell activation in aspirin provocation of aspirin-induced asthma. Allergy, 56(11), 1061-1067.

O'Sullivan, S., Dahlén, B., Dahlén, S. E., & Kumlin, M. (1996). Increased urinary excretion of the prostaglandin D 2 metabolite 9α, 11β-prostaglandin F 2 after aspirin challenge supports mast cell activation in aspirin-induced airway obstruction. Journal of Allergy and Clinical Immunology, 98(2), 421-432.

Togo, K., Suzuki, Y., Yoshimaru, T., Inoue, T., Terui, T., Ochiai, T., & Ra, C. (2009). Aspirin and salicylates modulate IgE-mediated leukotriene secretion in mast cells through a dihydropyridine receptor-mediated Ca 2+ influx. Clinical Immunology, 131(1), 145-156.

409   Noordenbos, T., Yeremenko, N., Gofita, I., van de Sande, M., Tak, P. P., Cañete, J. D., & Baeten, D. (2012). Interleukin-17–positive mast cells contribute to synovial inflammation in spondylarthritis. Arthritis & Rheumatism, 64(1), 99-109.

Keijsers, R. R., Joosten, I., Erp, P. E., Koenen, H. J., & Kerkhof, P. (2014). Cellular sources of IL-17 in psoriasis: a paradigm shift?. Experimental dermatology, 23(11), 799-803.

Lin, A. M., Rubin, C. J., Khandpur, R., Wang, J. Y., Riblett, M., Yalavarthi, S.,...& Bruce, A. T. (2011). Mast cells and neutrophils release IL-17 through extracellular trap formation in psoriasis. The Journal of Immunology, 187(1), 490-500.

Hueber, A. J., Asquith, D. L., Miller, A. M., Reilly, J., Kerr, S., Leipe, J.,...& McInnes, I. B. (2010). Cutting edge: mast cells express IL-17A in rheumatoid arthritis synovium. The Journal of Immunology, 184(7), 3336-3340.

Shin, K., Nigrovic, P. A., Crish, J., Boilard, E., McNeil, H. P., Larabee, K. S.,...& Lee, D. M. (2009). Mast cells contribute to autoimmune inflammatory arthritis via their tryptase/heparin complexes. The Journal of Immunology, 182(1), 647-656.

Henderson, W. R. (1994). The role of leukotrienes in inflammation. Annals of internal medicine, 121(9), 684-697.

410   Barcik, W., Pugin, B., Westermann, P., Perez, N. R., Ferstl, R., Wawrzyniak, M.,...& Akdis, C. A. (2016). Histamine-secreting microbes are increased in the gut of adult asthma patients. Journal of Allergy and Clinical Immunology, 138(5), 1491-1494.

Özoğul, F. (2004). Production of biogenic amines by Morganella morganii, Klebsiella pneumoniae and Hafnia alvei using a rapid HPLC method. European Food Research and Technology, 219(5), 465-469.

Pugin, B., Barcik, W., Westermann, P., Heider, A., Wawrzyniak, M., Hellings, P., ...& O'Mahony, L. (2017). A wide diversity of bacteria from the human gut produces and degrades biogenic amines. *Microbial ecology in health and disease*, *28*(1), 1353881.

411   Johnston, C. S., Retrum, K. R., & Srilakshmi, J. C. (1992). Antihistamine effects and complications of *supplemental* vitamin C. Journal of the American Dietetic Association (USA).
Bucca, C., Rolla, G., Oliva, A., & Farina, J. C. (1990). Effect of vitamin C on histamine bronchial responsiveness of patients with allergic rhinitis. Annals of allergy, 65(4), 311-314.

412   Healy, E., Newell, L., Howarth, P., & Friedmann, P. S. (2008). Control of salicylate intolerance with fish oils. *British Journal of Dermatology*, *159*(6), 1368-1369.

413   http://www.noarthritis.com/nightshades.htm

414   Afifi, L., Danesh, M. J., Lee, K. M., Beroukhim, K., Farahnik, B., Ahn, R. S., ...& Liao, W. (2017). Dietary behaviors in psoriasis: patient-reported outcomes from a US National Survey. *Dermatology and therapy*, *7*(2), 227-242.

415   Cantwell, M. (1996). A review of important facts about potato glycoalkaloids. Perishables Handling Newsletter, 87, 26-27.

416   Patel, B., Schutte, R., Sporns, P., Doyle, J., Jewel, L., & Fedorak, R. N. (2002). Potato glycoalkaloids adversely affect intestinal permeability and aggravate inflammatory bowel disease. Inflammatory bowel diseases, 8(5), 340-346.
Hashimoto, K., Kawagishi, H., Nakayama, T., & Shimizu, M. (1997). Effect of capsianoside, a diterpene glycoside, on tight-junctional permeability. Biochimica et Biophysica Acta (BBA)-Biomembranes, 1323(2), 281-290.

417   Patel, B., Schutte, R., Sporns, P., Doyle, J., Jewel, L., & Fedorak, R. N. (2002). Potato glycoalkaloids adversely affect intestinal permeability and aggravate inflammatory bowel disease. Inflammatory bowel diseases, 8(5), 340-346.

418   Hashimoto, K., Kawagishi, H., Nakayama, T., & Shimizu, M. (1997). Effect of capsianoside, a diterpene glycoside, on tight-junctional permeability. Biochimica et Biophysica Acta (BBA)-Biomembranes, 1323(2), 281-290.

419   Jensen-Jarolim, E., Gajdzik, L., Haberl, I., Kraft, D., Scheiner, O., & Graf, J. (1998). Hot spices influence permeability of human intestinal epithelial monolayers. The Journal of nutrition, 128(3), 577-581.
Isoda, H., Han, J., Tominaga, M., & Maekawa, T. (2001). Effects of capsaicin on human intestinal cell line Caco-2. Cytotechnology, 36(1-3), 155-161;

Tsukura, Y., Mori, M., Hirotani, Y., Ikeda, K., Amano, F., Kato, R., ... & Tanaka, K. (2007). Effects of capsaicin on cellular damage and monolayer permeability in human intestinal Caco-2 cells. Biological and Pharmaceutical Bulletin, 30(10), 1982-1986.

420   Nachbar, M. S., & Oppenheim, J. D. (1980). Lectins in the United States diet: a survey of lectins in commonly consumed foods and a review of the literature. The American journal of clinical nutrition, 33(11), 2338-2345;
Pramod, S. N., Venkatesh, Y. P., & Mahesh, P. A. (2007). Potato lectin activates basophils and mast cells of atopic subjects by its interaction with core chitobiose of cell-bound non-specific immunoglobulin E. Clinical & Experimental Immunology, 148(3), 391-401.

421   Pramod, S. N., Venkatesh, Y. P., & Mahesh, P. A. (2007). Potato lectin activates basophils and mast cells of atopic subjects by its interaction with core chitobiose of cell-bound non-specific immunoglobulin E. Clinical & Experimental Immunology, 148(3), 391-401.

422   Pramod, S. N., Venkatesh, Y. P., & Mahesh, P. A. (2007). Potato lectin activates basophils and mast cells of atopic subjects by its interaction with core chitobiose of cell-bound non-specific immunoglobulin E. Clinical & Experimental Immunology, 148(3), 391-401.

423   Kaushal, N., Jain, S., Kondaiah, P., & Tiwary, A. K. (2009). Influence of piperine on transcutaneous permeation of repaglinide in rats and on tight junction proteins in HaCaT cells: unveiling the mechanisms for enhanced permeation. Sci Pharm, 77, 877-897.

424   Feng, X., Liu, Y., Wang, X., & Di, X. (2014). Effects of piperine on the intestinal permeability and pharmacokinetics of linarin in rats. Molecules, 19(5), 5624-5633.
Jin, M. J., & Han, H. K. (2010). Effect of piperine, a major component of black pepper, on the intestinal absorption of fexofenadine and its implication on food–drug interaction. Journal of food science, 75(3), H93-H96.

Chapter 8. Anti-inflammatory Supplements

425   Milliken, S. V., Wassall, H., Lewis, B. J., Logie, J., Barker, R. N., Macdonald, H., ... & Ormerod, A. D. (2012). Effects of ultraviolet light on human serum 25-hydroxyvitamin D and systemic immune function. Journal of Allergy and Clinical Immunology, 129(6), 1554-1561.
Bryson, K. J., Nash, A. A., & Norval, M. (2014). Does vitamin D protect against respiratory viral infections?. Epidemiology and infection, 142(09), 1789-1801.

426   Webb, A. R., Kline, L., & Holick, M. F. (1988). Influence of season and latitude on the cutaneous synthesis of vitamin D3: exposure to winter sunlight in Boston and Edmonton will not promote vitamin

D3 synthesis in human skin. The journal of clinical endocrinology & metabolism, 67(2), 373-378.

427 Grazio, S., Grubišić, F., Kavanagh, H. S., Naglić, Đ. B., Anić, B., Bakula, M., . . . & Cvijetić, S. (2015). Vitamin D serum level, disease activity and functional ability in different rheumatic patients. The American journal of the medical sciences, 349(1), 46-49.

Holick, M. F. (2006, March). High prevalence of vitamin D inadequacy and implications for health. In Mayo Clinic Proceedings (Vol. 81, No. 3, pp. 353-373).

Rossini, M., Bongi, S. M., La Montagna, G., Minisola, G., Malavolta, N., Bernini, L., . . . & Adami, S. (2010). Vitamin D deficiency in rheumatoid arthritis: prevalence, determinants and associations with disease activity and disability. Arthritis research & therapy, 12(6), R216.

428 Ricceri F, Pescitelli L, Tripo L, Prignano F. Deficiency of serum concentration of 25-hydroxyvitamin D correlates with severity of disease in chronic plaque psoriasis. J Am Acad Dermatol. 2013;68:511–2

Grazio, S., Grubišić, F., Kavanagh, H. S., Naglić, Đ. B., Anić, B., Bakula, M., . . . & Cvijetić, S. (2015). Vitamin D serum level, disease activity and functional ability in different rheumatic patients. The American journal of the medical sciences, 349(1), 46-49.

Lin, J., Liu, J., Davies, M. L., & Chen, W. (2016). Serum vitamin D level and rheumatoid arthritis disease activity: review and meta-analysis. PloS one, 11(1), e0146351.

Cutolo, M., Otsa, K., Laas, K., Yprus, M., Lehtme, R., Secchi, M. E., . . . & Seriolo, B. (2006). Circannual vitamin D serum levels and disease activity in rheumatoid arthritis: Northern versus Southern Europe. Clin Exp Rheumatol, 24(6), 702-4.

Oelzner, P., Müller, A., Deschner, F., Hüller, M., Abendroth, K., Hein, G., & Stein, G. (1998). Relationship between disease activity and serum levels of vitamin D metabolites and PTH in rheumatoid arthritis. Calcified tissue international, 62(3), 193-198.

Patel, S., Farragher, T., Berry, J., Bunn, D., Silman, A., & Symmons, D. (2007). Association between serum vitamin D metabolite levels and disease activity in patients with early inflammatory polyarthritis. Arthritis & Rheumatism, 56(7), 2143-2149.

Lange, U., Jung, O., Teichmann, J., & Neeck, G. (2001). Relationship between disease activity and serum levels of vitamin D metabolites and parathyroid hormone in ankylosing spondylitis. Osteoporosis International, 12(12), 1031-1035.

429 Finamor, D. C., Sinigaglia-Coimbra, R., Neves, L. C., Gutierrez, M., Silva, J. J., Torres, L. D., . . . & Lopes, A. C. (2013). A pilot study assessing the effect of prolonged administration of high daily doses of

vitamin D on the clinical course of vitiligo and psoriasis. Dermato-endocrinology, 5(1), 222-234.

Morimoto, S., Yoshikawa, K., Kozuka, T., Kitano, Y., Imanaka, S., Fukuo, K., ... & Kumahara, Y. (1986). Treatment of psoriasis vulgaris by oral administration of 1α-hydroxyvitamin D 3—Open-design study. Calcified tissue international, 39(3), 209-212.

Smith, E. L., Pincus, S. H., Donovan, L., & Holick, M. F. (1988). A novel approach for the evaluation and treatment of psoriasis: oral or topical use of 1, 25-dihydroxyvitamin D3 can be a safe and effective therapy for psoriasis. Journal of the American Academy of Dermatology, 19(3), 516-528.

Takamoto, S., Onishi, T., Morimoto, S., Imanaka, S., Yu-kawa, S., Kozuka, T., ... & Kumahara, Y. (1986). Effect of 1α-hydroxycholecalciferol on psoriasis vulgaris: a pilot study. Calcified tissue international, 39(6), 360-364.

Perez, A., Raab, R., Chen, T. C., Turner, A., & HOLLCK, M. (1996). Safety and efficacy of oral calcitriol (1, 25-dihydroxyvitamin D3) for the treatment of psoriasis. British journal of dermatology, 134(6), 1070-1078.

430   Finamor, D. C., Sinigaglia-Coimbra, R., Neves, L. C., Gutierrez, M., Silva, J. J., Torres, L. D., ... & Lopes, A. C. (2013). A pilot study assessing the effect of prolonged administration of high daily doses of vitamin D on the clinical course of vitiligo and psoriasis. Dermato-endocrinology, 5(1), 222-234.

Morimoto, S., Yoshikawa, K., Kozuka, T., Kitano, Y., Imanaka, S., Fukuo, K., ... & Kumahara, Y. (1986). Treatment of psoriasis vulgaris by oral administration of 1α-hydroxyvitamin D 3—Open-design study. Calcified tissue international, 39(3), 209-212.

Smith, E. L., Pincus, S. H., Donovan, L., & Holick, M. F. (1988). A novel approach for the evaluation and treatment of psoriasis: oral or topical use of 1, 25-dihydroxyvitamin D3 can be a safe and effective therapy for psoriasis. Journal of the American Academy of Dermatology, 19(3), 516-528.

Takamoto, S., Onishi, T., Morimoto, S., Imanaka, S., Yu-kawa, S., Kozuka, T., ... & Kumahara, Y. (1986). Effect of 1α-hydroxycholecalciferol on psoriasis vulgaris: a pilot study. Calcified tissue international, 39(6), 360-364.

Perez, A., Raab, R., Chen, T. C., Turner, A., & HOLLCK, M. (1996). Safety and efficacy of oral calcitriol (1, 25-dihydroxyvitamin D3) for the treatment of psoriasis. British journal of dermatology, 134(6), 1070-1078.

431   Holick, M. F. (2006, March). High prevalence of vitamin D inadequacy and implications for health. In Mayo Clinic Proceedings (Vol. 81, No. 3, pp. 353-373). Elsevier.

432 Andjelkovic, Z., Vojinovic, J., Pejnovic, N., Popovic, M., Dujic, A., Mitrovic, D., . . . & Stefanovic, D. (1999). Disease modifying and immunomodulatory effects of high dose 1 (OH) D3 in rheumatoid arthritis patients. Clinical and experimental rheumatology, 17, 453-456.
GaáL, J., Lakos, G., Szodoray, P., Kiss, J., HORVáTH, I., Horkay, E., . . . & SzEGEDI, A. (2009). Immunological and clinical effects of alphacalcidol in patients with psoriatic arthropathy: results of an open, follow-up pilot study. Acta dermato-venereologica, 89(2), 140-144
Huckins, D., Felson, D. T., & Holick, M. (1990). Treatment of psoriatic arthritis with oral 1, 25-dihydroxyvitamin D3: a pilot study. Arthritis & Rheumatology, 33(11), 1723-1727

433 Holick, M. F. (2006, March). High prevalence of vitamin D inadequacy and implications for health. In Mayo Clinic Proceedings (Vol. 81, No. 3, pp. 353-373). Elsevier.

434 Lange, U., Jung, O., Teichmann, J., & Neeck, G. (2001). Relationship between disease activity and serum levels of vitamin D metabolites and parathyroid hormone in ankylosing spondylitis. Osteoporosis International, 12(12), 1031-1035.
Bianchi, M. L., Bardare, M., Caraceni, M. P., Cohen, E., Falvella, S., Borzani, M., & DeGaspari, M. G. (1990). Bone metabolism in juvenile rheumatoid arthritis. Bone and mineral, 9(2), 153-162.
Grossman, J. M., Gordon, R., Ranganath, V. K., Deal, C., Caplan, L., Chen, W., . . . & Volkmann, E. (2010). American College of Rheumatology 2010 recommendations for the prevention and treatment of glucocorticoid-induced osteoporosis. Arthritis care & research, 62(11), 1515-1526.

435 Grossman, J. M., Gordon, R., Ranganath, V. K., Deal, C., Caplan, L., Chen, W., . . . & Volkmann, E. (2010). American College of Rheumatology 2010 recommendations for the prevention and treatment of glucocorticoid-induced osteoporosis. Arthritis care & research, 62(11), 1515-1526.

436 Souberbielle, J. C., Body, J. J., Lappe, J. M., Plebani, M., Shoenfeld, Y., Wang, T. J., . . . & Gandini, S. (2010). Vitamin D and musculoskeletal health, cardiovascular disease, autoimmunity and cancer: recommendations for clinical practice. Autoimmunity reviews, 9(11), 709-715

437 Holick, M. F. (2006, March). High prevalence of vitamin D inadequacy and implications for health. In Mayo Clinic Proceedings (Vol. 81, No. 3, pp. 353-373). Elsevier.

438 Rossini, M., Bongi, S. M., La Montagna, G., Minisola, G., Malavolta, N., Bernini, L., . . . & Adami, S. (2010). Vitamin D deficiency in rheumatoid arthritis: prevalence, determinants and associations with disease

activity and disability. Arthritis research & therapy, 12(6), R216.

439   Souberbielle, J. C., Body, J. J., Lappe, J. M., Plebani, M., Shoenfeld, Y., Wang, T. J., ... & Gandini, S. (2010). Vitamin D and musculoskeletal health, cardiovascular disease, autoimmunity and cancer: recommendations for clinical practice. Autoimmunity reviews, 9(11), 709-715

440   Urashima, M., Segawa, T., Okazaki, M., Kurihara, M., Wada, Y., & Ida, H. (2010). Randomized trial of vitamin D supplementation to prevent seasonal influenza A in schoolchildren. The American journal of clinical nutrition, 91(5), 1255-1260.
Hyppönen, E., Läärä, E., Reunanen, A., Järvelin, M. R., & Virtanen, S. M. (2001). Intake of vitamin D and risk of type 1 diabetes: a birth-cohort study. The Lancet, 358(9292), 1500-1503.

441   Pavelká, K., Gatterová, J., Olejarová, M., Machacek, S., Giacovelli, G., & Rovati, L. C. (2002). Glucosamine sulfate use and delay of progression of knee osteoarthritis: a 3-year, randomized, placebo-controlled, double-blind study. Archives of Internal Medicine, 162(18), 2113-2123.
Reginster, J. Y., Deroisy, R., Rovati, L. C., Lee, R. L., Lejeune, E., Bruyere, O., ... & Gossett, C. (2001). Long-term effects of glu-cosamine sulphate on osteoarthritis progression: a randomised, placebo-controlled clinical trial. The Lancet, 357(9252), 251-256.

442   Reginster, J. Y., Deroisy, R., Rovati, L. C., Lee, R. L., Lejeune, E., Bruyere, O., ... & Gossett, C. (2001). Long-term effects of glu-cosamine sulphate on osteoarthritis progression: a randomised, placebo-controlled clinical trial. The Lancet, 357(9252), 251-256.

443   Sawitzke, A. D., Shi, H., Finco, M. F., Dunlop, D. D., Bingham, C. O., Harris, C. L., ... & Lane, N. E. (2008). The effect of glucosamine and/or chondroitin sulfate on the progression of knee osteoarthritis: a report from the glucosamine/chondroitin arthritis intervention trial. Arthritis & Rheumatology, 58(10), 3183-3191.

444   Cunnane, G., FitzGerald, O., Beeton, C., Cawston, T. E., & Bresni-han, B. (2001). Early joint erosions and serum levels of matrix metalloproteinase 1, matrix metalloproteinase 3, and tissue inhibitor of metalloproteinases 1 in rheumatoid arthritis. Arthritis & Rheu-matism, 44(10), 2263-2274.
Chen, J. J., Huang, J. F., Du, W. X., & Tong, P. J. (2014). Expression and significance of MMP3 in synovium of knee joint at different stage in osteoarthritis patients. Asian Pacific journal of tropical medicine, 7(4), 297-300.

445   Nakamura, H., Masuko, K., Yudoh, K., Kato, T., Kamada, T., & Kawa-hara, T. (2007). Effects of glucosamine administration on patients with rheumatoid arthritis. Rheumatology international, 27(3), 213-218.

446 Cunnane, G., FitzGerald, O., Beeton, C., Cawston, T. E., & Bresni-han, B. (2001). Early joint erosions and serum levels of matrix metalloproteinase 1, matrix metalloproteinase 3, and tissue inhibitor of metalloproteinases 1 in rheumatoid arthritis. Arthritis & Rheumatism, 44(10), 2263-2274.

Chen, J. J., Huang, J. F., Du, W. X., & Tong, P. J. (2014). Expression and significance of MMP3 in synovium of knee joint at different stage in osteoarthritis patients. Asian Pacific journal of tropical medicine, 7(4), 297-300.

447 Viswanath, V., Myles, A., Dayal, R., & Aggarwal, A. (2011). Levels of serum matrix metalloproteinase-3 correlate with disease activity in the enthesitis-related arthritis category of juvenile idiopathic arthritis. The Journal of rheumatology, 38(11), 2482-2487.

van Kuijk, A. W., Reinders-Blankert, P., Smeets, T. J., Dijkmans, B. A., & Tak, P. P. (2006). Detailed analysis of the cell infiltrate and the expression of mediators of synovial inflammation and joint destruction in the synovium of patients with psoriatic arthritis: implications for treatment. Annals of the rheumatic diseases, 65(12), 1551-1557.

Sarma, P. K., Misra, R., & Aggarwal, A. (2008). Elevated serum receptor activator of NFκB ligand (RANKL), osteoprotegerin (OPG), matrix metalloproteinase (MMP) 3, and ProMMP1 in patients with juvenile idiopathic arthritis. Clinical rheumatology, 27(3), 289-294.

448 Chan, P. S., Caron, J. P., & Orth, M. W. (2007). Effects of glucosamine and chondroitin sulfate on bovine cartilage explants under long-term culture conditions. American journal of veterinary research, 68(7), 709-715.

Dodge, G. R., & Jimenez, S. A. (2003). Glucosamine sulfate modulates the levels of aggrecan and matrix metalloproteinase-3 synthesized by cultured human osteoarthritis articular chondrocytes. Osteoarthritis and Cartilage, 11(6), 424-432.

Byron, C. R., Orth, M. W., Venta, P. J., Lloyd, J. W., & Caron, J. P. (2003). Influence of glucosamine on matrix metalloproteinase expression and activity in lipopolysaccharide-stimulated equine chondrocytes. American journal of veterinary research, 64(6), 666-671.

Nakamura, H., Shibakawa, A., Tanaka, M., Kato, T., & Nishioka, K. (2003). Effects of glucosamine hydrochloride on the production of prostaglandin E2, nitric oxide and metalloproteases by chondrocytes and synoviocytes in osteoarthritis. Clinical and experimental rheumatology, 22(3), 293-299.

449 Kim, L. S., Axelrod, L. J., Howard, P., Buratovich, N., & Waters, R. F. (2006). Efficacy of methylsulfonylmethane (MSM) in osteoarthritis pain of the knee: a pilot clinical trial. Osteoarthritis and Cartilage, 14(3), 286-294.

Debbi, E. M., Agar, G., Fichman, G., Ziv, Y. B., Kardosh, R., Halperin, N., ... & Debi, R. (2011). Efficacy of methylsulfonylmethane supplementation on osteoarthritis of the knee: a randomized controlled study. BMC complementary and alternative medicine, 11(1), 50.

450 Ziboh, V. A., & Fletcher, M. P. (1992). Dose-response effects of dietary gamma-linolenic acid-enriched oils on human polymorphonuclear-neutrophil biosynthesis of leukotriene B4. The American journal of clinical nutrition, 55(1), 39-45.
Surette, M. E., Swan, D. D., Fonteh, A. N., Johnson, M. M., & Chilton, F. H. (1996). Metabolism of gammalinolenic acid in human neutrophils. The Journal of Immunology, 156(8), 2941-2947.

451 Davidson, E. M., Rae, S. A., & Smith, M. J. (1983). Leukotriene B4, a mediator of inflammation present in synovial fluid in rheumatoid arthritis. Annals of the rheumatic diseases, 42(6), 677-679.

452 Iversen, L., Kragballe, K., & Ziboh, V. A. (1997). Significance of leukotriene-A4 hydrolase in the pathogenesis of psoriasis. Skin Pharmacology and Physiology, 10(4), 169-177.

453 Belch, J. J., & Hill, A. (2000). Evening primrose oil and borage oil in rheumatologic conditions. The American journal of clinical nutrition, 71(1), 352s-356s.

454 Leventhal, L. J., Boyce, E. G., & Zurier, R. B. (1993). Treatment of rheumatoid arthritis with gammalinolenic acid. Annals of Internal Medicine, 119(9), 867-873.
Zurier, R. B., Rossetti, R. G., Jacobson, E. W., Demarco, D. M., Liu, N. Y., Temming, J. E., ... & Laposata, M. (1996). Gamma-linolenic acid treatment of rheumatoid arthritis. A randomized, placebo-controlled trial. Arthritis & Rheumatism, 39(11), 1808-1817.

455 Ziboh, V. A., & Fletcher, M. P. (1992). Dose-response effects of dietary gamma-linolenic acid-enriched oils on human polymorphonuclear-neutrophil biosynthesis of leukotriene B4. The American journal of clinical nutrition, 55(1), 39-45.

456 Jäntti, J., Nikkari, T., Solakivi, T., Vapaatalo, H., & Isomäki, H. (1989). Evening primrose oil in rheumatoid arthritis: changes in serum lipids and fatty acids. Annals of the rheumatic diseases, 48(2), 124-127.

457 Barham, J. B., Edens, M. B., Fonteh, A. N., Johnson, M. M., Easter, L., & Chilton, F. H. (2000). Addition of eicosapentaenoic acid to γ-linolenic acid–supplemented diets prevents serum arachidonic acid accumulation in humans. The Journal of nutrition, 130(8), 1925-1931.

458 Ziboh, V. A., & Fletcher, M. P. (1992). Dose-response effects of dietary gamma-linolenic acid-enriched oils on human polymorpho-

nuclear-neutrophil biosynthesis of leukotriene B4. The American journal of clinical nutrition, 55(1), 39-45.

459 Jiang, Q. (2014). Natural forms of vitamin E: metabolism, antioxidant, and anti-inflammatory activities and their role in disease prevention and therapy. Free Radical Biology and Medicine, 72, 76-90.

460 Edmonds, S. E., Winyard, P. G., Guo, R., Kidd, B., Merry, P., Langrish-Smith, A.,...& Blake, D. R. (1997). Putative analgesic activity of repeated oral doses of vitamin E in the treatment of rheumatoid arthritis. Results of a prospective placebo controlled double blind trial. Annals of the rheumatic diseases, 56(11), 649-655.

Helmy, M., Shohayeb, M., Helmy, M. H., & El-Bassiouni, E. A. (2001). Antioxidants as adjuvant therapy in rheumatoid disease. Arzneimittelforschung, 51(04), 293-298.

Wittenborg, A., Petersen, G., Lorkowski, G., & Brabant, T. (1998). Effectiveness of vitamin E in comparison with diclofenac sodium in treatment of patients with chronic polyarthritis. Zeitschrift fur Rheumatologie, 57(4), 215-221.

Kolarz, G., Scherak, O., El Shohoumi, M., & Blankenhorn, G. (1990). Hochdosiertes Vitamin E bei chronischer Polyarthritis. Aktuelle Rheumatologie, 15(06), 233-237.

Kharaeva, Z., Gostova, E., De Luca, C., Raskovic, D., & Korkina, L. (2009). Clinical and biochemical effects of coenzyme Q 10, vitamin E, and selenium supplementation to psoriasis patients. Nutrition, 25(3), 295-302.

461 Kharaeva, Z., Gostova, E., De Luca, C., Raskovic, D., & Korkina, L. (2009). Clinical and biochemical effects of coenzyme Q 10, vitamin E, and selenium supplementation to psoriasis patients. Nutrition, 25(3), 295-302.

462 Hagfors, L., Leanderson, P., Sköldstam, L., Andersson, J., & Johansson, G. (2003). Antioxidant intake, plasma antioxidants and oxidative stress in a randomized, controlled, parallel, Mediterranean dietary intervention study on patients with rheumatoid arthritis. Nutrition journal, 2(1), 5.

463 Reiter, E., Jiang, Q., & Christen, S. (2007). Anti-inflammatory properties of α-and γ-tocopherol. Molecular aspects of medicine, 28(5), 668-691.

464 Kurd, S. K., Smith, N., VanVoorhees, A., Troxel, A. B., Badmaev, V., Seykora, J. T., & Gelfand, J. M. (2008). Oral curcumin in the treatment of moderate to severe psoriasis vulgaris: A prospective clinical trial. Journal of the American Academy of Dermatology, 58(4), 625-631.

465 Dcodhar, S. D., Sethi, R., & Srimal, R. C. (2013). Preliminary study on antirheumatic activity of curcumin (diferuloyl methane). Indian journal of medical research, 138(1).

Kurd, S. K., Smith, N., VanVoorhees, A., Troxel, A. B., Badmaev, V., Seykora, J. T., & Gelfand, J. M. (2008). Oral curcumin in the treatment of moderate to severe psoriasis vulgaris: A prospective clinical trial. Journal of the American Academy of Dermatology, 58(4), 625-631

466   Stohs, S. J., Ji, J., Bucci, L. R., & Preuss, H. G. (2018). A Comparative Pharmacokinetic Assessment of a Novel Highly Bioavailable Curcumin Formulation with 95% Curcumin: A Randomized, Double-Blind, Crossover Study. *Journal of the American College of Nutrition, 37*(1), 51-59.

467   Belcaro, G., Cesarone, M. R., Dugall, M., Pellegrini, L., Ledda, A., Grossi, M. G.,... & Appendino, G. (2010). Efficacy and safety of Meriva (R), a curcumin-phosphatidylcholine complex, during extended administration in osteoarthritis patients. *Altern Med Rev, 15*(4), 337-44.

468   Haroyan, A., Mukuchyan, V., Mkrtchyan, N., Minasyan, N., Gasparyan, S., Sargsyan, A.,... & Hovhannisyan, A. (2018). Efficacy and safety of curcumin and its combination with boswellic acid in osteoarthritis: a comparative, randomized, double-blind, placebo-controlled study. *BMC complementary and alternative medicine, 18*(1), 7.

469   Di Pierro Francesco, R. G., Eleonora, A. D. M., Giovanni, A., Federico, F., & Stefano, T. (2013). Comparative evaluation of the pain-relieving properties of a lecithinized formulation of curcumin (Meriva*), nimesulide, and acetaminophen. *Journal of pain research, 6*, 201.

470   Allegri, P., Mastromarino, A., & Neri, P. (2010). Management of chronic anterior uveitis relapses: efficacy of oral phospholipidic curcumin treatment. Long-term follow-up. *Clinical Ophthalmology (Auckland, NZ), 4*, 1201.

471   Kumar, S., Ahuja, V., Sankar, M. J., Kumar, A., & Moss, A. C. (2010). Curcumin for maintenance of remission in ulcerative colitis. *Cochrane Database of Systematic Reviews, 10*.

472   Antiga, E., Bonciolini, V., Volpi, W., Del Bianco, E., & Caproni, M. (2015). Oral curcumin (Meriva) is effective as an adjuvant treatment and is able to reduce IL-22 serum levels in patients with psoriasis vulgaris. *BioMed research international, 2015*.

473   Kurd, S. K., Smith, N., VanVoorhees, A., Troxel, A. B., Badmaev, V., Seykora, J. T., & Gelfand, J. M. (2008). Oral curcumin in the treatment of moderate to severe psoriasis vulgaris: A prospective clinical trial. Journal of the American Academy of Dermatology, 58(4), 625-631.

474   Cuomo, J., Appendino, G., Dern, A. S., Schneider, E., McKinnon, T. P., Brown, M. J.,... & Dixon, B. M. (2011). Comparative absorption

of a standardized curcuminoid mixture and its lecithin formulation. *Journal of natural products*, *74*(4), 664-669.

475   Ohno, M., Nishida, A., Sugitani, Y., Nishino, K., Inatomi, O., Sugimoto, M.,... & Andoh, A. (2017). Nanoparticle curcumin ameliorates experimental colitis via modulation of gut microbiota and induction of regulatory T cells. *PloS one*, *12*(10), e0185999.
Feng, W., Wang, H., Zhang, P., Gao, C., Tao, J., Ge, Z.,... & Bi, Y. (2017). Modulation of gut microbiota contributes to curcumin-mediated attenuation of hepatic steatosis in rats. *Biochimica et Biophysica Acta (BBA)-General Subjects*, *1861*(7), 1801-1812.
McFadden, R. M. T., Larmonier, C. B., Shehab, K. W., Midura-Kiela, M., Ramalingam, R., Harrison, C. A.,... & Ghishan, F. K. (2015). The role of curcumin in modulating colonic microbiota during colitis and colon cancer prevention. *Inflammatory bowel diseases*, *21*(11), 2483-2494.
Shen, L., Liu, L., & Ji, H. F. (2017). Regulative effects of curcumin spice administration on gut microbiota and its pharmacological implications. *Food & nutrition research*, *61*(1), 1361780.

476   Wang, J., Ghosh, S. S., & Ghosh, S. (2017). Curcumin improves intestinal barrier function: modulation of intracellular signaling, and organization of tight junctions. *American Journal of Physiology-Cell Physiology*, *312*(4), C438-C445.

477   Khajuria, A., Zutshi, U., & Bedi, K. L. (1998). Permeability characteristics of piperine on oral absorption-An active alkaloid from peppers and a bioavailability enhancer. Indian journal of experimental biology, 36, 46-50.
Kaushal, N., Jain, S., Kondaiah, P., & Tiwary, A. K. (2009). Influence of piperine on transcutaneous permeation of repaglinide in rats and on tight junction proteins in HaCaT cells: unveiling the mechanisms for enhanced permeation. Sci Pharm, 77, 877-897.
Feng, X., Liu, Y., Wang, X., & Di, X. (2014). Effects of piperine on the intestinal permeability and pharmacokinetics of linarin in rats. Molecules, 19(5), 5624-5633.
Jin, M. J., & Han, H. K. (2010). Effect of piperine, a major component of black pepper, on the intestinal absorption of fexofenadine and its implication on food–drug interaction. Journal of food science, 75(3), H93-H96.

478   Interlandi, J. (2016) Supplements Can Make You Sick. Dietary supplements are not regulated the same way as medications. This lack of oversight puts consumers' health at risk.
July 27, 2016. http://www.consumerreports.org/vitamins-supplements/supplements-can-make-you-sick/

479   Suskind, D. (2016). Nutrition in Immune Balance (NIMBAL) Therapy: Using Diet to Treat Inflammatory Bowel Disease. Seattle, Washington. Nimbal Publishing.

Chapter 9. The Science of Low-Dose Naltrexone

480   Gironi, M., Martinelli-Boneschi, F., Sacerdote, P., Solaro, C., Zaffaroni, M., Cavarretta, R.,...& Rodegher, M. E. (2008). A pilot trial of low-dose naltrexone in primary progressive multiple sclerosis. Multiple Sclerosis Journal, 14(8), 1076-1083.

481   Gironi, M., Martinelli-Boneschi, F., Sacerdote, P., Solaro, C., Zaffaroni, M., Cavarretta, R.,...& Rodegher, M. E. (2008). A pilot trial of low-dose naltrexone in primary progressive multiple sclerosis. Multiple Sclerosis Journal, 14(8), 1076-1083.

482   Cree, B. A., Kornyeyeva, E., & Goodin, D. S. (2010). Pilot trial of low-dose naltrexone and quality of life in multiple sclerosis. Annals of neurology, 68(2), 145-150.

483   Younger, J., Noor, N., McCue, R., & Mackey, S. (2013). Low-dose naltrexone for the treatment of fibromyalgia: Findings of a small, randomized, double-blind, placebo-controlled, counterbalanced, crossover trial assessing daily pain levels. Arthritis & Rheumatism, 65(2), 529-538.

484   Younger, J., Noor, N., McCue, R., & Mackey, S. (2013). Low-dose naltrexone for the treatment of fibromyalgia: Findings of a small, randomized, double-blind, placebo-controlled, counterbalanced, crossover trial assessing daily pain levels. Arthritis & Rheumatism, 65(2), 529-538.

485   Smith, J. P., Bingaman, S. I., Ruggiero, F., Mauger, D. T., Mukherjee, A., McGovern, C. O., & Zagon, I. S. (2011). Therapy with the opioid antagonist naltrexone promotes mucosal healing in active Crohn's disease: a randomized placebo-controlled trial. Digestive diseases and sciences, 56(7), 2088-2097.
Smith, J. P., Stock, H., Bingaman, S., Mauger, D., Rogosnitzky, M., & Zagon, I. S. (2007). Low-dose naltrexone therapy improves active Crohn's disease. The American journal of gastroenterology, 102(4), 820-828.
Smith, J. P., Field, D., Bingaman, S., Evans, R., & Mauger, D. (2013). Safety and tolerability of low dose naltrexone therapy in children with moderate to severe crohn's disease: a pilot study. Journal of clinical gastroenterology, 47(4), 339.

486   Smith, J. P., Bingaman, S. I., Ruggiero, F., Mauger, D. T., Mukherjee, A., McGovern, C. O., & Zagon, I. S. (2011). Therapy with the opioid antagonist naltrexone promotes mucosal healing in active Crohn's disease: a randomized placebo-controlled trial. Digestive diseases and sciences, 56(7), 2088-2097.

487   Jackson, B. D., Lewis, D. J., Beswick, L., Van Langenberg, D., Sparrow, M., & Gibson, P. R. (2013). Apparent efficacy and safety of low dose naltrexone in australian patients with active Crohn's disease.

Journal of Gastroenterology and Hepatology, 28, 99.

Shannon, A., Alkhouri, N., Mayacy, S., Kaplan, B., & Mahajan, L. (2010). Low-dose naltrexone for treatment of duodenal Crohn's disease in a pediatric patient. Inflammatory bowel diseases, 16(9), 1457.

488 Shannon, A., Alkhouri, N., Mayacy, S., Kaplan, B., & Mahajan, L. (2010). Low-dose naltrexone for treatment of duodenal Crohn's disease in a pediatric patient. Inflammatory bowel diseases, 16(9), 1457.

489 Lie, M. R., Giessen, J., Fuhler, G. M., Lima, A., Peppelenbosch, M. P., Ent, C., & Woude, C. J. (2018). Low dose Naltrexone for induction of remission in inflammatory bowel disease patients. *Journal of translational medicine, 16*(1), 55.

490 Jackson, B. D., Lewis, D. J., Beswick, L., Van Langenberg, D., Sparrow, M., & Gibson, P. R. (2013). Apparent efficacy and safety of low dose naltrexone in australian patients with active Crohn's disease. Journal of Gastroenterology and Hepatology, 28, 99.

491 Younger, J., Parkitny, L., & McLain, D. (2014). The use of low-dose naltrexone (LDN) as a novel anti-inflammatory treatment for chronic pain. Clinical rheumatology, 33(4), 451-459.

492 Wang, X., Zhang, Y., Peng, Y., Hutchinson, M. R., Rice, K. C., Yin, H., & Watkins, L. R. (2016). Pharmacological characterization of the opioid inactive isomers (+)-naltrexone and (+)-naloxone as antagonists of toll-like receptor 4. British journal of pharmacology, 173(5), 856-869.

Stevens, C. W., Aravind, S., Das, S., & Davis, R. L. (2013). Pharmacological characterization of LPS and opioid interactions at the toll-like receptor 4. British journal of pharmacology, 168(6), 1421-1429.

493 Hutchinson, M. R., Zhang, Y., Brown, K., Coats, B. D., Shridhar, M., Sholar, P. W.,...& Rice, K. C. (2008). Non-stereoselective reversal of neuropathic pain by naloxone and naltrexone: involvement of toll-like receptor 4 (TLR4). European Journal of Neuroscience, 28(1), 20-29.

494 Smith, R. L., Hébert, H. L., Massey, J., Bowes, J., Marzo-Ortega, H., Ho, P.,...& Warren, R. B. (2016). Association of Toll-like receptor 4 (TLR4) with chronic plaque type psoriasis and psoriatic arthritis. Archives of dermatological research, 308(3), 201-205.

Assassi, S., Reveille, J. D., Arnett, F. C., Weisman, M. H., Ward, M. M., Agarwal, S. K.,...& Mayes, M. D. (2011). Whole-blood gene expression profiling in ankylosing spondylitis shows upregulation of toll-like receptor 4 and 5. The Journal of rheumatology, 38(1), 87-98.

495 Xu, D., Yan, S., Wang, H., Gu, B., Sun, K., Yang, X.,...& Wang, X. (2015). IL-29 enhances LPS/TLR4-mediated inflammation in rheu-

matoid arthritis. Cellular Physiology and Biochemistry, 37(1), 27-34.

Yang, Z. X., Liang, Y., Zhu, Y., Li, C., Zhang, L. Z., Zeng, X. M., & Zhong, R. Q. (2007). Increased expression of Toll-like receptor 4 in peripheral blood leucocytes and serum levels of some cytokines in patients with ankylosing spondylitis. Clinical & Experimental Immunology, 149(1), 48-55.

Garcia–Rodriguez, S., Arias–Santiago, S., Perandrés–López, R., Castellote, L., Zumaquero, E., Navarro, P.,...& Zubiaur, M. (2013). Increased gene expression of Toll-like receptor 4 on peripheral blood mononuclear cells in patients with psoriasis. Journal of the European Academy of Dermatology and Venereology, 27(2), 242-250.

De Rycke, L., Vandooren, B., Kruithof, E., De Keyser, F., Veys, E. M., & Baeten, D. (2005). Tumor necrosis factor α blockade treatment down-modulates the increased systemic and local expression of toll-like receptor 2 and toll-like receptor 4 in spondylarthropathy. Arthritis & Rheumatology, 52(7), 2146-2158.

496   Hu, F., Li, Y., Zheng, L., Shi, L., Liu, H., Zhang, X.,...& Yang, Y. (2014). Toll-like receptors expressed by synovial fibroblasts perpetuate Th1 and th17 cell responses in rheumatoid arthritis. PLoS One, 9(6), e100266.

Begon, É., Michel, L., Flageul, B., Beaudoin, I., Jean-Louis, F., Bachelez, H.,...& Musette, P. (2007). Expression, subcellular localization and cytokinic modulation of Toll-like receptors (TLRs) in normal human keratinocytes: TLR2 up-regulation in psoriatic skin. European Journal of Dermatology, 17(6), 497-506.

497   Younger, J., Parkitny, L., & McLain, D. (2014). The use of low-dose naltrexone (LDN) as a novel anti-inflammatory treatment for chronic pain. Clinical rheumatology, 33(4), 451-459.

498   Younger, J., Noor, N., McCue, R., & Mackey, S. (2013). Low-dose naltrexone for the treatment of fibromyalgia: Findings of a small, randomized, double-blind, placebo-controlled, counterbalanced, crossover trial assessing daily pain levels. Arthritis & Rheumatism, 65(2), 529-538.

Gironi, M., Martinelli-Boneschi, F., Sacerdote, P., Solaro, C., Zaffaroni, M., Cavarretta, R.,...& Rodegher, M. E. (2008). A pilot trial of low-dose naltrexone in primary progressive multiple sclerosis. Multiple Sclerosis Journal, 14(8), 1076-1083.

499   Younger, J., Noor, N., McCue, R., & Mackey, S. (2013). Low-dose naltrexone for the treatment of fibromyalgia: Findings of a small, randomized, double-blind, placebo-controlled, counterbalanced, crossover trial assessing daily pain levels. Arthritis & Rheumatism, 65(2), 529-538.

Chapter 10: Putting It All Together

500   Ebringer, A., & Wilson, C. (1996). The use of a low starch diet in the treatment of patients suffering from ankylosing spondylitis. Clinical rheumatology, 15(1), 62-66.

Chapter 12. The Recipes

501   Hernandez, A. L., Kitz, A., Wu, C., Lowther, D. E., Rodriguez, D. M., Vudattu, N., ... & Hafler, D. A. (2015). Sodium chloride inhibits the suppressive function of FOXP3+ regulatory T cells. The Journal of clinical investigation, 125(11), 4212-4222.

Binger, K. J., Gebhardt, M., Heinig, M., Rintisch, C., Schroeder, A., Neuhofer, W., ... & Voelkl, J. (2015). High salt reduces the activation of IL-4–and IL-13–stimulated macrophages. The Journal of clinical investigation, 125(11), 4223-4238.

Salgado, E., Bes-Rastrollo, M., de Irala, J., Carmona, L., & Gomez-Reino, J. J. (2015). High sodium intake is associated with self-reported rheumatoid arthritis: a cross sectional and case control analysis within the SUN cohort. Medicine, 94(37), e0924.

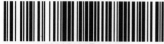

Made in the USA
Columbia, SC
04 September 2019